A Special Issue of
The European Journal of Cognitive Psychology

Ageing, Cognition, and Neuroscience

Guest Editors

Soledad Ballesteros
Universidad Nacional de Educación a Distancia, Madrid, Spain

Lars-Göran Nilsson
Stockholm University, Stockholm, Sweden

and

Patrick Lemaire
University of Provence, Aix-en-Provence, France

Psychology Press
Taylor & Francis Group
HOVE AND NEW YORK

First published 2009 by Psychology Press
27 Church Road, Hove, East Sussex, BN3 2FA

www.psypress.com

Simultaneously published in the USA and Canada
by Psychology Press
270 Madison Avenue, New York, NY 10016

Psychology Press is part of the Taylor & Francis Group, an Informa business

British Library Cataloguing in Publication Data
A catalogue record for this book is available from the British Library

ISBN 13: 978-1-84872-707-6
ISSN 0954-1446

Cover design by Anú Design, Tara, Co. Meath, Ireland
Typeset in India by Datapage International
Printed in the UK by Hobbs the Printers Ltd, Totton, Hampshire
Bound in the UK by TJ International Ltd, Padstow, Cornwall
The publication has been produced with paper manufactured to strict
environmental standards and with pulp derived from sustainable forests.

Contents*

(*continued overleaf*)

* This book is also a special issue of *The European Journal of Cognitive Psychology*, and comprises pp. 161–472 of Volume 21 (2009). The page numbers are taken from the journal and so begin with p. 161.

EUROPEAN JOURNAL OF COGNITIVE PSYCHOLOGY
2009, 21 (2/3), 161–175

Psychology Press
Taylor & Francis Group

Ageing, cognition, and neuroscience: An introduction

Soledad Ballesteros
Universidad Nacional de Educación a Distancia, Madrid, Spain

Lars-Göran Nilsson
Stockholm University, Stockholm, Sweden

Patrick Lemaire
University of Provence, Aix-en-Provence, France

The main goal of this special issue is to report new cognitive data in normal and pathological ageing that are related to neural data at different levels. Ageing is a universal complex process that profoundly affects mind and brain of all individuals. A number of psychological theories and theoretical approaches see ageing as a set of gains and losses. Cognitive research has relied upon behavioural measures of cognitive performance. We summarise briefly the large variety of topics dealt with in the articles that compose this special issue. This is organised in four main domains: (1) processing speed, inhibition, and executive processes in normal and pathological ageing; (2) implicit learning and memory in normal ageing; (3) cognitive flexibility and episodic memory; and (4) processing emotional information in the old age.

Keywords: Ageing; Cognition; Emotion; Neuroscience.

In December 2004, one of us organised in Madrid an international conference with the same title as this special issue, "Ageing, Cognition, and Neuroscience" (Ballesteros, 2006). Some of the contributors and guest editors to this special issue participated in that conference. The aim of the conference was to examine new breakthroughs in the understanding of the ageing mind and brain and how to use this knowledge to promote interdisciplinary research in the area. This is precisely the aim of this special issue.

Public interest in ageing has expanded greatly due, to a certain extent, by the global response given to the United Nations World Assemblies on ageing

Correspondence should be addressed to Soledad Ballesteros, Department of Basic Psychology II, Facultad de Psicología, Universidad Nacional de Educación a Distancia, Juan del Rosal, 10, 28040 Madrid, Spain. E-mail: mballesteros@psi.uned.es

http://www.psypress.com/ecp DOI: 10.1080/09541440802598339

convened the last one in Madrid in 2002. These global meetings concentrated on the problems and implications of the rapid and unprecedented growth of the number of ageing persons living in the society. The importance of relevant research to expand the knowledge and understanding of ageing was acknowledged. During the last decade the growth of research in this field has been enormous from many different levels including genetics, biology, psychology, neuroscience, and social sciences such as sociology, economy, and law (see Andrews, 2005).

Ageing is a universal complex multifaceted process that profoundly affects mind and brain of all individuals. The field of cognitive ageing is considered as a recent frontier of the human sciences, reflecting integrative influences from cognitive psychology and lifespan psychology (Dixon & Nilsson, 2004). Until quite recently, the cognitive and neural mechanisms of age-related changes in cognitive function were studied independently. However, the new discipline of cognitive neuroscience of ageing has emerged in recent years as a new and very exciting field with studies focusing on the relationships between the effects of ageing on cognitive processes and the brain function underlining them (see Cabeza, Nyberg, & Park, 2005).

Ageing is a diverse and complex phenomenon but a number of theoretical approaches and psychological theories consider ageing as a dynamic set of gains and losses as the "overall theory of successful (adaptative) psychological ageing" (Baltes, Freund, & Li, 2005). Cognitive research has relied until very recently upon behavioural measures of cognitive performance (mainly accuracy and response time). However, recent advances in neuroimaging techniques have allowed the investigation of the relations between cognitive performance and brain activity.

Resting-state structural neuroimaging measures suggest age-related grey and white matter decline with age with anterior regions showing greater decline than posterior regions (Raz et al., 2005; for a review, see Dennis & Cabeza, 2008). These results correlate with behavioural data showing larger performance declines in tasks mediated by the frontal lobes (Park et al., 2002; West, 1996). Functional imaging studies provide a posterior–anterior shift in old adults and a reduction in the asymmetry of brain activity. These consistent results suggest that the increase of activation in prefrontal cortex plays a compensatory role for age-related deficits occurring in other brain regions, suggesting that older adults are using other strategies than those put forwards by young in performing difficult tasks (Park & Gutchess, 2004; Reuter-Lorenz, 2002; Reuter-Lorenz & Lustig, 2005). The additional compensatory frontal recruitment suggests a great flexibility and reorganisation in neural networks with ageing (Park, Gutchess, Meade, & Stine-Morrow, 2007). Park and Reuter-Lorenz (in press) have just proposed the scaffolding theory of ageing and cognition (STAC) to account for the behavioural decline observed in a number of cognitive processes as well as the decrease in brain structure size and white matter integrity together with the increases observed in prefrontal activation. According to this theory, the increased frontal activation with age is a marker of brain adaptation. The old brain engages in scaffolding to compensate the decline of neural structures and function.

Important discoveries are being made at different levels of research on cognitive ageing: from the molecular/genetic level, to the cell, the synapse, the network, and the processing of information at the cognitive level. The ultimate goal in cognitive neuroscience is to understand this whole set of stages (e.g., Nilsson, 2006). We are not yet there. Most studies conducted so far have collected data at single levels only. However, great progress is being achieved in multiple fields. The main goal of this special issue is to report new cognitive data in normal and pathological ageing that are related to neural data at different levels.

Today it is well documented that important declines on a number of main cognitive functions take place during the ageing process (Baltes & Lindenberger, 1997; Nilsson, 2003; Park et al., 2002; Salthouse, 1996; see also Craik & Salthouse, 2000, 2008; Nilsson, 2003; Park & Schwarz, 2000; Park, Polk, Mikels, Taylor, & Marshuetz, 2001). However, this decline is not uniform across cognitive functions but follows different patterns of decline, stability, or even gains in some cases across lifespan (e.g., Ballesteros & Reales, 2004; Ballesteros, Reales, & Mayas, 2007; Fleischman & Gabrieli, 1998; Hedden & Gabrieli, 2004; Mitchell, 1989; Nilsson, 2003; Park et al., 2001; Rönnlund & Nilsson, 2006).

Cross-sectional (Nilsson, 2003; Park et al., 2002) as well as longitudinal studies (Rönnlund, Lövdén, & Nilsson, 2008; Rönnlund & Nilsson, 2006; Rönnlund, Nyberg, Bäckman, & Nilsson, 2005; Schaie, 1996) have shown different patterns that vary from decline to stability, and even growth across lifespan. First, comparisons between cross-sectional and longitudinal data reveal quite dramatic differences for the same functions. For example, Rönnlund et al. (2005) demonstrated an almost linear decline from 35 to 85 years of age for episodic memory on the basis of cross-sectional analyses with proper control for cohort effects. For longitudinal data with proper control for cohort effects and retest effects, however, the data pattern was completely different. Memory performance was stable from 35 to 65 years followed by a decline up to 85 years of age.

Although not as dramatic, the difference between cross-sectional and longitudinal data could also be seen for semantic memory. The longitudinal data, again with proper control for cohort effects and retest effects, revealed signs of an increase in performance from 35 to 60 years, stable performance between 65 and 75, and a slight decrease thereafter. Consistent differences between cross-sectional and longitudinal data have also been demonstrated

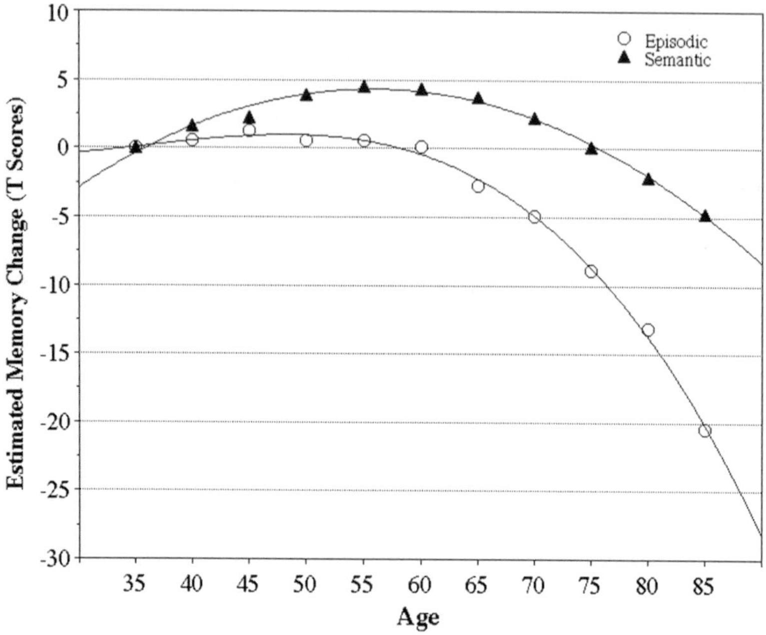

Figure 1. Estimated memory change across age (T scores) for the episodic and semantic memory factors on the basis of practice-adjusted longitudinal data. From M. Rönnlund, L. Nyberg, L. Bäckman, and L.-G. Nilsson (2005). Stability, growth, and decline in adult life-span development of declarative memory: Cross-sectional and longitudinal data from a population-based sample. *Psychology and Aging*, *20*, 3–18. Copyright 2005 by the American Psychological Association. Figure reprinted with permission from the authors and publisher.

in a Block Design task (Rönnlund & Nilsson, 2006) and a Tower of Hanoi task (Rönnlund et al., 2008).

Thus, performance patterns vary in several cognitive domains in cross-sectional and longitudinal data, respectively, when cohort effects and retest effects are adequately controlled. To the best of our knowledge, it is only for cognitive speed that similar patterns occur in cross-sectional (Salthouse, in press) and longitudinal data (Schaie, 1989). It is obvious from the papers cited that it is not only the type of design that matters when evaluating age trajectories, but also the particular cognitive domain that is assessed. As shown by Rönnlund et al. (2005), the difference between data patterns in episodic memory and semantic memory, respectively, is obvious.

Fortunately, not all cognitive processes deteriorate with age. Verbal abilities and world knowledge are spared or even show some improvement across lifespan (see Park et al., 2002). Implicit memory is another cognitive ability that appears stable with age (e.g., Ballesteros et al., this issue; Ballesteros & Reales, 2004; Ballesteros et al., 2007; Ballesteros, Reales,

Mayas, & Heller, 2008; LaVoie & Light, 1994; Mitchell, 1989; see Fleischman & Gabrieli, 1998). Implicit memory refers to better performance with previously experienced stimuli that do not require conscious or intended retrieval of previously encountered information (Graf & Schacter, 1985). Research on implicit memory has interested cognitive psychologists and neuroscientists for many years because empirical findings have shown consistently that this type of memory assessed by repetition priming is dissociable of explicit memory measures such a recognition or recall (e.g., Cooper, Schacter, Ballesteros, & Moore, 1992; Schacter, Wig, & Stevens, 2007; Tulving & Schacter, 1990).

Most of the information on the stability of repetition priming as a form of implicit memory with age proceeds from cross-sectional studies (Ballesteros & Reales, 2004; Ballesteros et al., 2007, 2008; LaVoie & Light, 1994; Mitchell, 1989). However, one 4-year longitudinal study (Fleischman, Wilson, Gabrieli, Bienias, & Bennett, 2004) has shown dissociations between implicit and explicit memory functions over a 4-year period in older healthy participants. Results showed that priming remained stable in this period while explicit memory declined significantly.

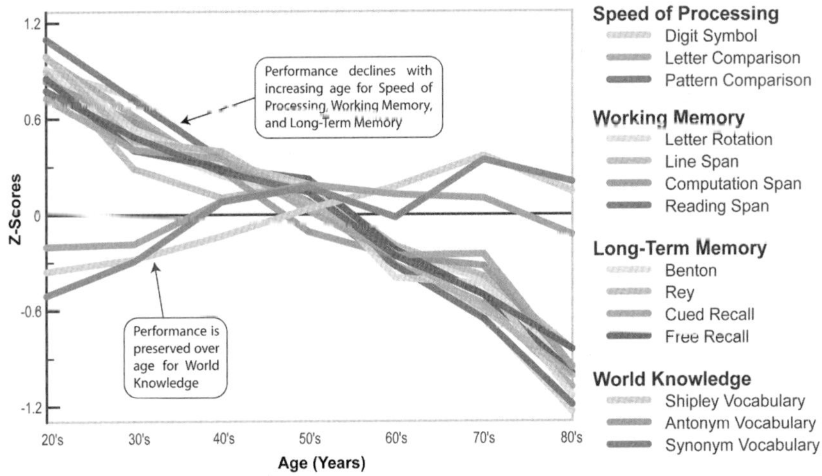

Figure 2. Cross-sectional ageing data showing behavioural performance on measures of speed of processing, working memory, long-term memory, and world knowledge. The figure shows that almost all measures of cognitive function show decline with age, except world knowledge that may even show some improvement with age. From D. C. Park, L. Davidson, G. Lautenschlager, A. D. Smith, P. Smith, & T. Hedden (2002). Models of visuospatial and verbal memory across the adult lifespan. *Psychology and Aging*, *17*, 299–320. Copyright 2002 by the American Psychological Association. Figure adapted with permission from the authors and publisher. To view this figure in colour, please visit the online version of the journal.

Next we summarise briefly the content of each paper in the special issue, organised within four main topics: (1) processing speed, inhibition, and executive processes in normal and pathological ageing; (2) implicit learning and memory in normal ageing; (3) cognitive flexibility and episodic memory; and (4) processing emotional information in old age.

PROCESSING SPEED, INHIBITION, AND EXECUTIVE PROCESSES IN NORMAL AND PATHOLOGICAL AGEING

Five papers in this special issue deal with differences in processing speed, inhibition or executive processes as a function of age. Meijer et al. examined whether differences in reaction time (RT) between younger (ranging from 25 to 35 years) and middle-aged (ranging from 50 to 60 years) healthy individuals increase with depth of processing. These researchers also examined whether this increase is less pronounced in higher educated individuals. Processing of words at the perceptual, phonological, and semantic level was induced by a case decision, an "e" detection, and a living/nonliving discrimination task, respectively. As shown in this paper, RTs increased with age and level of processing. The lack of interactions between age, task, and education suggest that different processing levels are equally sensitive to slowing in midlife and that education was not a moderating factor. Although no overall age by level of processing interaction was found, there was an age by stimulus type interaction in the deeper processing task. First, age-related differences in RT for words containing the letter "e" were smaller than for words without the letter "e", suggesting that middle-aged adults were slower than younger adults in performing a terminating search strategy. Second, age-related differences in RT for words referring to living items were smaller than for words referring to nonliving items. Meijer et al. suggested that middle-aged adults compared to younger adults have reduced access to specific semantic categories. The authors concluded that the results showed that vulnerability to age-related cognitive decline already exists in middle age.

Olk and Kingstone investigated the contribution of inhibition and response selection to the observed decline in processing speed and accuracy with age. In the study, young and aged adults were compared between conditions that required varying percentages of prosaccades, antisaccades, and no-go trials. The comparison between no-go (inhibition of a prosaccade) and antisaccade trials (inhibition of a prosaccade *and* selection of an antisaccade) showed significantly worse performance in the antisaccade task, especially for the older group, suggesting that they failed to select the antisaccade in a situation in which a competing, prepotent response is available. The results indicated that old participants experience pronounced difficulties when a situation requires the selection of a rare, less potent saccadic response that competes with a prepotent saccadic response that has to be inhibited. The present data are interpreted in the sense that the selection in the context of inhibition produces high error rates. Based on previous results the authors concluded that it may be the case that the older participants are less able to resolve the competition in favour of the antisaccade. Top-down signals reinforcing antisaccade generation and the activation of an antisaccade response may be weaker in the elderly or these commands may be given too slowly to avoid the execution of the faster erroneous prosaccade as suggested by Hutton and Ettinger (2006).

Andrés' study extended the research on part set cueing conducted in young adults into ageing. In the study included in this special issue, she investigated the involvement of inhibition as the explanatory factor of ageing using an incidental learning procedure to avoiding as much as possible retrieval strategies. The cues were presented either before (Experiment 1) or at recall (Experiment 2). The results showed clear and equivalent effects of part set cueing in young and older adults in both experiments. Andrés discussed these findings in relation to the Hasher and Zacks' (1988) inhibitory explanation of ageing as well as to the recent theoretical distinction between executive and automatic inhibition (Andrés, Guerrini, Phillips, & Perfect, 2008; Nigg, 2000). Andrés' study shows that both older and younger adults are affected by part set cueing in a similar way. These results parallel previous findings showing equivalent inhibitory effects in younger and older adults with tasks that do not require executive control (Andrés et al., 2008). Furthermore, her results confirm that non executive inhibition develops early in life as proposed by Zellner and Baulm (2005) and more importantly, remains unaffected by ageing.

Borella, Delaloye, Lecerf, Renaud, and de Ribaupierre used both correlational and experimental approaches and large samples of young and older adults to investigate the interference/inhibition issue in ageing. They also manipulated the salience of irrelevant information. The authors concluded that the differences between young and older adults in inhibition depend on the degree of activation involved in the tasks. A large number of young and older adults performed three different tasks involving inhibition/interference. These tasks were the classic Stroop colour task, the Hayling task, and a negative priming task embedded within the Stroop colour task. Borella and colleagues manipulated the level of activation of the irrelevant information. The study showed that interference effect was almost null in the negative priming task even when the irrelevant information was salient. In contrast, almost all young and older adults that participated in the study showed a significant interference effect in both, the Stroop colour and the Heyling tasks. Moreover, correlational analyses questioned the dimensionality of inhibition as the correlations between the indices of interference/inhibition were rather weak. The findings support previous results that have questioned the idea that inhibition is a unitary process and suggest that inhibition is a multifaceted concept.

McKinlay, Dalrymple-Alford, Grace, and Roger investigated the effect of attentional set-shifting, working memory, and processing speed on pragmatic language functioning in Parkinson's disease (PD) patients. In their study patients with PD were compared to matched controls on a number of measures such as pragmatic language functioning using the Test of Language Competence- Expanded (TLC-E), attentional set-shifting tasks, working memory, and processing speed measures. Overall, PD patients were impaired on aspects of language, working memory, and processing speed. Measures of cognition were significantly correlated with pragmatic language functioning. Path analyses revealed that deficits in pragmatic language functioning were mediated by verbal working memory and processing speed, but not attentional set-shifting. Regression analyses suggested that the relation between processing speed and pragmatic language performance was stronger than with verbal working memory. The authors concluded that pragmatic language deficits may be explained in terms of deficits in processing speed associated with the disease.

IMPLICIT LEARNING AND MEMORY IN NORMAL AGEING

Three papers in this special issue investigated implicit learning and memory in the old age. All the studies in this section suggest that certain types of processes referred as to implicit (implicit learning and implicit memory) are well preserved in the old age. Gaillard, Destrebecqz, Michiels, and Cleeremans investigated the effect of age and practice in sequence learning in three groups of participants ranging from young adults to older adults. In this study, participants first performed a serial reaction time (SRT) task, followed either by a short or a long training phase. Successive stimuli followed a repeating pattern although participants did not know it. After completing the training phase, participants performed a sequence generation task under inclusion and exclusion instructions. The study ended with a recognition task. SRT and generation data indicate both preserved learning and generation abilities in ageing, and beneficial effects of extended practice. By contrast, recognition results suggest that ageing tends to impair discrimination performance. Implications of these findings for understanding the effects of age and practice on the ability to control sequential knowledge are discussed in terms of the involvement of gradual representations of sequence structure. The present results open a promising "third way" in the domain of sequence learning in older adults. Middle-aged and older adults not only exhibited preserved learning abilities, but they also were just as able to control the acquired knowledge in a generation task as younger participants. Conversely, an age-related deficit in recognition was found, even though middle-aged and older adults were able to differentiate between old and new sequential fragments. The authors concluded that: (1) The generation task and recognition tasks may not tap the same processes and can be dissociated based on them, and (2) sequence learning tasks and implicit memory tasks, beyond their similarities, do differ from each other in significant ways.

Previous research with young adults has shown cross-modal repetition priming for familiar objects between vision and touch (e.g., Reales & Ballesteros, 1999). Not only within-modal implicit memory is preserved with age but also cross-modal implicit memory. In their paper, Ballesteros and colleagues examine whether cross-modal priming between vision and touch is preserved in older adults. They also investigated whether within-modal and cross-modal priming for ecological sounds and their corresponding pictures is preserved in the old age by comparing performance of younger and older adults. The results showed that the repetition priming exhibited by young adults was similar to that shown by the older participants. These behavioural findings on cross-modal visual, auditory, and haptic priming as well as other recent results from neuroimaging studies suggest the implication of areas in the occipital cortex that were previously considered modality specific. The results from these studies may indicate that cross modal facilitation might well occur in posterior extrastriate occipital areas that are well preserved not only in normal ageing but also in the first stage of Alzheimer's disease. These findings extend previous results with young adults (Reales & Ballesteros, 1999) showing that cross-modal priming was similar to within-modal priming when familiar objects were presented visually or haptically to the auditory events produced by objects and their corresponding pictures. The cross-modal facilitation observed here suggests that the representations supporting repetition priming are not modality specific and might depend on high-level structural features that define an object's shape and its spatiotemporal structure.

The results reported here suggest that repetition priming for objects presented to vision or touch, and the sounds produced by them, is not modality specific. Stimuli presented to a modality at study were identified faster and more accurately when the same stimuli were presented later at test to the other modality compared to new stimuli. The present results support the idea that vision, touch, and audition share common object representations. Moreover, young adults and older adults showed similar magnitudes of cross-modal priming, suggesting that not only within-modal priming, but also cross-modal priming is preserved in normal ageing. The findings support the multiple memory systems proposal (Tulving & Schacter, 1990) and have implications for theories of adult memory and cognitive ageing. Although the structural perceptual object system is spared with age, the episodic memory system that relies on the medial-temporal lobe is impaired. In contrast to the age-related decline on a number of cognitive functions, within-modal and cross-modal repetition priming (as a measure of implicit memory) is spared in older adults.

In their paper, Duñabeitia and colleagues investigate how elderly adults process morphologically complex words by using a compound word priming task to see whether it is affected by ageing. In the study, a group of healthy old adults was tested in a constituent priming study in which compound words served as targets (e.g., *BOOKSHOP*) and was briefly preceded by their first constituent lexeme (e.g., *book*), their second constituent lexeme (e.g., *shop*), or by an unrelated word (e.g., *house*). To test whether or not the elderly readers showed a morphological hyperpriming effect, young adults and older healthy adults were tested on a lexical decision task. Compound words were presented primed by their first constituent (*book-BOOKSHOP*), their second constituent (*shop-BOOKSHOP*), or by an unrelated word (*house-BOOKSHOP*). The results showed that morphological processing is fully preserved in the old as no difference was found in the magnitude of priming compared to young adults. As occurs with other incidental priming and learning tasks, morphological short-term priming is a process preserved in the old age suggesting that meaningful subword units forming transparent, solid compound words seem to be processed normally by aged participants.

COGNITIVE FLEXIBILITY AND EPISODIC MEMORY

Three papers in this special issue investigated the effect of ageing in voluntary and conscious long-term episodic memory. In their paper, Gutchess and Park reported the results from three experiments conducted to find out whether older adults show associative memory deficits compared to young adults using complex scenes as stimuli. The results usually showed that although memory for complex pictures seems to require the association of scene elements into one representation, this type of memory is often age-invariant. The authors speculated that the natural relationships contained in pictures may explain this distinction and that memory for scenes with novel relationships would be negatively affected with ageing. The results, however, did not confirm their predictions. The relatedness of scene elements does not differentially affect older compared to younger adults. The results suggest that the semantically rich associations contained in pictures need not rely on prior knowledge and experiences in order to support age-invariant picture memory. So, these results suggest that associative memory for complex pictures is another instance of a process little or not at all affected by age and that this type of associative memory may differ from memory for interitem associations more affected by ageing.

Taconnat and colleagues examine the effect of age on recall and clustering across successive trials in two samples of young and older adults using words as stimuli. Participants learnt a categorised word list that was later assessed by a recall test. To assess organisational strategy, the authors calculate a clustering index. Although recall for words was worse for old adults than for young adults, the clustering index for the old group was lower than that of younger adults but increased more across trials. Clustering was only associated with the recall scores for the younger adults. Participants were also administered cognitive tests (cognitive flexibility, cognitive speed, and categorical fluency) and young adults performed better on all the tests. Moreover, the variable most associated with clustering was cognitive flexibility. This finding supports the view that the age-related decrement in strategic organisation is due to a decrease in cognitive flexibility.

E. Nilsson and Wahlin used data collected in the Betula Prospective Cohort Study (see Nilsson et al., 1997, 2004) to investigate possible associations between diabetes and episodic memory performance under different levels of cognitive support at encoding and retrieval in participants with diabetes, without diabetes diagnosis but with elevated levels of glycosylated haemoglobin (HbA_{1c}), and persons without diabetes or elevated HbA_{1c}, ranging from 35 to 85 years of age. The results varied as a function of age and clinical conditions. Among participants 65 years of age and younger, diabetic patients performed worse than participants with elevated glysosylated haemoglobin and controls. In contrast, participants of 70 years of age or older, the group with elevated levels of glycosylated haemoglobin performed at the lowest level. These results indicate that undiagnosed diabetics are worse off than those who receive diagnosis and treatment. The differential results across age have important implications for future research in the sense that future studies of ageing and retrieval need to be performed with care.

PROCESSING EMOTIONAL INFORMATION IN OLD AGE

Two papers in the special issue deal with processing emotional information and ageing. Kensinger and Leclerc revised the outgrowing literature showing that older adults do not process emotional information as young adults do, as old adults seem to place more emphasis on pleasant information than on unpleasant information. The point is that age-related changes in emotional processing influence the types of information that are remembered best. Behavioural studies have shown that whereas young adults remember negative information well, older adults remember best positive information

(Mather, 2006; Mather & Carstensen, 2005). Kensinger and Leclerc considered closely in their paper the neural changes that may mediate these age-related changes. They suggest that changes in older adults' recruitment of prefrontal regions during emotional processing may reflect not only age-related changes in emotion regulation but also changes in self-referential processing. Because little research has examined the links between the neural networks supporting older adults' emotional and cognitive functioning, the authors concluded proposing a series of avenues for further research.

García and collaborators present the results of a study conducted to explore the role of spatial working memory in the identification of the six basic emotions, a process sensitive to normal and pathological (Alzheimer's disease, AD) ageing. They used as stimuli emotional faces expressing the six basic emotions as described by Ekman. The emotions were enacted by six 3-D virtual actors. In the study, young adults, AD patients and normal controls performed an emotional expression identification task in two different conditions. In a condition (the noninterference condition), participants performed just the identification task. In the interference condition, participants performed concurrently with the identification task a secondary task (the Corsi Block task). The results showed that performance was impaired in the three groups of participants in the interference condition. However, AD patients showed higher dual-task costs than older adults, suggesting that AD patients were more vulnerable to interference when they have to perform two tasks at once. The authors proposed a top-down control in emotional processing.

In summary, this overview anticipates that the field of ageing, cognition, and neuroscience is developing fast fertilised by the interdisciplinary collaboration between experts from several fields including psychology, neurology, radiology, and other medical specialties as well as Social Sciences and Engineering researchers. Understanding the interactions among neural, behavioural, cognitive, and social aspects of ageing is central to modelling and understanding normal and pathological ageing. This special issue includes papers dealing with normal and pathological ageing and a series of cognitive processes that do and do not decline as we get old, as well as its neurological implications.

REFERENCES

Andrews, G. R. (2005). Foreword. In M. L. Johnson (Ed.), *The Cambridge handbook of age and ageing* (pp. vii–xix). Cambridge, UK: Cambridge University Press.

Andrés, P., Guerrini, C., Phillips, L., & Perfect, T. (2008). Differential effects of aging on executive and automatic inhibition. *Developmental Neuropsychology, 33*, 101–123.

Ballesteros, S. (Ed.). (2006). *Ageing, cognition, and neuroscience.* Madrid: UNED.

Ballesteros, S., & Reales, J. M. (2004). Intact haptic priming in normal ageing and Alzheimer's disease: Evidence for dissociable memory systems. *Neuropsychologia, 44*, 1063–1070.

Ballesteros, S., Reales, J. M., & Mayas, J. (2007). Picture priming in ageing and dementia. *Psicothema, 19*, 239–244.

Ballesteros, S., Reales, J. M., Mayas, J., & Heller, M. A. (2008). Selective attention modulates visual and haptic repetition priming: Effects on ageing and Alzheimers' disease. *Experimental Brain Research, 189*, 473–483.

Baltes, P. B., Freund, A. M., & Li, S. C. (2005). The psychological science of human ageing. In M. L. Johnson (Ed.), *The Cambridge handbook of age and ageing* (pp. 47–71). Cambridge, UK: Cambridge University Press.

Baltes, P. B., & Lindenberger, U. (1997). Emergence of a powerful connection between sensory and cognitive functions across the adult lifespan: A new window to the study of cognitive aging? *Psychology and Aging, 12*, 12–21.

Cabeza, R., Nyberg, L., & Park, D. C. (2005). Cognitive neuroscience of ageing: Emergence of a new discipline. In R. Cabeza, L. Nyberg, & D. C. Park (Eds.), *Cognitive neuroscience of ageing* (pp. 3–15). Oxford, UK: Oxford University Press.

Cooper, L. A., Schacter, D. L., Ballesteros, S., & Moore, C. (1992). Priming and recognition of transformed three-dimensional objects: Effects of size and reflection. *Journal of Experimental Psychology: Learning, Memory, and Cognition, 18*, 43–57.

Craik, F. I., & Salthouse, T. A. (Eds.). (2000). *The handbook of aging and cognition.* Mahwah, NJ: Lawrence Erlbaum Associates, Inc.

Craik, F. I. M., & Salthouse, T. A. (Eds.). (2008). *The handbook of aging and cognition* (3rd ed.). New York: Psychology Press.

Dennis, N. A., & Cabeza, R. (2008). Neuroimaging of healthy cognitive aging. In F. I. M. Craik & T. A. Salthouse (Eds.), *The handbook of aging and cognition* (3rd ed., pp. 1–54). New York: Psychology Press.

Dixon, R. A., & Nilsson, L.-G. (2004). Don't fence us in: Probing the frontiers of cognitive ageing. In R. A. Dixon, L. Bäckman, & L.-G Nilsson (Eds.), *New frontiers in cognitive ageing* (pp. 4–15). Oxford, UK: Oxford University Press.

Fleischman, D. A., & Gabrieli, J. D. E. (1998). Repetition priming in normal aging and in Alzheimer's disease: A review of findings and theories. *Psychology and Aging, 13*, 88–119.

Fleischman, D. A., Wilson, R. S., Gabrieli, J. D. E., Bienias, J. L., & Bennett, D. A. (2004). A longitudinal study of implicit and explicit memory in old persons. *Psychology and Aging, 19*, 617–625.

Graf, P., & Schacter, D. L. (1985). Implicit and explicit memory for new associations in normal subjects and amnesic patients. *Journal of Experimental Psychology: Learning, Memory, and Cognition, 11*, 501–518.

Hasher, L., & Zacks, R. T. (1988). Working memory, comprehension, and aging: A review and a new view. In G. H. Bower (Ed.), *The psychology of learning and motivation* (Vol. 22, pp. 193–225). Orlando, FL: Academic Press.

Hedden, T., & Gabrieli, J. D. E. (2004). Insights into the aging mind: A view from cognitive neuroscience. *Nature Reviews Neuroscience, 5*, 87–97.

Hutton, S. B., & Ettinger, U. (2006). The antisaccade task as a research tool in psychopathology: A critical review. *Psychophysiology, 43*, 302–313.

La Voie, D., & Light, L. L. (1994). Adult age differences in repetition priming: A meta-analysis. *Psychology and Aging, 4*, 538–553.

Mather, M. (2006). Why memories may become more positive with age. In B. Uttl, N. Ohta, & A. L. Siegenthaler (Eds.), *Memory and emotion: Interdisciplinary perspectives* (pp. 135–159). Oxford, UK: Blackwell Publishing.

Mather, M., & Carstensen, L. L. (2005). Aging and motivated cognition: The positivity effect in attention and memory. *Trends in Cognitive Science*, *9*, 496–502.

Mitchell, D. B. (1989). How many memory systems? Evidence from ageing. *Journal of Experimental Psychology: Learning, Memory, and Cognition*, *15*, 31–49.

Nigg, J. T. (2000). On inhibition/disinhibition in developmental psychopathology: Views from cognitive and personality psychology and a working inhibition taxonomy. *Psychological Bulletin*, *126*, 200–246.

Nilsson, L.-G. (2003). Memory function in normal aging. *Acta Neurologica Scandinavica*, *107*, 7–13.

Nilsson, L.-G. (2006). Memory processes, ageing, cognitive decline and neurodegenerative diseases. *The European Psychologist*, *11*, 304–311.

Nilsson, L.-G., Adolfsson, R., Bäckman, L., de Frias, C., Molander., B., & Nyberg, L. (2004). Betula: A prospective cohort study on memory, health and aging. *Aging, Neuropsychology, and Cognition*, *11*, 134–148.

Nilsson, L.-G., Bäckman, L., Nyberg, L., Erngrund, K., Adolfsson, R., Bucht, G., et al. (1997). The Betula prospective cohort study: Memory, health, and aging. *Aging, Neuropsychology, and Cognition*, *4*, 1–32.

Park, D. C., Davidson, L., Lautenschlager, G., Smith, A. D., Smith, P., & Hedden, T. (2002). Models of visuospatial and verbal memory across the adult lifespan. *Psychology and Aging*, *17*, 299–320.

Park, D. C., & Gutchess, A. H. (2004). Long-term memory and aging: A cognitive neuroscience perspective. In R. Cabeza, L. Nyberg, & D. C. Park (Eds.), *Cognitive neuroscience of aging: Linking cognitive and cerebral aging* (pp. 218–245). New York: Oxford University Press.

Park, D. C., Gutchess, A. H., Meade, M. L., & Stine-Morrow, E. A. L. (2007). Improving cognitive function in older adults: Nontraditional approaches. *Journal of Gerontology*, *62B*, 45–52.

Park, D. C., Polk, T. A., Mikels, J. A., Taylor, S. F., & Marshuetz, C. (2001). Cerebral aging: Integration of brain and behavioural models of cognitive function. *Dialogues in Clinical Neuroscience*, *3*, 151–165.

Park, D. C., & Reuter-Lorenz, P. (in press). The adaptative brain: Aging and neurocognitive scaffolding. *Annual Review of Psychology.*

Park, D. C., & Schwarz, N. (Eds.). (2000). *Cognitive aging: A primer.* Philadelphia, PA: Psychology Press.

Raz, N., Lindenberger, U., Rodrigue, K. M., Kennedy, K. M., Head, D., Williamson, A., et al. (2005). Regional brain changes in aging healthy adults: General trends, individual differences and modifiers. *Cerebral Cortex*, *15*, 1676–1689.

Reales, J. M., & Ballesteros, S. (1999). Implicit and explicit representations of visual and haptic objects: A cross-modal study. *Journal of Experimental Psychology: Learning, Memory, and Cognition*, *20*, 1–25.

Reuter-Lorenz, P. A. (2002). New visions of the ageing mind and brain. *Trends in Cognitive Science*, *6*, 394–400.

Reuter-Lorenz, P. A., & Lustig, C. (2005). Brain aging: Reorganization discoveries about the ageing mind. *Current Opinion in Neurobiology*, *15*, 245–251.

Rönnlund, M., Lövdén, M., & Nilsson, L.-G. (2008). Cross-sectional versus longitudinal age gradients of Tower of Hanoi performance: The role of practice effects and cohort differences in education. *Aging, Neuropsychology, and Cognition*, *15*, 40–67.

Rönnlund, M., & Nilsson, L.-G. (2006). Adult life-span patterns in WAIS block design performance: Cross-sectional versus longitudinal age gradients and relations to demographic predictors. *Intelligence*, *34*, 63–78.

Rönnlund, M., Nyberg, L., Bäckman, L., & Nilsson, L.-G. (2005). Stability, growth, and decline in adult life-span development of declarative memory: Cross-sectional and longitudinal data from a population-based sample. *Psychology and Aging*, *20*, 3–18.

Salthouse, T. A. (1996). The processing-speed theory of adult age differences in cognition. *Psychological Review, 103*, 403–428.

Salthouse, T. A. (in press). When does cognitive decline begin? *Neurobiology of Aging.*

Schacter, D. L., Wig., G. S., & Stevens, W. D. (2007). Reductions in cortical activity during priming. *Current Opinions in Neurobiology, 17*, 171–176.

Schaie, K. W. (1989). Perceptual speed in adulthood: Cross-sectional and longitudinal studies. *Psychology and Aging, 4*, 443–453.

Schaie, K. W. (1996). *Intellectual development in adulthood: The Seattle Longitudinal Study.* Cambridge, MA: Cambridge University Press.

Tulving, E., & Schacter, D. L. (1990). Priming and human memory systems. *Science, 247*, 301–306.

West, R. L. (1996). An application of the prefrontal cortex theory to cognitive ageing. *Psychological Bulletin, 120*, 272–292.

Zellner, M., & Baulm, K. H. (2005). Intact retrieval inhibition in children's episodic recall. *Memory and Cognition, 33*, 396–404.

EUROPEAN JOURNAL OF COGNITIVE PSYCHOLOGY
2009, 21 (2/3), 176–191

Psychology Press
Taylor & Francis Group

Equivalent part set cueing effects in younger and older adults

Pilar Andrés

School of Psychology, University of Plymouth, Plymouth, UK

In a recall test, presenting some of the items as cues inhibits memory for the remaining items. This finding is known as the part set cueing effect. The aim of the current study was to extend the research on part set cueing into ageing. The involvement of inhibition as the explanatory factor for the part set cueing effect was maximised by using an incidental learning procedure where retrieval strategies could not be built up. The cues were presented either before or at recall (Experiments 1 and 2, respectively). The results showed clear and equivalent effects of part set cueing in young and older adults in both experiments. The findings are discussed in relation to Hasher and Zacks' (1988) inhibitory account of ageing and in relation to the recent theoretical distinction between executive and automatic inhibition (Andrés, Guerrini, Phillips, & Perfect, 2008; Nigg, 2000).

Over the past decades research has shown clear effects of ageing on central cognitive abilities such as attention, memory, and language. Hasher and Zacks (1988) provided evidence that a decrease in the ability to control for interfering information might be an important explanatory concept for understanding these age effects. This is known as the inhibitory hypothesis of ageing. However, recent research has shown that age-related differences in inhibitory tasks is far from universal and authors have claimed the existence of a family of specific types of inhibitory processes rather than a unitary mechanism (Hasher, Lustig, & Zacks, 2007; Hasher, Zacks, & May, 1999; Langley, Vivas, Fuentes, & Bagne, 2005; Maylor & Henson, 2000; Nigg, 2000).

Correspondence should be addressed to Pilar Andrés, School of Psychology, University of Plymouth, Portland Square, Drake Circus, Plymouth PL4 8AA, UK. E-mail: pandres @plymouth.ac.uk

I am grateful to Jo Cox, Ruth Moore, Rebecca Thompson, and Claire Summers for their help with data collection. Thanks are also due to Fabrice Parmentier for his comments on previous versions of this paper. Parts of this data were presented at the XIII Conference of the European Society for Cognitive Psychology, Granada, Spain, 17–20 September 2003.

http://www.psypress.com/ecp DOI: 10.1080/09541440802033980

In an attempt to capture the factors responsible for the specificity of age-related differences in inhibitory mechanisms, Andrés, Guerrini, Phillips, and Perfect (2008) suggested that one of the elements responsible for the specificity is the level of executive control involved in producing the inhibitory effect. More specifically, Andrés et al. showed that tasks such as the Stroop task and the stop signal task were affected by ageing to a greater extent than tasks such as negative priming, which only requires automatic inhibition. These findings led to the conclusion that *executive* or controlled inhibition tasks, which require the ability to deliberately inhibit dominant stimuli or responses, are more sensitive to ageing than tasks where participants are unaware of the need to inhibit stimuli to successfully complete the task.

So far, ageing research has concentrated on the effects of ageing on executive inhibitory control (i.e., Stroop task), with surprisingly little research on automatic inhibition (see, however, Maylor & Henson, 2000), particularly in the field of memory. This is even more surprising given the existence of basic memory phenomena such as retrieval inhibition, where recall of a subset of items hinders recall of the remaining items, and this without the participant's intention to forget them.

Part set cueing refers to the detrimental effect that presenting a subset of to-be-remembered items as cues for retrieval has on recall. This "inhibitory" effect occurs outside the participant's awareness, and hence is considered to be the consequence of an automatic process (Anderson, 2005). There have been two main explanations proposed for the part set cueing effect. The first is known as the competition at retrieval or inhibitory hypothesis, and suggests that recall of the items that are not presented as cues is impaired because the cued items have a tendency to be re-retrieved, thus blocking (inhibiting) access to the remaining items (Rundus, 1973; Tulving & Hastie, 1972). A second explanation has been suggested based on the assumption that when a list is presented for encoding, participants organise a strategy to aid recall (Basden & Basden 1995; Brown & Hall, 1979). The idea is that part set cueing occurs because the participant's initial retrieval strategy is disrupted by the unexpected presence of the cues at recall. This is known as the retrieval strategy disruption hypothesis. Finally, Bauml and Aslan (2006) have suggested that these two accounts are not incompatible, and have argued that part set cueing impairment may be caused by different mechanisms depending on the characteristics of the encoding situations. Part list cueing effects would be mediated by inhibitory mechanisms when no elaborated retrieval plans can be built up and by strategy disruption when associations between items and serial retrieval plans are established.

Only three published studies have been dedicated to the effect of ageing on part set cueing, and they have reported conflicting patterns of data. In the first experimental report of part set cueing and ageing, Hultsch and Craig

(1976) published a short report showing an absence of part set cueing in older adults. This would imply the presence of an inhibitory deficit in ageing, but with no means reported in their paper, this conclusion is tentative. In another study, Foos and Clark (2000) gave participants movie star names and US states to recall, either without or with exemplars as cues at recall. The part set cueing effect was not observed for US states in either age group and was only observed for the younger adults for the movie star names. The older adults actually benefited from the presence of cues in that latter study. Finally, Marsh, Dolan, Balota, and Roediger (2004) showed equivalent effects of part set cueing in younger and older participants in three experiments with the exception of a condition (in Experiment 3) where relatively few of the items were presented as cues at recall. However, as the learning phase was intentional and the cues were presented at recall, one cannot ascertain to what extent a possible disruption of retrieval strategies could explain the part set cueing effects observed.

Since the studies looking at part set cueing and ageing have been scarce and have yielded contradictory results, further research is needed to clarify the situation and investigate whether part set cueing is observed in old age or not. This was the aim of the present research. An incidental learning procedure was used for two reasons. The first and main reason was to prevent participants from creating retrieval strategies during encoding. As mentioned before, retrieval inhibition is more likely to account for the part set cueing effects when retrieval strategies cannot be created at encoding (Bauml & Aslan, 2006). The second reason was to minimise age effects on episodic memory at baseline, since the effects of ageing on memory are typically characterised by a decline of attentional resources impacting greatly on encoding processes (Anderson, 1999; Anderson, Craik, & Naveh-Benjamin, 1998; Craik, 1986; Fernandès & Moscovitch, 2000; Park, Smith, Duffley, & Lafronza, 1989). Incidental learning, on the other hand, is relatively well preserved in older adults (Craik & Jennings, 1992).

According to the hypothesis that age has little or no effect on automatic inhibitory processes (Andrés et al., 2008; Hasher & Zacks, 1979; Maylor & Henson, 2000), it was predicted that normal part set cueing effects would be observed in older adults.

EXPERIMENT 1

Method

Participants. Sixty people participated in this experiment. Thirty young adults between the ages of 18 and 25 ($M = 23.9$, $SD = 3.8$) from the University of Plymouth participated as part of course requirements and 30 older adults, over the age of 60 ($M = 73.3$, $SD = 5.7$) from a subject pool at the University of Plymouth volunteered in exchange of a small monetary reward.

Materials and design. There were two phases in this experiment (see Figure 1): a fragment completion phase (Phase 1) and a recall phase (Phase 2). The first consisted in the presentation of 30 incomplete names of movie stars (e.g., T O _ C R U _ _ _ for Tom Cruise). Participants were presented with these fragmented proper names on an A4 page and were asked to complete as many names as possible. They were not given a time limit, but were encouraged to complete them as quickly as they could without making any mistakes (see Appendix for instructions to participants). The 30 movie stars were selected in a way that they represented three different cinema eras. Ten were movie stars from a very past era (e.g., Charlie Chaplin), ten were from a more recent but still past era (e.g., Sean Connery), and ten were younger movie stars from the present (e.g., Brad Pitt). Names were organised so that movie stars from the three eras (present, middle, and past) were presented one after another repeatedly. The names and order of presentation were always the same for all participants.

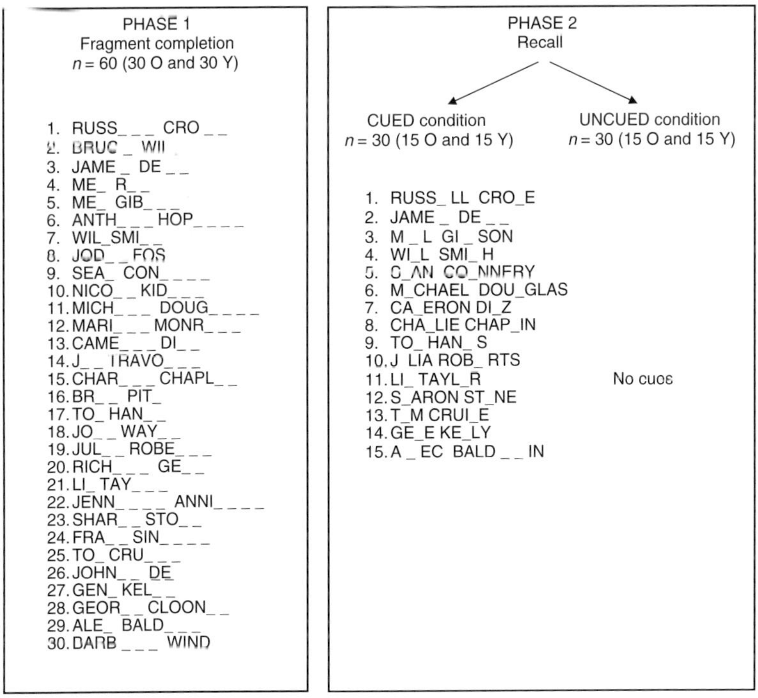

Figure 1. Experimental procedure and stimuli used in Experiment 1. "O" refers to older adults and "Y" refers to younger adults.

Following the fragment completion phase, participants were required to recall as many movie stars as possible (recall phase) from the initial phase. The procedural details of the recall phase varied between participants. Participants in the cued condition were provided, at the time of recall, with 15 of the movie star names as cues (those from the initial list located in odd numbered positions, i.e., 1, 3, . . . , 29, see Figure 1). They were asked to recall (write down) as many of the remaining movie star names as possible (maximum = 15). Participants in the uncued condition were not presented with any of the target names as cues. Their task was to recall as many movie star names as possible from the initial list. Participants were randomly allocated to the cued and uncued conditions so that 15 participants from each age group (younger and older) were allocated to the cued condition and 15 from each age group were allocated to the uncued condition.

All participants were administered the Mill Hill Vocabulary Test (Raven, Raven, & Court, 1998) after completing these tasks.

Results

The age and Mill Hill vocabulary scores for the two subgroups of participants assigned to the cued and uncued conditions are presented in Table 1. *T*-test comparisons showed that the subgroups of younger and older adults allocated to the cued and uncued conditions did not differ in their age or Mill Hill scores.

The Mill Hill results showed a significant effect of ageing for the cued, $t(28) = 5.03$, $p < .001$, and uncued, $t(28) = 5.09$, $p = .0001$, conditions, revealing better scores in the older than in the younger adults (see Table 1). The average number of names completed in the fragment completion phase (Phase 1, maximum = 30) is presented in Table 2, showing that older adults completed fewer items than younger adults in the cued,

TABLE 1
Experiment 1: Age and Mill Hill scores for participants from the cued and uncued conditions

	Cued	*Uncued*	
Age			
Younger	23.87 (3.40)	24.00 (4.20)	$t(28) = -0.09$
Older	74.53 (5.65)	72.10 (5.60)	$t(28) = 1.17$
Mill Hill			
Younger	16.90 (3.40)	18.40 (2.90)	$t(28) = -1.28$
Older	22.80 (3.00)	25.80 (4.80)	$t(28) = -2.04$

All *t*-tests have an associated significance level of $p > .05$.

TABLE 2
Experiment 1: Items completed in Phase 1 and items recalled in Phase 2 by younger and older adults from uncued and cued conditions

	Phase 1				*Phase 2*					
	Total completed items		*Completed never cued items*		*Total recall*		*Recall of never cued items*		*Final recall score*	
	Uncued	*Cued*	*Uncued*	*Cued*	*Uncued*	*Cued*	*Uncued*	*Cued*	*Uncued*	*Cued*
Older	20.70 (6.90)	19.50 (6.20)	10.40 (3.80)	9.93 (3.40)	9.70 (5.00)	2.93 (2.50)	5.60 (2.70)	2.93 (2.50)	0.53 (0.18)	0.27 (0.17)
Younger	28.00 (3.70)	27.90 (3.70)	13.80 (1.90)	13.90 (20.00)	15.10 (3.90)	5.30 (1.60)	7.90 (2.30)	5.30 (1.60)	0.56 (0.12)	0.37 (0.09)

Number of movie star names completed in Phase 1 by participants from the uncued and cued conditions (total completed items; maximum = 30); number of never cued names completed in Phase 1 by participants from the uncued and cued conditions (completed never cued items; maximum = 15); total number of names of movie stars recalled in Phase 2 by participants from the uncued and cued conditions (total recall; maximum = 30 for uncued condition, maximum = 15 for cued condition); number or items recalled that were never presented as cues by participants from the uncued and cued conditions (recall of never cued items; maximum = 15); score resulting from dividing the number of never cued items recalled in Phase 2 by the number of never cued items filled in during Phase 1 for participants from the uncued and cued conditions (final recall score).

$t(28) = -4.44$, $p < .0001$, and uncued, $t(28) = -3.61$, $p = .001$, conditions. Table 2 also presents the total number of names recalled in the recall phase (Phase 2) by older and younger participants from the cued (maximum = 30) and uncued (maximum = 15)[1] conditions, and the number of names recalled other than the 15 names presented as cues (thereafter referred to as "never cued names", maximum = 15 in both conditions). In order to control for the difference between the age groups in the number of fragments completed in Phase 1 and to compare the cued and uncued conditions on the same basis, the dependent variable (final recall score) was the proportion of the number of never cued names recalled relative to the number of these never cued names completed by participants during Phase 1. A 2 (age) × 2 (condition) ANOVA showed a general tendency for older adults to recall fewer items, $F(1, 56) = 3.403$, $MSE = 0.073$, $p = .07$. The effect of condition was significant, $F(1, 56) = 34.925$, $MSE = 0.746$, $p < .0001$, indicating that both younger and older adults recalled fewer uncued names in the cued condition than in the uncued condition. There was, however, no interaction between age and condition, $F(1, 56) = 1.091$, $MSE = 0.023$.

Discussion

The aim of this experiment was to ascertain whether part set cueing effects were observed in younger and older adults in a task where learning was incidental, and therefore no retrieval strategies were created at encoding. Under these circumstances, retrieval inhibition is more likely to explain the part set cueing effect (Bauml & Aslan, 2006). The results showed that when presented with cues, both younger and older adults recalled fewer of the remainder of the list, which confirms Peynircioglu and Moro's (1995) finding that part set cueing can be induced by incidental learning procedures. Additionally, the equivalent part set cueing effect in younger and older adults supports the hypothesis that automatic inhibitory processes in memory are not affected by age.

Experiment 1 used an incidental learning procedure to rule out the possible disruption, at recall, of a strategy prepared during the encoding. However, it remains possible that the construction of an output strategy may be disrupted by cues at the time of recall too. The procedure used in Experiment 1 does not rule out that possibility. In order to reduce the possibility of attributing the part set cueing effect to non inhibitory processes, Experiment 2, where the cueing phase was introduced before

[1] In this condition, as participants are presented with cues at recall, only uncued names are left to recall and therefore maximum recall is 15. Hence, total recall and recall of never-cued items are equivalent (see Table 2).

the recall phase, was carried out. If the findings from Experiment 1 were to be replicated in Experiment 2, this would provide additional support to the idea that age does not affect part set cueing, even when inhibitory processes are most likely to underpin the effect.

EXPERIMENT 2

Method

Participants. Eighty people participated in this experiment. Forty young adults between the ages of 18 and 25 ($M = 20.0$, $SD = 1.5$) from the University of Plymouth participated as part of course requirements and 40 older adults over the age of 60 ($M = 73.8$, $SD = 5.7$) from the University of Plymouth ageing database volunteered in exchange of a small monetary reward.

Materials and design. There were three phases in this experiment (see Figure 2). The fragment completion phase (Phase 1) was exactly the same as in Experiment 1. Following the name completion phase, participants took part in a second fragment completion task (Phase 2) where a list of 15 incomplete words was presented. The items presented during this phase varied between participants. For participants in the cued condition, 15 of the names from Phase 1 were presented and participants were asked to complete the names. For participants in the uncued condition, 15 animal names, for example, H O R _ E (horse), were presented and participants were asked to complete these fragments. Participants were randomly assigned to either the cued or uncued condition so that 20 participants from each age group (younger and older) were allocated to the cued condition and 20 from each age group were allocated to the uncued condition. During the final recall phase (Phase 3), a free recall task was presented to all participants: Participants were asked to write down as many movie star names from Phase 1 as they could and were not provided with any cues (see Appendix for instructions given to participants).

All participants were administered the Mill Hill Vocabulary Test (Raven et al., 1998) after completing these tasks.

Results

The age and Mill Hill vocabulary scores for the two subgroups of participants allocated to the cued and uncued conditions are presented in Table 3. *T*-test comparisons showed that the two subgroups of younger and

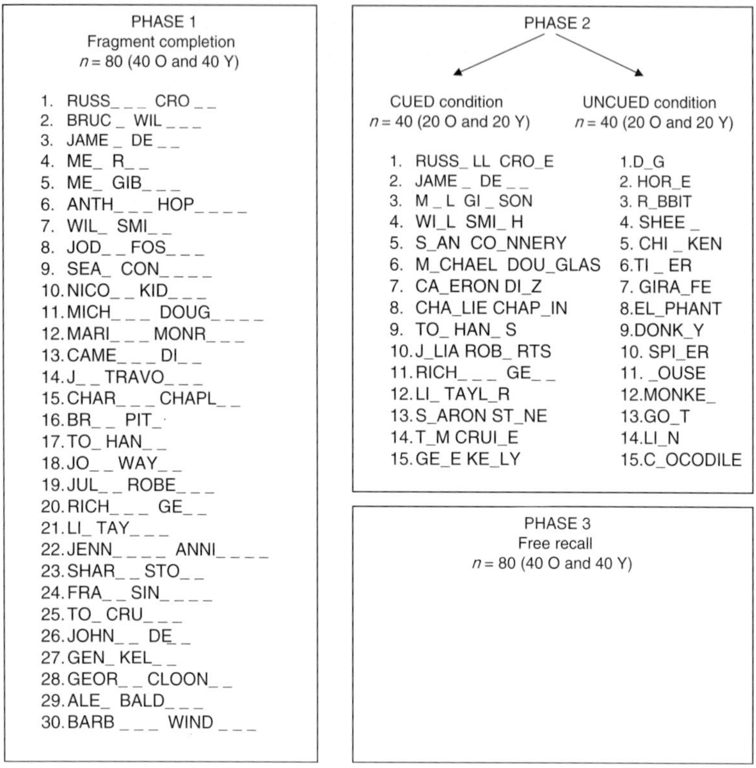

Figure 2. Experimental procedure and stimuli used in Experiment 2. "O" refers to older adults and "Y" refers to younger adults.

older adults assigned to the cued and uncued conditions did not differ in their age or Mill Hill scores.

The Mill Hill results showed a significant effect of ageing for the cued, $t(38) = 5.90$, $p < .0001$, and uncued, $t(38) = 8.01$, $p = .0001$, conditions, revealing better scores in the older than in the younger adults (see Table 3).

The average number of names of movie stars completed during the fragment completion phase (Phase 1, maximum = 30) is presented in Table 4. As in Experiment 1, older adults completed fewer items in this phase than younger adults, and this for the cued, $t(38) = -5.39$, $p < .0001$, and uncued, $t(38) = -2.8$, $p < .001$, conditions. Table 4 also presents the total number of movie star names recalled in Phase 3 by older and younger participants from the cued and uncued conditions (both maximum = 30) and the number of these items that were never presented as cues in Phase 2 for the cued and

TABLE 3
Experiment 2: Age and Mill Hill scores for participants from the cued and uncued conditions

	Cued	*Uncued*	
Age			
Younger	20.15 (1.53)	19.90 (1.50)	$t(38) = 0.52$
Older	74.65 (6.32)	72.45 (5.83)	$t(38) = 1.14$
Mill Hill			
Younger	15.15 (3.80)	15.75 (3.50)	$t(38) = 0.52$
Older	24.15 (5.70)	25.50 (4.20)	$t(38) = 0.86$

All t-tests have an associated significance level of $p > .05$.

uncued conditions (both maximum = 15). In order to control for the difference between the age groups in the number of fragments completed in Phase 1 and to compare the cued and uncued conditions on the same basis, the dependent variable (final recall score) was the proportion of the number of never cued names recalled (maximum = 15) relative to the number of these uncued names completed by participants during the fragment completion phase (maximum = 15). A 2 (age) × 2 (condition) ANOVA showed a main effect of age, $F(1, 76) = 9.352$, $MSE = 0.197$, $p < .005$, indicating that older adults recalled globally fewer movie stars than younger adults and a main effect of condition, $F(1, 76) = 32.185$, $MSE = 0.679$, $p < .0001$, indicating that younger and older adults recalled fewer movie stars in the cued than in the uncued condition. There was, however, no interaction between age and condition, $F(1, 76) = 0.303$, $MSE = 0.006$.

The number of movie stars recalled that had been presented as cues during Phase 2 was also analysed to investigate whether participants from the cued condition recalled more cued movie stars than those from the uncued condition. Average recall was 5.6 ($SD = 2.3$) in the uncued condition and 7.7 ($SD = 2.8$) in the cued condition. A t-test showed a significant difference between these two conditions, $t(78) = 3.71$, $p < .01$, indicating that participants from the cued condition recalled more movie star names that had been cued than the participants from the uncued condition. Finally, in order to investigate a possible effect of age on this beneficial effect, the recall of movie stars that had been presented as cues during Phase 2 divided by the number of cued movie stars that were successfully completed during Phase 2 of younger and older adults were compared. The results showed that the facilitation effect induced by the cueing in Phase 2 was equivalent in younger (score = 0.55, $SD = 0.20$) and older (score = 0.58, $SD = 0.43$) adults, $t(78) = 0.317$, $p = .752$.

TABLE 4
Experiment 2: Items completed in Phase 1 and items recalled in Phase 3 by younger and older adults from uncued and cued conditions

	Phase 1				*Phase 3*					
	Total completed items		*Completed never cued items*		*Total recall*		*Recall of never cued items*		*Final recall score*	
	Uncued	*Cued*	*Uncued*	*Cued*	*Uncued*	*Cued*	*Uncued*	*Cued*	*Uncued*	*Cued*
Older	24.20 (6.00)	20.90 (5.10)	12.00 (3.34)	10.95 (2.90)	0.80 (4.20)	9.20 (4.30)	5.80 (2.90)	3.05 (2.20)	0.47 (0.17)	0.27 (0.16)
Younger	28.10 (1.80)	27.90 (2.50)	14.00 (1.20)	14.00 (1.40)	14.00 (3.30)	14.60 (3.50)	7.80 (2.00)	5.30 (1.60)	0.55 (0.14)	0.39 (0.09)

Number of movie star names completed in Phase 1 by participants from the uncued and cued conditions (total completed items; maximum = 30); number of never cued names completed in Phase 1 by participants from the uncued and cued conditions (completed never cued items; maximum = 15); total number of names of movie stars recalled in Phase 3 by participants from the uncued and cued conditions (total recall; maximum = 30); number of never cued items recalled by participants from the uncued and cued conditions (recall of never cued items; maximum = 15); score resulting from dividing the number of never cued items recalled by the number of never cued items filled in during Phase 1 for participants from the uncued and cued conditions (final recall score).

Discussion

The aim of this experiment was to explore whether part set cueing could be observed in young and older adults by using a methodology that excludes as much as possible the possibility that recall strategies may be disrupted by the unexpected presence of cues and so to maximise the involvement of inhibitory processes in the part set cueing effect. The method used clearly strengthened the cued items (and hence blocked the uncued items; Rundus, 1973) by introducing the cueing in a phase previous to recall. This contention is further supported by the observation that participants from the cued condition recalled significantly more movie star names that were presented as cues than participants from the uncued condition.

The results from this experiment show robust and equivalent effects of part set cueing in young and older participants, which supports the hypothesis that when the inhibitory effect investigated does not depend on the executive and conscious control of the participant, it is resistant to ageing (Andrés et al., 2008).

GENERAL DISCUSSION

The aim of this study was to look at the possible effects of ageing on part set cueing. The mechanisms responsible for part set cueing may depend on the methodology used. In this study, retrieval strategy disruption (e.g., Basden & Basden, 1995, Basden, Basden, & Galloway, 1977) was unlikely to be at play as an incidental learning procedure was used, so no clear retrieval strategy could have been formed (e.g., Bauml & Aslan, 2006). Moreover, in Experiment 2, cues were presented in an intermediate phase, not at recall; therefore disruption of recall strategies was very unlikely. The most likely explanation of the part set cueing effect in our study is the competition at retrieval hypothesis (Rundus, 1973), which claims that the strengthening of a subset of items results in a weakening of the remaining items of the list and involves inhibitory mechanisms.

Following the hypothesis that automatic inhibition should be resistant to ageing (Andrés et al., 2008; see also Maylor & Henson, 2000), it was predicted that equivalent part set cueing effects would be observed in young and older adults. The results confirm our prediction by showing robust effects of part set cueing in both groups. These findings are similar to the findings in Marsh et al.'s (2004) study. It is important to note that in Marsh et al.'s study participants were explicitly required to learn the list of words for later recall. Also, cues were presented at recall in all experiments, so the possibility that some kind of disruption occurred either at encoding or at recall cannot be completely ruled out. In that sense, our study confirms and extends Marsh et al.'s findings to a situation where inhibitory mechanisms must be more heavily involved in the part set cueing effect.

Previous studies have found an absence of part set cueing effects in older adults (Hultsch & Craig, 1976) or even a benefit from the presence of cues in older adults (Foos & Clark, 2000). As mentioned earlier, it is difficult to evaluate the findings from Hultsch and Craig's study due to the lack of detail provided in their short report. As for Foos and Clark's study, the benefit from part set cueing in older adults was observed in a task where there was no distinction between learning and cueing phases. In what was considered to be the part set cueing condition, participants were given a set of 25 movie stars and were told to study them because it could help them later when asked to name as many movie stars as possible. However, given that older adults have longer life experience, they must have undoubtedly encoded more movie stars during their lives. As the lists were open set (rather than belonging to a particular learning episode), older adults could remember as many movie stars as possible without any restriction. Moreover, there is evidence showing that cues may help facilitate recall and not hinder when the list is too long to be spontaneously recalled unaided (e.g., Basden & Basden, 1995; Roediger, 1974; Slamecka, 1968). This would not have occurred in the present study.

In the current research, the presentation of cues at recall had the effect of heightening the awareness of these items, whilst reducing the accessibility of the never cued items. This process was defined as automatic as it occurred without the awareness of the participants and therefore the part set cueing effect was not seen to discriminate between the two different age groups, though it had a detrimental effect on all. Consistent with our findings on part set cueing, Aslan, Bauml, and Pastotter (2007) found normal retrieval induced forgetting in older adults, a reduction in recall provoked by an intermediate episode of recall where a subset of items are recalled at a practice phase. This inhibitory effect is also considered to be automatic in nature (Anderson, 2005), and is beyond the awareness of participants. Maylor and Henson (2000) also found no age differences in the Ranschburg effect, an inhibitory effect observed in short-term memory that does not require executive inhibition. At the other end of the lifespan, robust part set cueing effects have also been observed in children by Zellner and Bauml (2005). All together, these results show that the inhibitory processes involved in part set cueing develop very early in life and remain resistant to the effects of ageing. This would support the idea that there are different inhibitory mechanisms (Friedman & Miyake, 2004; Harnishfeger, 1995; Nigg, 2000; Zacks & Hasher, 1997), rather than a unitary "inhibition" function, and that when the inhibitory effect is not under the participant's executive control, the effect is equivalent in young and older adults (Andrés et al., 2008).

This type of phenomena may have implications in older people's everyday life situations such as compliance with medicines. For example, when a general practitioner or family member reminds an older adult to take a medicine, it might have a negative impact on remembering other necessary medicines. Also, this study produces practical implications for writing cues, for example writing only some of the items down from any given list assuming that the person would remember the other items. Our findings suggest writing only some cues and not all would prevent remembering the rest of the items and this would occur with younger and older adults to the same extent.

In conclusion, the results from the current study show that both older and younger adults are affected by part set cueing. These results parallel previous findings showing equivalent inhibitory effects in younger and older adults with tasks that do not require executive control (Andrés et al., 2008), and confirm that nonexecutive inhibition develops early in life (Zellner & Bauml, 2005) and remains unaffected by ageing.

REFERENCES

Anderson, M. C. (2005). The role of inhibitory control in forgetting unwanted memories: A consideration of three methods. In C. MacLeod & B. Uttl (Eds.), *Dynamic cognitive processes* (pp. 159–190). Tokyo: Springer-Verlag.

Anderson, N. D. (1999). The attentional demands of encoding and retrieval in younger and older adults: 2. Evidence from secondary task reaction time distributions. *Psychology and Aging*, *14*, 645–655.

Anderson, N. D., Craik, F. I., & Naveh-Benjamin, M. (1998). The attentional demands of encoding and retrieval in younger and older adults: 1. Evidence from divided attention costs. *Psychology and Aging*, *13*, 405–423.

Andrés, P., Guerrini, C., Phillips, L., & Perfect, T. (2008). Differential effects of aging on executive and automatic inhibition. *Developmental Neuropsychology*, *33*, 101–123.

Aslan, A., Bauml, K., & Pastotter, B. (2007). No inhibitory deficit in older adults' episodic memory. *Psychological Science*, *18*, 72–78.

Basden, D. R., & Basden, B. H. (1995). Some tests of the strategy disruption interpretation of part list cueing inhibition. *Journal of Experimental psychology: Learning, Memory, and Cognition*, *21*, 1656–1669.

Basden, D. R., Basden, B. H., & Galloway, B. C. (1977). Inhibition with part list cueing: Some tests of the item strength hypothesis. *Journal of Experimental Psychology: Human Learning and Memory*, *1*, 100–108.

Bauml, K., & Aslan, A. (2006). Part-list cuing can be transient and lasting: The role of encoding. *Journal of Experimental Psychology: Learning, Memory, and Cognition*, *32*, 33–43.

Brown, A. S., & Hall, L. A. (1979). Part-list cuing inhibition in semantic memory structures. *American Journal of Psychology*, *92*, 351–362.

Craik, F. I. M. (1986). A functional account of age differences in memory. In F. Klix & H. Hagendorf (Eds.), *Human memory and cognitive capabilities, mechanisms, and performance* (pp. 409–422). Amsterdam: Elsevier Science Publishers.

Craik, F. I. M., & Jennings, J. M. (1992). Human memory. In F. I. M. Craik & T. A. Salthouse (Eds.), *The handbook of aging and cognition* (pp. 51–110). Hillsdale, NJ: Lawrence Erlbaum Associates, Inc.

Fernandes, M. A., & Moscovitch, M. (2000). Divided attention and memory: Evidence of substantial interference effects at retrieval and encoding. *Journal of Experimental Psychology: General, 129*, 155–176.

Foos, P. W., & Clark, M. C. (2000). Old age, inhibition and the part set cueing effect. *Educational Gerontology, 26*, 155–160.

Friedman, N. P., & Miyake, A. (2004). The relations among inhibition and interference control functions: A latent variable analysis. *Journal of Experimental Psychology: General, 133*, 101–135.

Harnishfeger, K. (1995). The development of cognitive inhibition: Theories, definitions, and research evidence. In F. K. Dempster & C. J. Brainerd (Eds.), *Interference and inhibition in cognition* (pp. 176–206). London: Academic Press.

Hasher, L., Lustig, C., & Zacks, R. T. (2007). Inhibitory mechanisms and the control of attention. In A. Conway, C. Jarrold, M. Kane, A. Miyake, & J. Towse (Eds.), *Variation in working memory* (pp. 227–249). New York: Oxford University Press.

Hasher, L., & Zacks, R. T. (1979). Automatic and effortful processes in memory. *Journal of Experimental Psychology: General, 108*, 356–388.

Hasher, L., & Zacks, R. T. (1988). Working memory, comprehension, and aging: A review and a new view. In G. H. Bower (Ed.), *The psychology of learning and motivation* (Vol. 22, pp. 193–225). Orlando, FL: Academic Press.

Hasher, L., Zacks, R. T., & May, C. P. (1999). Inhibitory control, circadian arousal, and age. In D. Gopher & A. Koriat (Eds.), *Attention and performance XVII: Cognitive regulation of performance: Interaction of theory and application* (pp. 653–675). Cambridge, MA: MIT Press.

Hultsch, D. F., & Craig, E. R. (1976). Adult age differences in the inhibition of recall as a function of retrieval cues. *Developmental Psychology, 12*, 83–84.

Langley, L., Vivas, A., Fuentes, L., & Bagne, A. G. (2005). Differential age effects on attention-based inhibition: Inhibitory tagging and inhibition of return. *Psychology and Aging, 20*, 356–360.

Marsh, E. J., Dolan, P. O., Balota, D. A., & Roediger, H. L. (2004). Part-set cueing effects in younger and older adults. *Psychology and Aging, 19*, 134–144.

Maylor, E., & Henson, R. (2000). Aging and the Ranschburg effect: No evidence of reduced response suppression in old age. *Psychology and Aging, 15*, 657–670.

Nigg, J. T. (2000). On inhibition/disinhibition in developmental psychopathology: Views from cognitive and personality psychology and a working inhibition taxonomy. *Psychological Bulletin, 126*, 200–246.

Park, D. C., Smith, A. D., Duddley, W. N., & Lafronza, V. N. (1989). Effects of age and a divided attention task presented during encoding and retrieval on memory. *Journal of Experimental Psychology: Learning, Memory, and Cognition, 15*, 1185–1191.

Peynircioglu, Z., & Moro, C. (1995). Part-set cuing in incidental and implicit memory. *American Journal of Psychology, 108*, 1–11.

Raven, J. C., Raven, J., & Court, J. H. (1988). *Mill Hill Vocabulary Scale.* Oxford, UK: Oxford Psychology Press.

Roediger, H. L. (1974). Inhibition effects of recall. *Memory and Cognition, 2*, 261–269.

Rundus, D. (1973). Negative effects of using list items as recall cues. *Journal of Verbal Learning and Verbal Behaviour, 12*, 43–50.

Slamecka, N. J. (1968). An examination of trace storage in free recall. *Journal of Experimental Psychology, 76*, 504–513.

Tulving, E., & Hastie, R. (1972). Inhibition effects of intralist repetition in free recall. *Journal of Experimental Psychology, 92*, 297–304.

Zacks, R., & Hasher, L. (1997). Cognitive gerontology and attentional inhibition: A reply to Burke and McDowd. *Journal of Gerontology: Psychological Sciences, 52B*, 274–283.
Zellner, M., & Bauml, K. H. (2005). Intact retrieval inhibition in children's episodic recall. *Memory and Cognition, 33*, 396–404.

APPENDIX: Instructions

Experiment 1

Phase 1. In this task, you will be presented with a list of movie stars. Each name on the list will have missing letters. The aim of the study is to see how many movie star names you can complete. Please fill in as many as you can and as quickly as you can without making mistakes.

Phase 2, cued condition. Please recall as many movie stars as possible from the list you initially completed. To help you, here are some of the movie star names from the previous task.

Phase 2, uncued condition. Please recall as many movie stars as possible from the previous task.

Experiment 2

Phase 1. In this task, you will be presented with a list of movie stars. Each name on the list will have missing letters. The aim of the study is to see how many movie star names you can complete. Please fill in as many as you can and as quickly as you can without making mistakes.

Phase 2, cued and uncued conditions. This task is similar to the first one. You will be presented with a list of words with missing letters. Please fill in as many as you can.

Phase 3. Please recall as many movie stars as possible from the list you initially completed.

EUROPEAN JOURNAL OF COGNITIVE PSYCHOLOGY
2009, 21 (2/3), 192–215

Psychology Press
Taylor & Francis Group

Age-related changes in the neural mechanisms supporting emotion processing and emotional memory

Elizabeth A. Kensinger and Christina M. Leclerc
Department of Psychology, Boston College, Boston, MA, USA

Older adults process emotional information differently than young adults, placing more emphasis on pleasant information. Age-related changes in emotional processing have downstream effects on the types of information that are remembered best; whereas young adults remember negative information well, older adults often show greater mnemonic benefits for positive information. Although these cognitive changes have been discussed previously (Mather, 2006; Mather & Carstensen, 2005), here we review the neural changes that may mediate these age-related changes. We suggest that changes in older adults' recruitment of prefrontal regions during emotional processing may reflect not only age-related changes in emotion regulation but also changes in self-referential processing. Because little research has examined the links between the neural networks supporting older adults' emotional and cognitive functioning, we conclude with a discussion of avenues meriting further research.

Though cognitive changes with ageing often have been focused on to the exclusion of affective changes, research over the last two decades has begun to examine age-related differences in the processing of emotional information. By emotional information, we refer to information that elicits a response-tendency including a subjective feeling state as well as changes in behaviour, motivation, and physiology (see, for recent debates regarding the construct of emotion, Barrett, 2006; Frijda & Sundararajan, 2007; Izard, 2007; Panksepp, 2007). Behavioural research has revealed significant developmental changes in the processing of emotional information, with affect information taking on increased importance as individuals advance from young adulthood (usually considered to be the late teenage years through the early thirties) and into old age (usually considered to begin in

Correspondence should be addressed to Elizabeth A. Kensinger, Department of Psychology, Boston College, McGuinn Hall, 140 Commonwealth Ave., Chestnut Hill, MA 02467, USA. E-mail: Elizabeth.kensinger@bc.edu

Preparation of this manuscript was supported by grants to EAK from the National Science Foundation, the American Federation for Aging Research, and the Dana Foundation.

http://www.psypress.com/ecp DOI: 10.1080/09541440801937116

the early to mid-sixties; reviewed by Carstensen & Mikels, 2005; Mather & Carstensen, 2005). As adults age, they derive additional pleasure from emotionally gratifying activities, and their emotional well-being begins to take centre stage in influencing their decision making. Older adults are more likely to spend time with close friends and family (Fung, Carstensen, & Lutz, 1999), they resonate with advertisements focusing on emotional goals (e.g., "Capture those special moments"; Fung & Carstensen, 2003), and they tend to categorise people based upon their emotional characteristics (Fredrickson & Carstensen, 1990). Laura Carstensen and colleagues have proposed that these motivational shifts occur with ageing because individuals begin to perceive time as limited (Carstensen, Isaacowitz, & Charles, 1999).

Probably because of the increased importance that older adults place on emotional gratification, they tend to focus more on positive information than do young adults. Older adults sustain attention on positive information longer than young adults (Isaacowitz, Wadlinger, Goren, & Wilson, 2006) and they are faster to divert their attention away from negative information (Isaacowitz et al., 2006; Mather & Carstensen, 2003). They remember their prior choices in a more positive light (Mather & Johnson, 2000), and they are more likely to remember events that elicited positive affect and less likely to remember those that elicited negative affect (e.g., Grühn, Scheibe, & Baltes, 2007; Kennedy, Mather, & Carstensen, 2004). This change in the types of emotional information most likely to be remembered has been referred to as a "positivity shift", and it exists both when information is attended and retained over the short term (reviewed by Carstensen & Mikels, 2005) and also when memory is assessed after long delays (reviewed by Mather & Carstensen, 2005).

These age-related changes in emotional processing and emotional memory are in opposition with older adults' structural preservation of the limbic structures associated with emotional processing. In contrast to vast age-related changes in regions traditionally associated with "cold" cognition (e.g., lateral prefrontal and hippocampal areas), regions associated with affect, including the medial prefrontal cortex and amygdala, seem relatively preserved with ageing (reviewed by Chow & Cummings, 2000). This contrast between relatively preserved structure, but altered behaviour, suggests that the age-related changes may be happening not at the level of brain *structure* but rather at the level of brain *function*.

Indeed, as will be described later, evidence has begun to suggest that there are fundamental age-related changes in the types of information that elicit the strongest responses in regions throughout the limbic system. This review highlights the recent studies that have revealed such changes and discusses how these age-related changes may be tied to older adults' regulation of emotion and their tendency to process information in a self-referential fashion. We then turn our attention to how memory for emotional information is impacted by these changes in neural response, paying particular attention to new research suggesting a link between older adults' engagement of regions implicated in self-referential processing and their heightened ability to remember positive information. Because research into the neural processes supporting older adults' emotional processing and emotional memory still is sparse, we conclude with a discussion of implications and directions for future research, including the need to pay attention to individual differences in emotion processing and to consider how changes in emotion processing may contribute to older adults' performance in other domains, such as decision making.

EMOTIONAL PROCESSING IN AGEING

As mentioned earlier, ageing is associated with a "positivity shift" (Carstensen & Mikels, 2005; Mather & Carstensen, 2005): Older adults focus their attention on positive information more often than on negative information. This shift appears to be characterised both by enhanced attention towards positive information and by a withdrawal from negative information. Not only do older adults look longer at positive images than younger adults (Isaacowitz et al., 2006), they also tend to avoid processing negative information (Isaacowitz et al., 2006; Mather & Carstensen, 2003).

Some of these age-related changes may result from alterations in amygdala function. Older adults tend to show reductions in amygdala activation to negative images (Mather et al., 2004) and facial expressions (e.g., Gunning-Dixon et al., 2003; Iidaka et al., 2002) as compared to young adults (see Table 1). However, although these findings initially were interpreted as indicating general age-related disruption of amygdala function, this interpretation has begun to be rethought. The amygdala is not always less active in older adults than in young adults. Rather, it seems more accurate to conclude that, in older adults, the amygdala responds to different types of stimuli than in younger adults. For one, amygdala activation in older adults tends to be more sensitive to changes in novelty; thus, when faces are both novel and fearful, older adults show as robust an amygdala response as young adults (Wright et al., 2006; Wright, Dickerson, Feczko, Negeira, & Williams, 2007). Second, in older adults the amygdala appears to be more responsive to positive things than in younger adults. When young and older adults were shown positive, negative, or neutral photographs (from the IAPS set; Lang, Bradley, & Cuthbert, 1997) while undergoing an event-related functional magnetic resonance imaging scan, young adults showed similarly high levels of amygdala activity for negative and positive images. Older adults, in contrast, showed more amygdala activity for positive than for negative images (Mather et al., 2004). Thus, the neural data parallel the behavioural findings: As compared to young adults, older adults attend more to positive than to negative images and their amygdala activation is greater for positive images but can be diminished for negative images.

Amygdala activation often is associated with the relatively automatic processing of emotional information. By automatic processing we refer to a fast operating, hard-wired, relatively unconscious system that quickly codes for the attributes and evaluative implications of stimuli and behaviours (see, for discussion of the neural processes supporting such automatic functions, Esslen, Pascual-Marqui, Hell, Kochi, & Lehmann, 2004; Jansma, Ramsey, Slagter, & Kahn, 2001; Kalisch, Wiech, Critchley, & Dolan, 2006; Satpute & Lieberman, 2006). Amygdala function has been linked to a person's ability to rapidly detect emotional information presented with a rapid stream of stimuli (Anderson & Phelps, 1998). Amygdala activity also has been tied to a person's ability to detect emotional stimuli even when attentional resources are taxed (reviewed by Dolan & Vuilleumier, 2003), suggesting that its role in emotional processing is not heavily dependent on the availability of extensive cognitive resources (though see Pessoa, 2005, for evidence that some awareness of stimuli may be required for normal amygdala responsivity).

Because of this link between amygdala activity and relatively automatic emotional processing, altered amygdala function with ageing might be considered to reflect age-related changes in the rapid detection or automatic processing of emotional information in the environment. However, behavioural evidence is mounting to suggest that this is not the case. On tasks assessing the automatic detection of emotional information, older adults tend to perform quite similarly to young adults. On visual search tasks, older adults detect negative arousing information just as quickly as they detect positive arousing information (Leclerc & Kensinger, in press a), and they show as much facilitation for detecting negative arousing information as do young adults (Leclerc & Kensinger, in press a; Mather & Knight, 2006). Both age groups also tend to focus on arousing information within a complex scene (Kensinger, Gutchess, & Schacter, 2007) and to first fixate upon an emotional stimulus in a two-stimulus array (Hahn, Carlson, Singer, & Gronlund, 2006; Knight et al., 2007). Thus, age differences in emotional processing do not appear to reflect changes in the automatic detection of emotional information.

If age differences in emotional processing do not reflect changes in the types of information initially detected, then what do they reflect? A plausible hypothesis is that age differences exist not at relatively automatic stages of processing, but rather in the more controlled or strategic processing of emotional information (see Mather, 2006; Mather & Carstensen, 2005). By controlled processing, we refer to the attention-demanding processes that allow a person to hold motivational goals in mind and to use prior knowledge or contextual information to guide or alter the inferences made

TABLE 1
Summary of neuroimaging studies comparing young and older adults' emotional processing

Study	Age range (years)	Stimulus type	Task design *(stimulus duration)*	Key findings regarding age changes in emotion processing
Event-related functional magnetic resonance imaging				
Gutchess, Kensinger, & Schacter (2007)	YA = 18–28 OA = 61–80	words	Decide whether positive or negative adjectives describe you, describe Albert Einstein, or are written in upper case font (4 s/jittered ITI).	OA (not YA) show increased activity in the dorsal prefrontal cortex for positive relative to negative adjectives.
Leclerc & Kensinger (in press b)	YA = 19–31 OA = 61–80	coloured photo-objects	Make a size decision about positive, negative, or neutral objects (1 s/jittered ITI).	Age-related valence reversal in response of ventromedial PFC and precuneus (greater response to negative than positive items in YA; opposite pattern in OA); similar arousal responses in YA and OA.
Mather et al. (2004)	YA = 18–29 OA = 70–90	coloured pictures	Rate arousal of positive, negative, and neutral pictures (3 s/jittered ITI).	Both age groups show greater amygdala activity to emotional items (collapsing across positive and negative) than neutral items. Only OA show more amygdala activity to positive than to negative images.
Blocked design functional magnetic resonance imaging				
Fischer et al. (2005)	YA = 20–30 OA = 70–80	faces	View blocks of either angry or neutral faces (200 ms/300 ms ITI).	For angry faces, amygdala activity greater in YA than in OA and insula activity greater in OA than in YA.

Table 1 (*Continued*)

Study	Age range (years)	Stimulus type	Task design (*stimulus duration*)	Key findings regarding age changes in emotion processing
Gunning-Dixon et al. (2003)	YA = 19–29 OA = 57–79	faces	View blocks of faces expressing a single emotion (4 s/no ITI).	Amygdala activity greater in YA than in OA. Left PFC activity greater in OA than in YA.
Iidaka et al. (2002)	YA = 19–39 OA = 62–72	faces	Judge gender of faces with negative, positive, or neutral expressions (2.5 s/0.2 s ITI).	Amygdala activity greater in YA than in OA for negative faces.
Tessitore et al. (2005)	YA = 20–29 OA = 60–80	faces	Match angry or fearful face cue with a face target displaying the correct emotion (5 s/no ITI).	Amygdala activity greater in YA than in OA. Ventrolateral and medial PFC activity greater in OA than in YA.
Wedig et al. (2005)	YA = 21–27 OA = 62–84	faces	Measure habituation by comparing activity early in a block of repeated faces to activity late in the block (200 ms/300 ms ITI).	YA and OA show similar amounts of amygdala habituation overall, but with laterality effects (more left hemisphere habituation in OA; more right hemisphere habituation in YA).
Williams et al. (2006)	Teen = 12–19 YA = 20–29 Middle = 30–49 OA = 50–79	faces	Attend to blocks of happy, fearful, or neutral faces (500 ms/300 ms ITI).	YA show greater amygdala and caudate activity for fear and happy faces than OA; OA show greater medial PFC activity to fear than YA and less medial PFC activity to happy than YA.
Wright et al. (2006, 2007a)	YA = 21–27 OA = 62–72	faces	View blocks of familiar neutral or novel fearful faces (200 ms/300 ms ITI).	Amygdala activity greater for fearful than for neutral faces in both age groups; no age differences.

Table 1 (*Continued*)

Study	Age range (years)	Stimulus type	Task design (*stimulus duration*)	Key findings regarding age changes in emotion processing
Event-related potentials				
Kisley et al. (2007)	18–81 continuous	coloured pictures	Same as Wood & Kisley (2006).	LPP amplitude for negative images correlates negatively with age; no correlation with age for positive or neutral images.
Williams et al. (2006)	Teen = 12–19 YA = 20–29 Middle = 30–49 OA = 50–79	faces	Attend to blocks of happy, fearful, or neutral faces (500 ms/300 ms ITI).	OA show more late-onset medial PFC activity to fearful faces and more early onset PFC activity to happy faces than YA.
Wood & Kisley (2006)	YA = 19–22 OA = 56–81	coloured pictures	Categorise blocks of positive, negative, and neutral images; some images are inconsistent with the other images presented in a block (e.g., a negative image intermixed with neutral images) (1 s/1.2 s ITI).	For YA, late positive potential (LPP) waveform greatest for inconsistent negative images; for OA, LPP waveform equally great for negative and positive images.

YA = young adults, OA = older adults, ITI = intertrial interval, PFC = prefrontal cortex.

about stimuli or behaviours. Such processes are slow operating and require working memory resources, and they will include both regulatory and elaborative components (for more discussion of controlled emotional processing and the neural substrates that may support such processing, see Kalisch et al., 2006; Leventhal & Scherer, 1987; Robinson, 1998; Satpute & Lieberman, 2006). Indeed, the types of tasks that most reliably show age-related changes are those that focus not on automatic detection but rather on sustained attention or on elaborative processing (Mather, 2006). Although young and older adults both fixate initially on the same types of stimuli, older adults are more likely than young adults to dwell on the positive images and to disengage from the negative ones (e.g., Isaacowitz et al., 2006). Older adults also can show a greater positivity shift when they are asked to remember stimuli that benefit primarily from controlled processing (e.g., low arousal information) rather than stimuli that benefit from more automatic processing (e.g., high arousal information; Kensinger, in press). Older adults also may be more likely to engage elaborative processes when asked to reflect upon how positive information relates to themselves, whereas young adults may employ these controlled processes more for negative information (Gutchess, Kensinger, & Schacter, 2007).

The most convincing behavioural evidence to support the role of controlled processing in older adults' "positivity shift" has come from studies of divided attention. When older adults are able to devote full attention towards the processing of emotional information, they show a robust positivity shift. In contrast, when their attention is divided as they process the information, they do not show a positivity shift (Knight et al., 2007). Rather, their attentional focus parallels that of young adults (Mather & Knight, 2005). Although it may seem surprising that divided attention manipulations can diminish or reverse older adults' positivity shift, it is exactly this pattern of results that would be expected if older adults' shift arises from controlled processing. When older adults have the cognitive resources to devote to emotional processing, they engage in the controlled processing of emotional information, leading them to show a positivity shift; however, as soon as their cognitive resources are depleted, they cannot deploy those controlled processes and their positivity shift disappears (reviewed by Mather, 2006). Further evidence to suggest a link between the positivity shift and controlled processing has come from studies demonstrating that the older adults with the best cognitive control ability are the ones who show the strongest shift. In contrast, older adults with poor cognitive control ability show no positivity shift (Mather & Knight, 2005).

The neuroimaging data also support the interpretation that older adults may engage more controlled processing than young adults when they encounter emotional information. In particular, many of the same studies that revealed reduced amygdala activation in older adults also revealed increased prefrontal activation in the older individuals (see Table 1). The prefrontal regions revealed in those studies (e.g., ventrolateral prefrontal cortex; Tessitore et al., 2005) are thought to be brought online during the controlled maintenance and manipulation of information (reviewed by Courtney, Petit, Haxby, & Ungerleider, 1998). Therefore, older adults' increased engagement of those regions during emotion processing, and their reduced engagement of the amygdala during emotion processing, could signify an age-related shift from relatively automatic to more controlled emotion processing.

CHANGES IN OLDER ADULTS' REGULATION OF EMOTIONAL PROCESSING

If age-related differences in emotional processing arise from changes in controlled processing, a likely contributor to the effect would be age-related changes in emotion regulation. Emotion regulation refers to a person's ability to control which emotions they have, in what context and for how long they have them, and how intensely they experience them (Gross, 1998). When emotional cues are attended to and evaluated, these cues trigger a series of emotional response tendencies that involve experiential, behavioural, and physiological systems (Gross & John, 2003). These response tendencies may be modulated in a number of ways, but Gross and his colleagues discuss in depth two major emotion regulation strategies: antecedent- and response-focused regulation strategies. Antecedent-focused strategies, such as cognitive reappraisal, are those that take place before the emotion response tendencies become fully activated and before they begin to influence behavioural and physiological responses. In contrast, response-focused strategies, such as expressive suppression, take place once an emotion is already underway and after the response tendencies have been generated (Gross, in press).

Older adults often report using emotion regulation strategies to a greater degree than do younger adults (Gross et al., 1997; Labouvie-Vief & Medler, 2002; Lawton, Kleban, Rajagopal, & Dean, 1992). More specifically, research suggests that older adults make greater use of antecedent-based emotion regulation strategies, such as cognitive reappraisal, than do young adults. In contrast, this same research indicates that younger adults make greater use of less healthy response-focused emotion regulation strategies, such as suppression (Gross & John, 2002). Part of this shift towards antecedent-based strategies with advancing age may be due to changing contextual factors, such as retirement, that alter the types of emotion regulation strategies best suited to a person's daily environment. For example, younger adults may require suppression in the workplace, whereas older adults' environments may not elicit the same need for suppression of felt emotions. Older adults also may learn, over the course of their lifetime, that antecedent-based strategies are more effective, healthier, and less cognitively demanding than response-focused ones (John & Gross, 2004). Overall, this age-related research suggests that older adults' shifts to antecedent-based emotion regulation strategies, such as cognitive reappraisal, serves the broader motivational goals of this population, including conserving cognitive resources, ensuring consistent emotional demands, and heightening positive emotional experience (Carstensen et al., 1999).

Paradoxically, research has found that even though emotion regulation requires an exertion of cognitive resources, older adults, whose cognitive processing resources are reduced compared to younger adults (reviewed by Braver & Barch, 2002; Braver & West, in press; Park & Payer, 2006), may be more successful in regulating emotion because they devote a larger portion of their available resources to this task (reviewed by Mather, 2006). It has been proposed that due to their view of a limited future time perspective, emotion regulation goals become chronically activated at an unconscious level for older adults, whereas in younger adults, these goals are only activated in limited situations (Carstensen et al., 1999; Labouvie-Vief & Medler, 2002; Lawton et al., 1992; Mather & Knight, 2005). Thus, older adults seem to prioritise emotion regulation and to devote a greater proportion of their cognitive resources to emotion regulation than young adults, thereby allowing them to succeed at their regulation attempts despite overall age-related declines in cognitive control.

Given this extensive literature, it would make good sense that changes in older adults' processing of emotional information would stem from differences in how they are regulating their emotional responses to information. Indeed, recent evidence using eyetracking methods supports the suggestion that age differences in emotional processing may stem from older adults' attempts at emotion regulation. When young adults are instructed to regulate their emotions as they view images, they display eye gaze patterns similar to those of older adults: They gaze less at negative images and more at positive images. In contrast, when young adults are given no instructions to regulate their reactions to the images, they show no such effects of valence on viewing time (Xing & Isaacowitz, 2006). Thus, when young adults' emotion regulation goals are active, they display the same attentional patterns as older adults display spontaneously. These findings support the hypothesis that older adults' emotion regulation goals are chronically active, and that this focus on emotional regulation is linked to their positivity shift.

Neuroimaging evidence also has begun to suggest a link between emotion regulation processes and older adults' "positivity shift". Williams et al. (2006) used a combination of event-related potential and functional magnetic resonance imaging methods to examine the neural responses of individuals aged 12–79 as they viewed blocks of fearful or happy faces. The critical finding was that older adults showed greater medial prefrontal activity in response to negative emotional images at late stages of processing (more than 200 ms after stimulus presentation) than did young adults. Medial prefrontal activity often is associated with emotion regulation; when the medial prefrontal cortex is brought online, it appears to modulate the functioning of the amygdala (either downregulating or upregulating its response; Ochsner et al., 2004). This modulation of the amygdala by prefrontal processes occurs not only in young adults (e.g., Ochsner, 2004) but also in older adults (Urry et al., 2006). Therefore, it makes sense that older adults' enhanced recruitment of medial prefrontal regions might signify their increased exertion of control over the processing of negative stimuli. By contrast, the young adults may not show this prefrontal recruitment because they are less likely to control their affective responses to negative information. Further evidence for the use of controlled regulatory processing of negative information has come from event-related potential studies demonstrating that older adults show a greater late-onset evoked potential in response to negative stimuli than do young adults. By contrast, age differences are minimal at earlier points in time (Kisley, Wood, & Burrows, 2007; Wood & Kisley, 2006). These neuroimaging findings suggest that age differences in emotion processing may occur not at relatively early or automatic stages of processing but rather at later stages that involve more controlled, regulatory processes.

Within this context, it is worth pointing out that the neuroimaging studies revealing no effects of ageing on amygdala activity typically have assessed the processing of rapidly-presented stimuli (e.g., Wright et al., 2006, presented faces for only 200 ms each). In contrast, the studies that revealed robust age-related changes usually were those that gave participants extensive time (i.e., many seconds) to view the images (see Table 1). It is plausible that the changes in amygdala response to positive versus negative images did not reflect age-related changes in amygdala reactivity per se, but rather changes in top-down modulation of the amygdala by cortical regions including the prefrontal cortex. A plausible hypothesis (although one that needs to be tested directly) is that when given sufficient time for top-down processes implemented within the prefrontal cortex to modulate amygdala activity, older adults may show reductions in amygdala response to negative information. However, when time (or cognitive capacity) is insufficient for such top-down regulation, amygdala activation to negative information may be just as strong for older adults as it is for young adults.

This hypothesis could be addressed in at least two ways. The duration of stimulus presentation (or the intertrial interval) could be varied (e.g., from very brief presentations to very long presentations) and neural activity could be compared for the long-trial presentations versus the short-trial presentations. If the amygdala initially has a robust response to negative stimuli in both older and young adults, but then shows disengagement in the older adults due to engagement of controlled processes, then amygdala activity should be comparable in the two age groups when stimuli are presented only briefly (or when analyses focus on amygdala response immediately after stimulus presentation), whereas divergent patterns of amygdala activity may emerge with long-trial presentations (or with analyses that focus on amygdala activity that lags with the onset of the stimulus). Another way to examine the link between engagement of controlled processes and age-related change in amygdala responsivity would be to ask participants to perform a secondary task while they processed some of the items. If the engagement of controlled processes are what lead to age differences in the amygdalar response to affective stimuli, then such differences should be mitigated when older adults' attention is divided (i.e., when cognitive resources are depleted). By contrast, the differences should be pronounced when older adults can devote those resources toward emotion regulation. In fact, when processing is brief, or when cognitive resources are depleted, there might be a complete reversal of the age effect, with older adults showing more, rather than less, amygdala activity to negative items. As Mather and colleagues have elegantly discussed (reviewed in Mather, 2006), older adults may be particularly savvy in detecting negative information, because detection is a requisite precursor for emotional regulation. If a person does not detect negative information, there is no way for that person to avoid that information or to regulate his reaction to it. Thus, it might be expected that older adults' amygdala engagement in response to negative stimuli should be strong initially, but it might dissipate over time due to modulation by controlled emotion processing regions (such as those implemented by prefrontal cortex). It will be important for future studies to follow-up on the validity of this hypothesis.

EMOTIONAL MEMORY IN AGEING

Though we have focused so far on the evidence for age-related changes in emotional processing, it is well known that the way in which information is processed initially can influence the likelihood of later retrieval (e.g., Craik & Lockhart, 1972); attending to information, and elaborating upon it, increases the likelihood that it is remembered (e.g., Schacter, 1999). Thus, it makes sense that age-related changes in emotional processing would have implications for the types of information that older adults remember over short- and long-term delays. Indeed, there are differences in the types of information that young and older adults remember best, with older adults often showing a "positivity shift" in memory: Whereas young adults often are no more likely to remember positive items than they are to remember neutral items, older adults tend to show large mnemonic benefits for positive items (reviewed by Carstensen & Mikels, 2005; Mather & Carstensen, 2005). In fact, older adults sometimes show better memory for positive items than they do for negative ones (Charles, Mather, & Carstensen, 2003; Kennedy et al., 2004; Leigland, Schulz, & Janowsky, 2004; Mather & Knight, 2005). Moreover, whereas older adults often show poorer memory for neutral or negative information than do young adults, their memory deficits can be reduced—or even eliminated—for positive information (Kensinger, Garoff-Eaton, & Schacter, 2007; Kensinger, O'Brien, Swanberg, Garoff-Eaton, & Schacter, 2007).

The positivity shift appears to be critically impacted by the way in which information is initially encoded. If older adults are asked to attend specifically to the emotional content of the information, they usually do not show a positivity shift. In contrast, if they are asked to process information in a more open-ended fashion, or if they are asked to attend to nonemotional features of the information, the positivity shift often is observed (reviewed by Mather, 2006). Importantly, however, the positivity shift does not appear to be influenced by lower-level processes, such as the detection of emotional information. Even when older adults are equally likely to detect negative and positive emotional information, they still show a positivity shift in memory (Thomas & Hasher, 2006). Moreover, individuals who show the best ability to detect positive information are not necessarily the individuals who show the greatest positivity shift.

SELF-REFERENTIAL PROCESSING IN AGEING: LINKS TO EMOTIONAL MEMORY

Rather than arising from differences in the likelihood that information is detected, older adults' positivity shift in memory seems to arise from differences in how older adults process the positive information once they notice its presence (discussed by Mather, 2006; Mather & Carstensen, 2005). Though it has been proposed that age differences in controlled processing mediate older adults' positivity shift (discussed by Mather, 2006; Mather & Carstensen, 2005), here we review recent evidence suggesting that, within the general realm of controlled processing, an important specific contributor to older adults' positivity shift may be their increased likelihood of processing positive information in a self-referential fashion.

Older adults are more likely to focus upon their thoughts and feelings about stimuli than are young adults (reviewed by Kensinger, 2008). In fact, while young adults tend to remember primarily external attributes of events (e.g., the sights, sounds, smells), older adults are more likely to remember the internal thoughts and feelings generated by the event (Comblain, D'Argembeau, & van der Linden, 2005; Hashtroudi, Johnson, & Chrosniak, 1990; Schaefer & Philippot, 2005). In other words, older adults are more likely to think about how an event impacts them and to remember those self-relevant details.

It is widely accepted that relating information to oneself is a successful encoding strategy. People remember more information that they have been asked to process in a self-referent fashion than information that they have been asked to process in other semantic ways or in relation to another person (e.g., Rogers, Kuiper, & Kirker, 1977; Symons & Johnson, 1997). These mnemonic benefits appear to arise because of specialised elaborative processes that are engaged when individuals process information in relation to themselves (see Craik et al., 1999; Kelley et al., 2002; Macrae, Moran, Heatherton, Banfield, & Kelley, 2004), and older adults appear to benefit from these processes to the same extent as young adults (Gutchess, Kensinger, Yoon, & Schacter, 2007; Mueller, Wonderlich, & Dugan, 1986). Thus, it makes sense that there would be mnemonic consequences for older adults' enhanced reliance on self-referential encoding processes.

There has been increasing evidence to suggest that older adults are more likely to engage self-referential processes for positive information as compared to negative information. In particular, age-related reversals in the valence of information that elicits the most activity within self-referential processing regions have been revealed. In one event-related fMRI study (Leclerc & Kensinger, in press b), young and older adults were asked to view objects. Some objects elicited positive emotion (e.g., a box of chocolates, a wedding dress), others elicited negative emotion (e.g., a snake, a grenade), and others were neutral (e.g., a canoe, a barometer). There were not age differences in the regions that responded equally strongly to positive and negative objects, consistent with proposals that ageing does not impact the general effects of arousal on emotional processing (e.g., Mather, 2006; Kensinger, in press). However, there were fundamental effects of age in the regions that showed valence-based responses, responding more to positive objects than to negative ones, or vice versa. In particular, a number of regions—including the ventromedial prefrontal cortex and anterior cingulate gyrus, the precuneus, and the angular gyrus—showed an age-related valence reversal in their responsiveness. Young adults showed more activity in these regions during the processing of negative compared to positive objects, consistent with suggestions that young adults are particularly likely to process negative information in reference to themselves (Baumeister, Bratslavsky, Finkenauer, & Vohs, 2001). But older adults showed the opposite pattern of results, engaging these regions more during the processing of positive information than during the processing of negative information. A similar reversal within the prefrontal cortex was also demonstrated in an event-related functional magnetic resonance imaging study that asked young and older adults to process adjectives and to decide whether or not the adjective was a good self-descriptor (Gutchess, Kensinger, & Schacter, 2007).

The regions that have shown these valence reversals are those that frequently have been associated with self-referential processing. For example, in a meta-analysis, Northoff & Bermpohl (2004) discussed the key role that cortical midline structures, including regions of the ventromedial prefrontal cortex, anterior and posterior portions of the cingulate gyrus, and precuneus, play in processing information in reference to the self. Additional studies have implicated the angular gyrus and the thalamus in self-referential processing, particularly as it relates to body perception (Blanke, Ortigue, Landis, & Seeck, 2002; Craig, 2002, Panksepp, 2005). Thus, it seems likely that age differences in engagement of these regions correspond with differences in the likelihood that individuals connect the information to themselves.

The extent of recruitment of these self-referential processing regions also corresponds with older adults' ability to remember positive information. The positive items that are associated with the strongest engagement of cortical midline structures are those items that older adults are most likely to later remember (Kensinger & Schacter, in press), consistent with evidence that engagement of these self-referential processes boosts the efficacy of encoding operations (Kelley et al., 2002; Macrae et al., 2004). Moreover, it tends to be the case that the older adults who show the greatest recruitment of self-referential processes during the encoding of positive items are also those individuals who show the greatest mnemonic advantage for positive as compared to neutral information. These findings provide intriguing evidence that older adults' positive shift arises from changes in the types of elaborative processes engaged during the encoding of emotional information.

SUMMARY AND CONCLUSIONS

As has been noted previously (e.g., Mather, 2006), ageing seems to have little impact on the relatively automatic processing of emotional information. Older adults are just as capable as young adults at detecting emotional information, and the neural processes associated with automatic, arousal-based, processing appear to be relatively preserved with ageing In contrast, ageing seems to result in large changes in the more controlled processing of emotional information, which seem particularly tied to changes in older adults' emotion regulation goals and in the likelihood that they process information in a self-relevant fashion. These changes in controlled and elaborative processes have consequences not only for the way in which emotional information initially is processed but also for the types of information that are most likely to be remembered. At a neural level, valence reversals in the types of information that elicit the most activity in cortical midline structures seem to be an important mediator of older adults' positivity shift. Because of these regions' roles in self-referential processing, it seems plausible that older adults' positivity shift in memory stems, at least in part, from older adults' increased tendency to recruit self-referential processes (Grady, Springer, Honwanishkul, McIntosh, & Winocur, 2006; Lustig et al., 2003), particularly for positive information.

DIRECTIONS FOR FURTHER INVESTIGATION

Investigations of the effects of ageing on emotional processing and emotional memory are in their infancy, and there is much to be learned. For example, although the positivity shift is critically impacted by how emotional information is processed initially, retrieval processes also may contribute. It is nearly impossible, within a behavioural experiment, to reveal at what mnemonic stage emotion is exerting its effect. However, event-related neuroimaging methods provide a means to tease apart those processes that correspond with the successful encoding of emotional information and those that relate to the successful retrieval of emotional information. It will therefore be important for future research to take advantage of these neuroimaging methods to examine whether ageing impacts the processes recruited during retrieval of emotional information.

We also lack knowledge about the consistency of the positivity shift across individuals. Although cognitive control ability is known to influence the magnitude of the shift (Mather & Knight, 2005), it is not clear whether other personality or environmental factors may influence the degree to which a person shows a positivity shift. At least in young adults, personality traits such as extraversion or neuroticism can affect the amygdala's responsiveness to happy or fearful facial expressions, with extroverts showing stronger amygdala activity to happy faces and neurotics showing stronger activity to fearful faces (reviewed by Canli, 2004). Although this research has not yet been extended to older adults, it seems plausible that these personality variables may influence neural responses to stimuli throughout the adult lifespan, perhaps in turn affecting the magnitude of the positivity shift demonstrated. For instance, older adults high in neuroticism may show less of a positivity shift, or may require more cognitive resources to elicit such a shift, than older adults low in neuroticism (and see Wright, Feczko, Dickerson, & Williams, 2007, for evidence that personality can affect the neural processes associated with older adults' processing of emotional information). It will be important for future research to examine not only the instances in which the positivity shift is demonstrated consistently across older adults but also those instances that may give rise to a stronger positivity shift in some older adults.

We believe that a particularly interesting avenue for future research will be an examination of how age-related changes in the neural processes supporting emotion processing correspond with changes in decision making. Although research on decision making traditionally has focused on "cold" cognition, philosophers always have placed a great deal of importance on the relationship between how we feel and how we think. In fact, affect has been shown to be intimately involved in the decision making process, with factors such as mood playing an important role in determining how people respond (e.g., Clore & Tamir, 2002; Schwarz, 2001; Sechrist, Swim, & Mark, 2003). Neuroanatomically, there is evidence that emotion–cognition interactions may be robust within prefrontal regions typically associated with working memory and executive control, lending credence to the idea that affective state may influence the efficacy of decision-making processes (e.g., Fellows, in press; Gray, 2001).

The vast majority of research examining affect's influence on decision making has focused on how college-age adults decide, with little attention paid to the developmental process. However, it is increasingly clear that quality and length of life are dependent on the decisions ageing individuals make regarding their diets, healthcare, social relationships, and living arrangements. Particularly given the growing size of our older population and the increasing number of complex choices that older adults must make, it is critical to understand how older adults make decisions in light of their changing cognitive functioning capacities.

There are a few reasons to believe that affect may be central to older adults' decision-making processes. First, ageing is associated with declines in the efficiency of controlled processing mechanisms, such as working memory (MacPherson, Phillips, & Della Sala, 2002; Salthouse, 1994), processing speed (Salthouse, 1996), and inhibition of task-irrelevant information (Hasher & Zacks, 1979). There also are prominent age-related volumetric and functional declines in the prefrontal regions (e.g., dorsolateral prefrontal cortex) typically recruited during performance of these tasks (Daigneault, Braun, & Whitaker, 1992; Mittenberg, Seidenburg, O'Leary, & DiGiulio, 1989; Moscovitch & Winocur, 1995; Parkin, 1997; Raz, 1996; Shimamura, 1994; West, 1996). Because affect processing regions such as the amygdala and ventromedial prefrontal cortex are relatively preserved with ageing (at least as compared to regions such as the dorsolateral prefrontal cortex; reviewed by Chow & Cummings, 2000; Mather, 2003), older adults may rely more on affective information when making decisions. Put another way, older adults may devote more of their cognitive resources towards monitoring and regulating their emotional responses and fewer of them towards strategic decision making. Thus, older adults may rely more on feelings to decide whether a decision is appropriate (see Blanchard-Fields, 1998, for discussion).

Second, as discussed earlier, ageing results in an increased emphasis on social goals and on emotional fulfilment, whereas young adults are more focused on knowledge seeking (Carstensen, 1993; Ebner, Freund, & Baltes, 2006). This shift may mean that older adults' decision making is based more upon a decision's congruency with these goals and less on whether the decision is optimal across a number of dimensions. For example, although older adults generate fewer potential solutions to a given problem than young adults (McCrae, Arenberg, & Costa, 1987), this difference may not reflect age-related decline but rather may signify older adults' ability to rely on somatic markers (Damasio, 1994) to quickly and automatically reject options not consistent with their affective goals.

Third, as individuals age, their experience with the use of affective information (and with the use of affect as a source of information) expands, which may result in the more efficient and frequent use of this information by older adults compared to younger adults. Older adults seem to be particularly good at making decisions in familiar environments (reviewed by Fisk & Rogers, 2000) and in domains about which they have expertise (Kim & Hasher, 2005; Tentori, Osherson, Hasher, & May, 2001). Thus, it would make sense that older adults could benefit from a lifetime's experience using affect to aid in decision making. Indeed, there is evidence to suggest that older adults may do a better job than young adults in making decisions that allow them to reach their ultimate goals, in part because of their ability to set reachable intermediate goals (Riediger, Freund, & Baltes, 2005)

Cognitive neuroscience methods will provide a particularly fruitful means to address these hypotheses regarding older adults' decision making. If older adults rely less on "cold" cognition and more on affective processes when making decisions, then the neural circuitry they recruit during their attempts at decision making should showcase this shift. More broadly, cognitive neuroscience methods will shed light on the ways in which older adults' affective and cognitive processes interface. For instance, as alluded to earlier, the finding that older adults are better at emotion regulation than young adults seems at odds with the finding that older adults have more difficulty deploying controlled processes to modify their behaviour than do young adults. Neuroimaging methods are likely to shed light on the basis for this seeming contradiction. For example, it is plausible that the neural networks recruited for top-down control of affect and those recruited for top-down control of other behaviours are dissociable and that the pathways recruited for top-down control of affect may be relatively preserved in ageing.

Alternately, it is possible that it is the same pool of cognitive control resources that exert control over all forms of behaviour, and that ageing shifts the proportion of those resources devoted to affective regulation versus to more cognitive executive functions. By combining neuroimaging methods with rigorous behavioural testing, these sorts of alternatives can be adjudicated. The implications of this research are likely to be far reaching, holding promise for understanding how older adults remember information in everyday life and how they make decisions that affect their well-being.

REFERENCES

Anderson, A. K., & Phelps, E. A. (1998). Intact recognition of vocal expressions of fear following bilateral lesions of the human amygdala. *Neuroreport, 9*, 3607–3613.

Barrett, L. F. (2006). Are emotions natural kinds? *Perspectives on Psychological Science, 1*, 28–58.

Baumeister, R. F., Bratslavsky, E., Finkenauer, C., & Vohs, K. D. (2001). Bad is stronger than good. *Review of General Psychology, 5*, 323–370.

Blanchard-Fields, F. (1998). The role of emotion in social cognition across the adult life span. In K. W. Schaie & L. M. Powell (Eds.), *Annual review of gerontology and geriatrics: Focus on emotion and adult development* (Vol. 17, pp. 238–265)). New York: Springer.

Blanke, O., Ortigue, S., Landis, T., & Seeck, M. (2002). Stimulating illusory own-body perceptions. *Nature, 6904*, 269–270.

Braver, T. S., & Barch, D. M. (2002). A theory of cognitive control, aging cognition, and neuromodulation. *Neuroscience and Biobehavioral Reviews, 26*, 809–817.

Braver, T. S., & West, R. (in press). Working memory, executive control and aging. In F. I. M. Craik & T. A. Salthouse (Eds.), *The handbook of aging and cognition* (3rd ed.). New York: Psychology Press.

Canli, T. (2004). Functional brain mapping of extraversion and neuroticism: Learning from individual differences in emotion processing. *Journal of Personality, 72*, 1105–1132.

Carstensen, L. L. (1993). Motivation for social contact across the life span: A theory of socioemotional selectivity. In J. E. Jacobs (Ed.), *Nebraska symposium on motivation: 1992. Developmental perspectives on motivation* (Vol. 40 (pp. 209–254)). Lincoln, NE: University of Nebraska Press.

Carstensen, L. L., Isaacowitz, D., & Charles, S. T. (1999). Taking time seriously: A theory of socioemotional selectivity. *The American Psychologist, 54*, 165–181.

Carstensen, L. L., & Mikels, J. A. (2005). At the intersection of emotion and cognition: Aging and the positivity effect. *Current Directions in Psychological Science, 14*(3), 117–121.

Charles, S., Mather, M., & Carstensen, L. L. (2003). Aging and emotional memory: The forgettable nature of negative images for older adults. *Journal of Experimental Psychology: General, 132*, 310–324.

Chow, T. W., & Cummings, J. L. (2000). The amygdala and Alzheimer's disease. In J. P. Aggleton (Ed.), *The amygdala: A functional analysis* (pp. 656–680). Oxford, UK: Oxford University Press.

Clore, G. L., & Tamir, M. (2002). Affect as embodied information. *Psychological Inquiry, 13*, 37–45.

Comblain, C., D'Argembeau, A., & van der Linden, M. (2005). Phenomenal characteristics of autobiographical memories for emotional and neutral events in older and younger adults. *Experimental Aging Research, 31*, 173–189.

Courtney, S. M., Petit, L., Haxby, J. V., & Ungerleider, L. G. (1998). The role of prefrontal cortex in working memory: Examining the contents of consciousness. *Philosophical Transactions of the Royal Society London, Series B, 353*, 1819–1828.

Craig, A. D. (2002). How do you feel? Interoception: The sense of the physiological condition of the body. *Nature Reviews Neuroscience, 3*, 655–666.

Craik, F. I. M., & Lockhart, R. (1972). Levels of processing: A framework for memory research. *Journal of Verbal Learning & Verbal Behavior, 11*, 671–684.

Craik, F. I. M., Moroz, T. M., Moscovitch, M., Stuss, D. T., Winocur, G., Tulving, E., & Kapur, S. (1999). In search of the self: A positron emission tomography study. *Psychological Sciences, 10*, 26–34.

Daigneault, S., Braun, C. M. J., & Whitaker, H. A. (1992). Early effects of normal aging in perseverative and non-perseverative prefrontal measures. *Developmental Neuropsychology, 8*, 99–114.

Damasio, A. R. (1994). *Descartes' error: Emotion, reason, and the human brain.* New York: Avon.

Dolan, R. J., & Vuilleumier, P. (2003). Amygdala automaticity in emotional processing. *Annals of the New York Academy of Sciences, 985*, 348–355.

Ebner, N. C., Freund, A. M., & Baltes, P. B. (2006). Developmental changes in personal goal orientation from young to late adulthood: From striving for gains to maintenance and prevention of losses. *Psychology and Aging, 21*, 664–678.

Esslen, M., Pascual-Marqui, R. D., Hell, D., Kochi, K., & Lehmann, D. (2004). Brain areas and time course of emotional processing. *NeuroImage, 21*, 1189–1203.

Fellows, L. K. (in press). The role of orbitofrontal cortex in decision making: A component process account. *Annals of the New York Academy of Sciences.*

Fischer, H., Sandblom, J., Gavazzeni, J., Fransson, P., Wright, C. I., & Bäckman, L. (2005). Age-differential patterns of brain activation during perception of angry faces. *Neuroscience Letters, 386*, 99–104.

Fisk, A. D., & Rogers, W. A. (2000). Influence of training and experience on skill acquisition and maintenance in older adults. *Journal of Aging and Physical Activity, 8*, 373–378.

Fredrickson, B. L., & Carstensen, L. L. (1990). Choosing social partners: How old age and anticipated endings make us more selective. *Psychology and Aging, 5*, 335–347.

Frijda, N. H., & Sundararajan, L. (2007). Emotion refinement: A theory inspired by Chinese poetics. *Perspectives on Psychological Science, 2*, 227–241.

Fung, H., & Carstensen, L. L. (2003). Sending memorable messages to the old: Age differences in preferences and memory for advertisements. *Journal of Personality and Social Psychology, 85*, 163–178.

Fung, H. H., Carstensen, L. L., & Lutz, A. (1999). The influence of time on social preferences: Implications for life-span development. *Psychology and Aging, 14*, 595–604.

Grady, C. L., Springer, M. V., Honwanishkul, D., McIntosh, A. R., & Winocur, G. (2006). Age-related changes in brain activity across the adult lifespan. *Journal of Cognitive Neuroscience, 18*, 227–241.

Gray, J. R. (2001). Emotional modulation of cognitive control: Approach-withdrawal states double-dissociate spatial from verbal two-back task performance. *Journal of Experimental Psychology: General, 130*, 436–452.

Gross, J. J. (1998). Antecedent- and response-focused emotion regulation: Divergent consequences for experience, expression, and physiology. *Journal of Personality and Social Psychology, 74*, 224–237.

Gross, J. J. (in press). Emotion regulation. In M. Lewis, J. M. Haviland-Jones, & L. F. Barrett (Eds.), *Handbook of emotions* (3rd ed.). New York: Guilford Press.

Gross, J. J., Carstensen, L. L., Pasupathi, M., Tsai, J., Skorpen, C. G., & Hsu, A. Y. C. (1997). Emotion and aging: Experience, expression, and control. *Psychology and Aging, 12*, 590–599.

Gross, J. J., & John, O. P. (2002). Wise emotion regulation. In L. Feldman Barrett & P. Salovey (Eds.), *The wisdom of feelings: Psychological processes in emotional intelligence* (pp. 297–318). New York: Guilford Press.

Gross, J. J., & John, O. P. (2003). Individual differences in two emotion regulation processes: Implications for affect, relationships, and well-being. *Journal of Personality and Social Psychology, 85*, 348–362.

Grühn, D., Scheibe, S., & Baltes, P. B. (2007). Reduced negativity effect in older adults' memory for emotional pictures: The heterogeneity-homogeneity list paradigm. *Psychology and Aging, 22*, 644–649.

Grühn, D., Smith, J., & Baltes, P. B. (2005). No aging bias favoring memory for positive material: Evidence from a heterogeneity-homogeneity list paradigm using emotionally toned words. *Psychology and Aging, 20*, 579–588.

Gunning-Dixon, F. M., Gur, R. C., Perkins, A. C., Schroder, L., Turner, T., Turetsky, B. I., et al. (2003). Age-related differences in brain activation during emotional face processing. *Neurobiology of Aging, 24*, 285–295.

Gutchess, A. H., Kensinger, E. A., & Schacter, D. L. (2007). Aging, self-referencing, and medial prefrontal cortex. *Social Neuroscience, 2*, 117–133.

Gutchess, A. H., Kensinger, E. A., Yoon, C., & Schacter, D. L. (2007). Aging and the self-reference effect in memory. *Memory, 15*, 822–837.

Hahn, S., Carlson, C., Singer, S., & Gronlund, S. D. (2006). Aging and visual search: Automatic and controlled attentional bias to threat faces. *Acta Psychologica, 123*, 312–336.

Hasher, L., & Zacks, R. T. (1979). Automatic and effortful processes in memory. *Journal of Experimental Psychology, 108*, 356–388.

Hashtroudi, S., Johnson, M. K., & Chrosniak, L. D. (1990). Aging and qualitative characteristics of memories for perceived and imagined complex events. *Psychology and Aging, 5*, 119–126.

Iidaka, T., Okada, T., Murata, T., Omori, M., Kosaka, H., Sadato, N., & Yonekura, Y. (2002). Age-related differences in the medial temporal lobe responses to emotional faces as revealed by fMRI. *Hippocampus, 12*, 352–362.

Isaacowitz, D. M., Wadlinger, H. A., Goren, D., & Wilson, H. R. (2006). Selective preference in visual fixation away from negative images in old age? An eye-tracking study. *Psychology of Aging, 21*, 40–48.

Izard, C. E. (2007). Basic emotions, natural kinds, emotion schemas, and a new paradigm. *Perspectives on Psychological Science, 2*, 260–280.

Jansma, J. M., Ramsey, N. F., Slagter, H. A., & Kahn, R. S. (2001). Functional anatomical correlates of controlled and automatic processing. *Journal of Cognitive Neuroscience, 13*, 730–743.

John, O. P., & Gross, J. J. (2004). Healthy and unhealthy emotion regulation: Personality processes, individual differences, and life span development. *Journal of Personality, 72*, 1301–1333.

Kalisch, R., Wiech, K., Critchley, H. D., & Dolan, R. J. (2006). Levels of appraisal: A media prefrontal role in high-level appraisal of emotional material. *NeuroImage, 30*, 1458–1466.

Kelley, W. M., Macrae, C. N., Wyland, C. L., Caglar, S., Inati, S., & Heatherton, T. F. (2002). Finding the self? An event-related fMRI study. *Journal of Cognitive Neuroscience, 14*, 785–794.

Kennedy, Q., Mather, M., & Carstensen, L. L. (2004). The role of motivation in the age-related positive bias in autobiographical memory. *Psychological Science, 15*, 208–214.

Kensinger, E. A. (2008). How emotion affects older adults' memories for event details. *Manuscript submitted for publication.*

Kensinger, E. A. (in press). Age differences in memory for arousing and nonarousing emotional words. *Journal of Gerontology: Psychological Sciences.*

Kensinger, E. A., Garoff-Eaton, R. J., & Schacter, D. L. (2007). Effects of emotion on memory specificity in young and older adults. Journals of Gerontology. *Series B: Psychological Sciences and Social Sciences, 62*, P208–P215.

Kensinger, E. A., Gutchess, A. H., & Schacter, D. L. (2007). Effects of aging and encoding instructions on emotion-induced memory trade-offs. *Psychology and Aging, 22*, 781–795.

Kensinger, E. A., O'Brien, J., Swanberg, K., Garoff-Eaton, R. J., & Schacter, D. L. (2007). The effects of emotional content on reality-monitoring performance in young and older adults. *Psychology and Aging*, *22*, 752–764.

Kensinger, E. A., & Schacter, D. L. (in press). Neural processes supporting young and older adults' emotional memories. *Journal of Cognitive Neuroscience.*

Kim, S., & Hasher, L. (2005). The attraction effect in decision making: Superior performance by older adults. *Quarterly Journal of Experimental Psychology*, *58A*, 120–133.

Kisley, M. A., Wood, S., & Burrows, C. L. (2007). Looking at the sunny side of life: Age-related change in an event-related potential measure of the negativity bias. *Psychological Science*, *18*, 838–843.

Knight, M., Seymour, T. L., Gaunt, J. T., Baker, C., Nesmith, K., & Mather, M. (2007). Aging and goal-directed emotional attention: Distraction reverses emotional biases. *Emotion*, *7*, 705–714.

Labouvie-Vief, G., & Medler, M. (2002). Affect optimization and affect complexity: Modes and styles of regulation in adulthood. *Psychology and Aging*, *17*, 571–588.

Lang, P. J., Bradley, M. M., & Cuthbert, B. N. (1997). Motivated attention: Affect, activation, and action. In P. J. Lang, R. F. Simons, & M. Balaban (Eds.), *Attention and orienting: Sensory and motivational processes* (pp. 97–135). Mahwah, NJ: Lawrence Erlbaum Associates, Inc.

Lawton, M. P., Kleban, M. H., Rajagopal, D., & Dean, J. (1992). Dimensions of affective experience in three age groups. *Psychology and Aging*, *7*, 171–184.

Leclerc, C. M., & Kensinger, E. A. (in press a). Effects of age on detection of emotional information. *Psychology and Aging.*

Leclerc, C. M., & Kensinger, E. A. (in press b). Age-related differences in medial prefrontal activation in response to emotional images. *Cognitive, Affective, and Behavioral Neuroscience.*

Leigland, L. A., Schulz, L. E., & Janowsky, J. S. (2004). Age related changes in emotional memory. *Neurobiology of Aging*, *25*, 1117–1124.

Leventhal, H., & Scherer, K. R. (1987). The relationship of emotion to cognition: A functional approach to a semantic controversy. *Cognition and Emotion*, *1*, 3–28.

Lustig, C., Snyder, A. Z., Bhakta, M., O'Brien, K. C., McAvoy, M., Raichle, M. E., et al. (2003). Functional deactivations: Change with age and dementia of the Alzheimer type. *Proceedings of the National Academy of Sciences, USA*, *100*, 14504–14509.

MacPherson, S. E., Phillips, L. H., & Della Sala, S. (2002). Age, executive function, and social decision-making: A dorsolateral prefrontal theory of cognitive aging. *Psychology and Aging*, *17*, 598–609.

Macrae, C. N., Moran, J. M., Heatherton, T. F., Banfield, J. F., & Kelley, W. M. (2004). Medial prefrontal activity predicts memory for self. *Cerebral Cortex*, *14*, 647–654.

Mather, M. (2003). Aging and emotional memory. In D. Reisberg & P. Hertel (Eds.), *Memory and emotion* (pp. 272–307). London: Oxford University Press.

Mather, M. (2006). Why memories may become more positive with age. In B. Uttl, N. Ohta, & A. L. Siegenthaler (Eds.), *Memory and emotion: Interdisciplinary perspectives* (pp. 135–159). Oxford, UK: Blackwell Publishing.

Mather, M., Canli, T., English, T., Whitfield, S., Wais, P., Ochsner, K., et al. (2004). Amygdala responses to emotionally valenced stimuli in older and younger adults. *Psychological Science*, *15*, 259–263.

Mather, M., & Carstensen, L. L. (2003). Aging and attentional biases for emotional faces. *Psychological Science*, *14*, 409–415.

Mather, M., & Carstensen, L. L. (2005). Aging and motivated cognition: The positivity effect in attention and memory. *Trends in Cognitive Science*, *9*, 496–502.

Mather, M., & Johnson, M. K. (2000). Choice-supportive source monitoring: Do our decisions seem better to us as we age? *Psychology and Aging*, *15*, 596–606.

Mather, M., & Knight, M. (2005). Goal-directed memory: The role of cognitive control in older adults' emotional memory. *Psychology and Aging*, *20*, 554–570.

Mather, M., & Knight, M. R. (2006). Angry faces get noticed quickly: Threat detection is not impaired among older adults. *Journals of Gerontology, Series B: Psychological Sciences and Social Sciences, 61*, P54–P57.

McCrae, R. R., Arenberg, D., & Costa, P. T. (1987). Declines in divergent thinking with age: Cross-sectional, longitudinal, and cross-sequential analyses. *Psychology and Aging, 2*, 130–137.

Mittenberg, W., Seidenburg, M., O'Leary, D. S., & DiGiulio, D. V. (1989). Changes in cerebral functioning associated with normal aging. *Journal of Clinical and Experimental Neuropsychology, 11*, 918–932.

Moscovitch, M., & Winocur, G. (1995). Frontal lobes, memory, and aging. *Annals of the New York Academy of Sciences, 769*, 119–150.

Mueller, J. H., Wonderlich, S., & Dugan, K. (1986). Self-referent processing of age-specific material. *Psychology and Aging, 1*, 293–299.

Northoff, G., & Bermpohl, F. (2004). Cortical midline structures and the self. *Trends in Cognitive Science, 8*, 102–107.

Ochsner, K. N., Ray, R. D., Cooper, J. C., Robertson, E. R., Chopra, S., Gabrieli, J. D., & Gross, J. J. (2004). For better or for worse: Neural systems supporting the cognitive down- and up-regulation of negative emotion. *Neuroimage, 23*, 483–499.

Panksepp, J. (2005). Affective consciousness: Core emotional feelings in animals and humans. *Consciousness and Cognition, 14*, 30–80.

Panksepp, J. (2007). Neurologizing the psychology of affects: How appraisal-based constructivism and basic emotion theory can coexist. *Perspectives on Psychological Science, 2*, 281–296.

Park, D. C., & Payer, D. (2006). Working memory across the adult lifespan. In E. Bialystock & F. Craik (Eds.), *Lifespan cognition: Mechanisms of change* (pp. 128–142). New York: Oxford University Press.

Parkin, A. J. (1997). Normal age-related memory loss and its relation to frontal lobe dysfunction. In P. M. A. Rabbitt (Ed.), *Methodology of frontal and executive function* (pp. 177–190). Hove, UK: Psychology Press.

Pessoa, L. (2005). To what extent are emotional visual stimuli processed without attention and awareness? *Current Opinion in Neurobiology, 15*, 188–196.

Raz, N. (1996). Neuroanatomy of the aging brain observed in vivo: A review of structural MRI findings. In E. D. Bigler (Ed.), *Neuroimaging II: Clinical applications* (pp. 153–184). New York: Plenum Press.

Riediger, M., Freund, A. M., & Baltes, P. B. (2005). Managing life through personal goals: Intergoal facilitation and intensity of goal pursuits in younger and older adulthood. *Journal of Gerontology, Series B: Psychological and Social Sciences, 60*, 84–91.

Robinson, M. D. (1998). Running from William James' bear: A review of preattentive mechanisms and their contribution to emotional experience. *Cognition and Emotion, 12*, 667–696.

Rogers, T. B., Kuiper, N. A., & Kirker, W. S. (1977). Self-reference and the encoding of personal information. *Journal of Personality and Social Psychology, 35*, 677–688.

Salthouse, T. A. (1994). The nature of the influence of speed on adult age differences in cognition. *Developmental Psychology, 30*, 240–259.

Salthouse, T. A. (1996). The processing-speed theory of adult age differences in cognition. *Psychological Review, 103*, 403–428.

Satpute, A. B., & Lieberman, M. D. (2006). Integrating automatic and controlled processes into neurocognitive models of social cognition. *Brain Research, 1079*, 86–97.

Schacter, D. L. (1999). The seven sins of memory: Insights from psychology and cognitive neuroscience. *The American Psychologist, 54*, 182–203.

Schaefer, A., & Philippot, P. (2005). Selective effects of emotion on the phenomenal characteristics of autobiographical memories. *Memory, 13*, 148–160.

Schwarz, N. (2001). Feelings as information: Implications for affective influences on information processing. In L. L. Martin & G. L. Clore (Eds.), *Theories of mood and cognition: A user's guidebook* (pp. 159–176). Mahwah, NJ: Lawrence Erlbaum Associates, Inc.

Sechrist, G. B., Swim, J. K., & Mark, M. M. (2003). Mood as information in making attributions to discrimination. *Personality and Social Psychology Bulletin, 29*, 524–531.

Shimamura, A. P. (1994). Neuropsychological perspectives on memory and cognitive decline in normal human aging. *Seminars in the Neurosciences, 6*, 387–394.

Symons, C. S., & Johnson, B. T. (1997). The self-reference effect in memory: A meta-analysis. *Psychological Bulletin, 121*, 371–394.

Tentori, K., Osherson, D., Hasher, L., & May, C. P. (2001). Wisdom and aging: Irrational preferences in college students but not older adults. *Cognition, 81*, 87–96.

Tessitore, A., Hariri, A. R., Fera, F., Smith, W. G., Das, S., Weinberger, D. R., & Mattay, V. S. (2005). Functional changes in the activity of brain regions underlying emotion processing in the elderly. *Psychiatry Research, 139*, 9–18.

Thomas, R. C., & Hasher, L. (2006). The influences of emotional valence on age differences in early processing and memory. *Psychology and Aging, 21*, 821–825.

Urry, H. L., van Reekum, C. M., Johnstone, T., Kalin, N. H., Thurow, M. E., Schaefer, H. S., et al. (2006). Amygdala and ventromedial prefrontal cortex are inversely coupled during regulation of negative affect and predict the diurnal pattern of cortisol secretion among older adults. *Journal of Neuroscience, 26*, 4415–4425.

Wedig, M. M., Rauch, S. L., Albert, M. S., & Wright, C. I. (2005). Differential amygdala habituation to neutral faces in young and elderly adults. *Neuroscience Letters, 385*, 114–119.

West, R. L. (1996). An application of prefrontal cortex function theory to cognitive aging. *Psychological Bulletin, 120*, 272–292.

Williams, L. M., Brown, K. J., Palmer, D., Liddell, B. J., Kemp, A. H., Olivieri, G., et al. (2006). The mellow years? Neural basis of improving emotional stability over age. *Journal of Neuroscience, 26*, 6422–6430.

Wood, S., & Kisley, M. A. (2006). The negativity bias is eliminated in older adults: Age-related reduction in event-related brain potentials associated with evaluative categorization. *Psychology and Aging, 21*, 815–820.

Wright, C. I., Dickerson, B. C., Feczko, E., Negeira, A., & Williams, D. (2007a). A functional magnetic resonance imaging study of amygdala responses to human faces in aging and mild Alzheimer's disease. *Biological Psychiatry, 62*, 1388–1395.

Wright, C. I., Feczko, E., Dickerson, B., & Williams, D. (2007b). Neuroanatomical correlates of personality in the elderly. *NeuroImage, 35*, 263–272.

Wright, C. I., Wedig, M. M., Williams, D., Rauch, S. L., & Albert, M. S. (2006). Novel fearful faces activate the amygdala in healthy young and elderly adults. *Neurobiology of Aging, 27*, 361–374.

Xing, C., & Isaacowitz, D. M. (2006). Aiming at happiness: How motivation affects attention to and memory for emotional images. *Motivation and Emotion, 30*, 249–256.

EUROPEAN JOURNAL OF COGNITIVE PSYCHOLOGY
2009, 21 (2/3), 216–234

Psychology Press
Taylor & Francis Group

Level of processing and reaction time in young and middle-aged adults and the effect of education

Willemien A. Meijer and Renate H. M. de Groot
European Graduate School of Neuroscience, Maastricht University, The Netherlands

Pascal W. M. van Gerven
Department of Neurocognition, Maastricht University, Maastricht, The Netherlands

Martin P. J. van Boxtel and Jelle Jolles
European Graduate School of Neuroscience, and Department of Neurocognition, Maastricht University, Maastricht, The Netherlands

The first aim was to examine whether differences in reaction time (RT) between younger (25–35 years) and middle-aged (50–60 years) individuals increase with depth of processing. The second aim was to examine whether this increase is less pronounced in higher educated individuals. Processing of words at the perceptual, phonological, and semantic level was induced by a case decision, an "e" detection, and a living/nonliving discrimination task, respectively. RTs increased with age and level of processing. However, there were no interactions between age, task, and education, suggesting that different processing levels are equally sensitive to slowing in midlife and that education was not a moderating factor. Although no overall age by level of processing interaction was found, there were age by stimulus type interactions in the deeper processing tasks. First, age-related differences in RT for words containing the letter "e" were smaller than for words without the letter "e", suggesting that middle-aged adults were slower than younger adults in performing a terminating search strategy. Second, age-related differences in RT for words referring to living items were smaller than for words referring to nonliving items. This suggests that middle-aged adults compared to younger adults have reduced access to specific semantic categories. Taken together, the results show that vulnerability to age-related cognitive decline already exists in middle age.

Keywords: Ageing; Education; Reaction time.

Correspondence should be addressed to R. H. M. de Groot, School for Mental Health and Neuroscience (MHeNS), Department of Psychiatry and Neuropsychology, Maastricht University, PO Box 616, 6200 MD Maastricht, The Netherlands. E-mail: rhm.degroot@np.unimaas.nl

http://www.psypress.com/ecp DOI: 10.1080/09541440802091780

Although most of the work on cognitive ageing has compared older adults (above 65 years) to young adults, some longitudinal and cross-sectional studies have examined cognitive functioning throughout adulthood (Dixon, de Frias, & Maitland, 2001; Houx & Jolles, 1993; Houx, Jolles, & Vreeling, 1993; Schaie, 1996). Results have shown that some aspects of cognitive functioning are maintained or even improved in midlife (Schaie, 1996). These include the pragmatic aspects of functioning, such as knowledge that depends on experience (Baltes, Staudinger, & Lindenberger, 1999; Sternberg, Grigorenko, & Oh, 2001). In contrast, mechanical aspects of cognition, including speed of processing and working memory, begin to show declines in midlife (Baltes et al., 1999). These early changes may reflect age-related structural changes in the prefrontal cortex, which have already been detected around the age of 35 years (Haug, 1985; Tisserand et al., 2002). Because of these declines, middle-aged adults may need to invest more cognitive effort in daily life to achieve the same performance as young adults, especially in cognitively demanding situations in which information must be processed under time pressure. In contrast to the more established literature on standard neuropsychological task performance across adulthood, very few experimental studies have included middle-aged persons as a reference group. In the present experimental study, the hypothesis is tested that middle-aged adults are cognitively less efficient than young adults, particularly in resource-demanding situations. For that purpose, an experimental paradigm is needed that involves variations in processing demands and includes a measure of cognitive efficiency. Such a paradigm can be based on the notion that various processing levels are involved in visual word recognition (Borowsky & Besner, 1993; Ellis & Young, 1996; Seidenberg & McClelland, 1989). Recent studies have indicated that tasks involving different types of decisions about words could be used to evoke different levels of visual word processing. Relevant levels are the orthographic level at which visual features are integrated to form orthographic patterns, the lexical level at which the phonological (and possibly the whole-word orthographic) representation of the printed word is activated, and the semantic level at which the meaning of the word is accessed (Bentin, Mouchetant-Rostaing, Giard, Echallier, & Pernier, 1999; Proverbio, Vecchi, & Zani, 2004).

Previous studies have compared processing of printed words at different levels between young and old adults in order to investigate which levels of word processing are most vulnerable to age-related slowing. An early study (Petros, Zehr, & Chabot, 1983) suggested that deeper processing stages involving the activation of semantic information are more vulnerable to age-related slowing than more shallow processing stages in which the word is only visually processed. That is, when different types of judgements regarding word pairs were made (i.e., whether two words were physically identical, similar in name, or belonged to the same semantic category), there was a disproportionate increase in older adults' reaction time in the semantic category judgements compared to the more shallow processing conditions. However, as pointed out by Madden (1985), comparison and decision processes are important factors when two words have to be compared. A particular interaction between response selection load and processing level may have led to the disproportional slowing in the semantic activation that was found by Petros et al.

In contrast to the relatively intact shallow processing in older adults, as was found in the study by Petros et al. (1983), more recent studies of age-related effects on lexical decision performance (i.e., speed of word/nonword discrimination) suggest that the shallow processing stages of visual encoding are more vulnerable to age-related slowing than the deeper stages of semantic processing. The effects of word frequency and semantic priming on reaction time, for example, have been found to be equal for young and older adults (Allen, Madden, Weber, & Groth, 1993; Madden, Pierce, & Allen, 1993). Other variables, such as stimulus quality (e.g., spacing between letters or case type), can lead to disproportionate slowing of older adults' responses (Allen et al., 1993; Madden, 1992; Madden et al., 1993). However, shallow and deeper levels of processing were not directly induced in these studies, but were inferred from the effects of stimulus quality (shallow processing) and word frequency or semantic priming (deep processing) on lexical decision performance. In addition, because these effects were assessed in different experiments, an actual differential effect of age on levels of processing may not have been established.

Because previous studies yielded equivocal results, differences in reaction time (RT) on tasks requiring a decision about a single word and inducing various levels of processing were compared in the present study. A comparison was drawn between a young and middle-aged group in order to examine whether middle-aged adults process information less efficiently than young adults in more resource-demanding conditions. Deeper, semantic processing is assumed to incorporate shallower perceptual and phonological processing stages. Therefore, the number of processing steps may increase with depth of processing, which would be reflected in longer RTs on tasks that induce deeper levels of processing. According to the information loss model of Myerson, Hale, Wagstaff, Poon, and Smith (1990), every processing step takes more time in older than in younger adults to compensate for loss of information. Because compensation for information loss is insufficient in older adults, processing time increases disproportionately with the number of processing steps (Myerson et al., 1990). A similar pattern is predicted by Salthouse's (1996) processing-speed theory. If complex processing operations are dependent on the products of simpler operations, and fewer of those products are available because of a lower processing speed, we may expect that the effects of age-related slowing are most pronounced in complex information processing. A first purpose of the present study is to examine if the implications of these cognitive ageing theories also apply to middle age. A disproportionate increase of RTs with depth of processing in middle-aged adults compared to younger adults would then be predicted.

Within the field of cognitive ageing, relatively limited attention has been given to factors influencing the level of cognitive abilities in midlife (Willis & Schaie, 2005). There are several arguments to support the notion that a high level of education serves as a protective factor for age-related cognitive change that occurs already in midlife. First, continuous mental stimulation associated with a high level of education may have a positive effect on neuronal growth and the complexity of neural networks (Coffey, Saxton, Ratcliff, Bryan, & Lucke, 1999). Second, highly educated persons are more likely to have an active and healthy lifestyle (e.g., in terms of nutrition and hygiene) that is associated with a lower risk of cognitive and neural dysfunction (Gold et al., 1995). Third, educational experience may provide cognitive reserve capacity in the form of a more elaborate set of basic skills or cognitive strategies (Stern, 2002).

Indeed, a high educational level has been shown to attenuate age-related cognitive decline (e.g., Bosma, van Boxtel, Ponds, Houx, & Jolles, 2003; van der Elst, van Boxtel, van Breukelen, & Jolles, 2006b). Others, however, have questioned the idea that more highly educated and more intelligent individuals show decelerated cognitive ageing with respect to individuals with lower mental ability (Rabbitt, Chetwynd, & McInnes, 2003). Recent studies (Christensen et al., 2007; van Dijk, van Gerven, van Boxtel, van der Elst, & Jolles, 2008) did show that the protective influence of education on cognitive ageing is limited. This may be a general limitation, but the influence of education may also depend on the cognitive domain or the age-range under investigation. In a review of 14 studies reporting on the effect of education on cognitive change (Anstey & Christensen, 2000), only three studies included persons younger than 55 years and two of these studies used the Mini-Mental State Examination (Farmer, Kittner, Rae, Bartko, & Regier, 1995). All seven studies using mental status measures found a protective effect of education. It is already known that the range of scores of mental status scales such as the MMSE is restricted at the upper end of the scoring distribution due to a ceiling effect (Tombaugh & McIntyre, 1992). The scales are therefore insensitive to cognitive decline in highly educated people (Christensen et al., 1997). In this regard, finding a reduced decline on the MMSE in higher compared to lower educated persons might overestimate the protective effect of education.

In persons older than 65 years, four of the seven studies that included measures of memory showed protective effects (Colsher & Wallace, 1991;

Evans et al., 1993; Schmand, Smit, Geerlings, & Lindeboom, 1997; Shichita, Hatano, Ohashi, Shibata, & Matuzaki, 1986). In comparison, none of the studies using measures of reasoning and information processing speed found protective effects of education. In light of this differential protective effect of education in persons older than 65 years, an interesting issue is whether age differences in visual word processing, which involves rather basic information processing, are smaller in higher educated persons who are younger than 65 years. In addition, making a semantic judgement involves access to semantic memory, which may be more efficient in higher educated persons than in lower educated persons (van der Elst, van Boxtel, van Breukelen, & Jolles, 2006a). A possible disproportionate increase of RT with depth of processing in middle-aged adults compared to younger adults may therefore be smaller in higher educated persons. Hence, the second purpose of the present study was to examine whether level of education moderates age-related differences in RT on the decision tasks.

We compared differences in RTs between younger and middle-aged individuals with low and high educational attainment on three decision tasks, each designed to induce processing at a particular level: Deciding whether words are written in lower or uppercase letters was assumed to induce shallow *perceptual/orthographic* processing (Bentin et al., 1999; Daselaar, Veltman, Rombouts, Raaijmakers, & Jonker, 2003). Deciding whether words contain the letter "e" was assumed to induce more elaborate *orthographic/phonological* processing (Proverbio et al., 2004). Finally, deciding whether words refer to a living or a nonliving item was assumed to invoke deep *semantic* processing (Daselaar et al., 2003; Tisserand, McIntosh, van der Veen, Backes, & Jolles, 2005). In addition to the different levels of processing, these tasks may also vary in the amount and type of search processes that are involved. In contrast to the case decision task, which hardly involves any search process, the "e" detection and semantic decision tasks involve visual search and search of semantic memory respectively. Differences in RT between the responses on the two possible stimulus types within each decision task may provide insight into the use of search strategies. For instance, if the RT for the words containing the letter "e" is shorter than for the words not containing an "e", this would suggest that a terminating search strategy is used, rather than an exhaustive search (Schneider & Shiffrin, 1977). Furthermore, it has been suggested that living things are processed in specialised semantic subsystems (Caramazza & Shelton, 1998). Mahon and Caramazza (2003) argue that evolutionary pressure has resulted in specialised systems only for those categories for which rapid and efficient identification could have had survival and reproductive advantages, such as living things. Thus living things should be processed faster than nonliving things (Shapiro & Olson, 2005). In this context, a shorter RT may be expected for the words referring to living things than to words referring to nonliving things. As a third goal of this study we compared the use of search strategies per level of processing between young and middle-aged adults and between persons with low and high educational levels, by examining the effects of age and education on response times of words in lowercase versus words in uppercase, words containing the letter “e” versus words without the letter “e”, and words referring to living items versus words referring to nonliving items.

METHOD

Participants

Eighty adults who were divided over two age groups and stratified according to sex and educational level (low and high) participated in the study. The younger group consisted of 20 people with a low educational level and 20 higher educated people aged between 25 and 35 years (mean age = 29.0 years, *SD* = 2.8). The middle-aged group consisted of 20 people with a low educational level and 20 people with a high educational level aged between 50 and 60 (mean age = 56.1 years, *SD* = 3.4). Participants were recruited by advertisements in local newspapers and posters at different locations (schools, clubs, etc.). There was a preliminary screening by telephone in order to exclude persons with health-related conditions known to interfere with normal cognitive functioning. Exclusion criteria were cerebrovascular pathology, psychiatric disturbances, neurological disorders, dyslexia, serious medical conditions with known impact on brain function such as renal dialysis, excessive use of alcohol (> 21 consumption/week), use of psychoactive medication or drugs, clinically overt visual or auditory deficits, and prior participation in cognitive studies. The Ethics Committee of the Department of Psychology, Maastricht University, approved the study and participants gave their written informed consent.

Level of education was assessed by classifying formal schooling according to a system commonly used in the Netherlands (de Bie, 1987), which is comparable to the International Standard Classification of Education (UNESCO, 1976). Educational level was scored in eight ordinal categories: (1) primary education, (2) lower vocational education, (3) intermediate secondary education, (4) intermediate vocational education, (5) higher secondary education, (6) higher vocational education, (7) higher professional education, and (8) university degree. In many western countries, persons between 50 and 60 are—generally—lower educated than persons between 25 and 35. Thus, the median educational level in the population differs for the age ranges used in the present study (Mares, 2004). We attempted to deal with this cohort effect by adjusting the classification into a low and a high educational level according to the median educational level in the population. A low level of education was defined in the young group as a maximum of intermediate vocational education (equivalent to a maximum of 13 years of education), and in the middle-aged group as a maximum of intermediate secondary education (equivalent to a maximum of 10 years of education).

The characteristics of the sample are shown in Table 1. This table shows that the lower educated persons were older than the highly educated persons in both the young, $F(1, 38) = 4.4$, $p < .05$, and the middle-aged group, $F(1, 38) = 6.0$, $p < .05$. Because the difference was at most 2.5 years, this was not considered to be a problem. The young and middle-aged participants did not perform differently on a 20-item multiple-choice Dutch vocabulary test, which is used as a measure of Verbal Intelligence (Luteijn & van der Ploeg, 1983), $F(1, 76) = 3.1$, $p = .09$. The vocabulary scores of the highly educated participants were higher than those for the poorly educated participants, $F(1, 76) = 33.1$, $p < .01$.

Design

A cross-sectional design was used with two age groups (younger and middle-aged) and two educational levels (low and high). All participants received three conditions, which yielded a 3 × 2 × 2 full-factorial design with decision type (case decision, "e" detection, and semantic decision) as the within-groups variable and age group and educational level as the between-groups factors.

TABLE 1
Participant characteristics

	Young (25–35 years)		*Middle-aged (50–60 years)*	
	Low educational level	*High educational level*	*Low educational level*	*High educational level*
N	20	20	20	20
Age: mean (*SD*)	29.9 (0.64)	28.1 (0.57)	57.4 (0.61)	54.9 (0.82)
Male/female ratio (*n*/*n*)	10/10	10/10	10/10	10/10
Vocabulary (*SEM*)	11.7 (0.49)	14.9 (0.49)	12.9 (0.49)	15.3 (0.49)
Left-/right-handedness (*n*/*n*)	17/3	16/4	20/0	19/1

Materials and procedure

There were three task conditions with 16 words presented in each condition. In the first condition, in which eight words were presented in uppercase and eight words in lowercase, the participants were asked to make a decision about the case of the letters. In the second condition, participants had to indicate whether or not the words contained the letter "e". In the last condition, participants were asked whether the words referred to a living or a nonliving item. The order in which the conditions were presented was randomised within each age group per educational level. The words used in the experiment were mono- or disyllabic, varying in length between five and seven letters, and with a value of six or higher on a Dutch 7-point normative scale for imagery (van Loon-Vervoorn, 1985). Words were centrally presented one at a time in white against black background on a computer screen (font: Arial, 50 pt.), using E-prime presentation software (Schneider, Eschman, & Zuccolotto, 2002). The three conditions involved three word lists that were matched for word frequency, word length, and that all contained eight living items and eight words containing the letter "e".

Participants were seated in front of a 17-inch monitor at a normal viewing distance of approximately 60 cm (25 inch), and responded with either their left or right index finger using two response buttons. A right buttonpress indicated "uppercase", "containing e", and "living" for the three conditions, respectively. The words were presented on the screen until a response was given, with a maximum of 1500 ms, and a fixed interval of 2000 ms between the appearance of one word and the appearance of the next word. Participants were instructed to respond as quickly and accurately as possible. Although accuracy measures were also recorded, reaction time was the main dependent variable.

Data analysis

The number of correct responses (range 0–16) and reaction times corresponding to correct responses were checked for normality (Kolmogorov-Smirnov test) and homogeneity of variance. Based on this information, data transformation was not considered necessary. Repeated-measures ANOVAs were used to analyse between and within-group differences with sex as covariate. Statistically significant main effects of decision type were further analysed following Fisher's LSD procedure. In order to analyse differential age and education effects on reaction times of different stimulus types, a repeated-measures ANOVA was conducted per decision type with stimulus type as within-groups factor, and age group and educational level as between-groups factors. Significant interactions were investigated by simple contrasts following Fisher's LSD procedure. Post hoc power analyses on the number of participants (Buchner, Faul, & Erdfelder, 1992) using a medium critical effect size of 0.25 and an alpha level of .05 resulted in a power of 0.99 for the within-groups effects and 0.75 for the between-groups effects.

RESULTS

Accuracy

The average accuracy was high for both age groups, i.e., more than 88%, although the older participants were somewhat less accurate than the young participants, $F(1, 75) = 7.3$, $p < .05$ (means are 14.8 and 14.2 for the young and middle-aged groups, respectively). The accuracy scores of the highly educated persons were higher than those for the poorly educated persons, $F(1, 75) = 5.8$, $p < .05$ (means are 14.8 and 14.3 for the highly and poorly educated groups, respectively). Accuracy was not significantly affected by decision type, $F(2, 150) = 0.06$, $p > .9$. Furthermore, age group did not interact with decision type, $F(2, 150) = 2.3$, $p > .1$. No Age × Decision type × Education, Education × Age, and Education × Decision type interactions were found (Fs < 1.5, ps > .2).

RT in different decision tasks

In Figure 1 the mean reaction times corresponding to correct responses are presented per age group and decision task. A main effect of age was found, indicating that younger individuals outperformed older individuals, $F(1, 75) = 14.8$, $p < .01$, partial $\eta^2 = .17$ (mean RTs over all conditions are 690 and 769 ms for the young and middle-aged groups, respectively). A main effect of decision type and significant contrasts between the three types indicated that people had longer reaction times in the semantic decision task than in the "e" detection task, and longer RTs in the "e" detection task than in the case decision task, $F(2, 150) = 24.5$, $p < .01$, partial $\eta^2 = .25$ (means are 828, 724, and 635 ms for the semantic decision, "e" detection, and case decision tasks, respectively). No Age × Decision type interaction was found, indicating that the age-related differences in RT performance were equal across decision tasks, $F(2, 150) = 1.8$, $p > .1$.

A main effect of education was found, indicating that people with a high educational level had shorter reaction times than people with a low educational level, $F(1, 75) = 11.5$, $p < .01$, partial $\eta^2 = .13$ (means are 764 and 695 ms for low and high educational levels, respectively). No Age × Decision type × Education, Education × Age, and Education × Decision

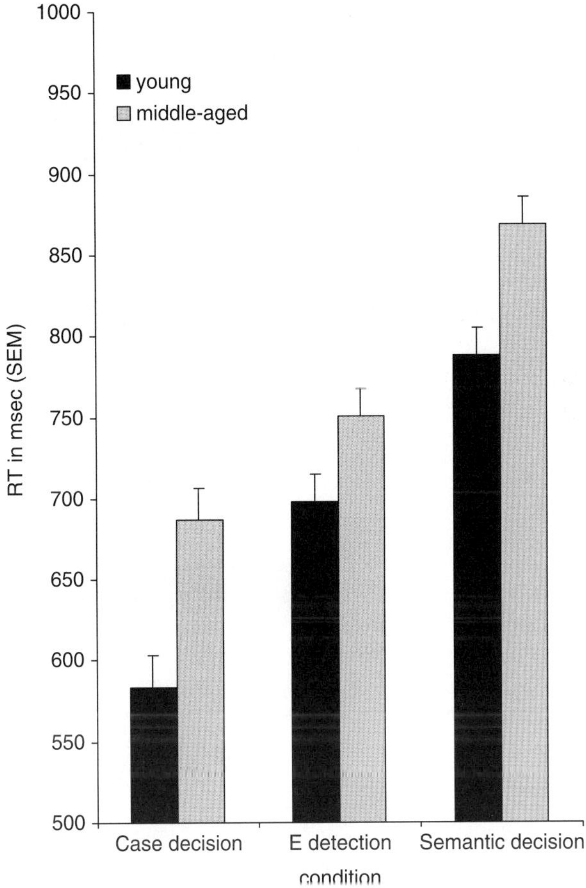

Figure 1. Mean reaction time as a function of age and level of processing. Error bars represent standard errors of the mean.

type interactions were found (*F*s < 1, *p*s > .6). Results were essentially the same when left-handed participants were excluded from the analyses.

RT split by stimulus type per decision task

In Figure 2 the mean reaction times are presented per age group and stimulus type, for each decision task. With respect to case decision, no difference in RT was found between response on uppercase and lowercase words, $F(1, 75) = 0.08$, $p > .8$. Main effects of age, $F(1, 75) = 12.4$, $p < .01$, and education, $F(1, 75) = 8.4$, $p < .01$ (means are 673 and 593 ms for low and

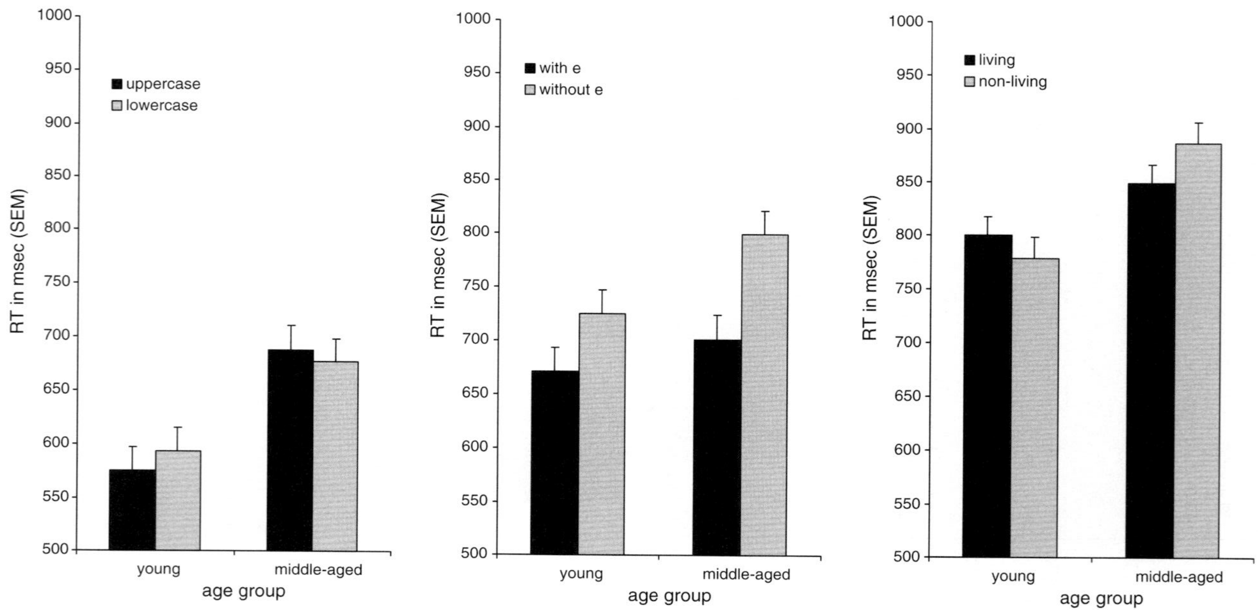

Figure 2. Mean reaction time as a function of (a) age and case, (b) age and presence of the letter "e", and (c) age and semantic dimension. Error bars represent standard errors of the mean.

high educational levels, respectively), but no interactions with stimulus type ($Fs < 2$, $ps > .19$) were found. Within the "e" detection task, a main effect of stimulus type was found, $F(1, 75) = 7.4$, $p < .05$, partial $\eta^2 = .09$, indicating that the RT for the words containing the letter "e" is shorter than for the words without "e". Besides a main effect of age, $F(1, 75) = 5.0$, $p < .05$, and education, $F(1, 75) = 7.8$, $p < .01$ (means are 756 and 691 ms for low and high education, respectively), an interaction between age and stimulus type was found, $F(1, 75) = 6.7$, $p < .05$, partial $\eta^2 = .08$. This indicates that the difference in RT between words with and without "e" was larger in the old group. Regarding the semantic decision task, no main effect of stimulus type was found, $F(1, 75) = 0.02$, $p > .8$, indicating that there was no difference in RT between living and nonliving words. However, in addition to a main effect of age, $F(1, 75) = 10.4$, $p < .01$, and education, $F(1, 75) = 6.0$, $p < .05$ (means are 858 and 798 ms for low and high educational levels, respectively), an interaction between age and stimulus type was found, $F(1, 75) = 8.4$, $p < .01$, partial $\eta^2 = .1$, indicating that the age difference in RT is larger for nonliving than for living words. No Age × Stimulus type × Education, Education × Age, and Education × Stimulus type interactions were found ($Fs < 2$, $ps > .15$). The results were essentially the same when left-handed participants were excluded from the analyses.

DISCUSSION

The first purpose of this study was to investigate whether middle-aged adults process information less efficiently than young adults in more resource-demanding conditions. We assessed age differences in RT on decision tasks that induce various levels of processing. The results indicate that middle-aged and young adults of both educational levels had longer reaction times in the semantic decision than in the "e" detection, and longer reaction times in the "e" detection than in the case decision task. This main effect of decision type suggests that the task conditions varied in their relative demands on the different components of visual word processing. Because the semantic decision task (deep processing) is assumed to incorporate shallow processing stages, this condition can be considered more complex than the shallower conditions. The effect of decision type on RT is in accordance with recent ERP studies using decision tasks to induce processing at a particular level. For instance, the findings in a study by Bentin et al. (1999) indicate that a size decision task induces visual/orthographic processing in which visual features are integrated to represent orthographic patterns. A rhyme decision task reflects the activation of a phonological representation of the printed word. Finally, a semantic decision task reflects accessing the meaning of a word.

Most importantly, the results of the present study showed no age by decision type interaction, that is, RT differences between age groups did not vary across decision tasks. This finding suggests that different levels of word processing are equally sensitive to slowing in middle age. Thus, the implications of the theories proposed by Myerson et al. (1990) and Salthouse (1996), which predict a disproportionate increase of RT in older adults as a function of the number of processing steps, do not apply to middle age. A straightforward explanation for this result is that the ageing process in adults of middle age is in such an early stage that a disproportional effect cannot be detected yet. It is possible that elderly (over 65 years of age) relative to young adults show a disproportionate increase of RT as a function of processing depth. It should be noted that the participants in the present sample consisted of persons in the age range between college age and retirement age. They were carefully screened for health problems to exclude potential age-extrinsic confounders. Furthermore, we did not rely on college students as the source of young participants, which is common practice in contemporary cognitive ageing research. To the extent that college students are not representative of their cohort in terms of intellectual ability, lifestyle, socioeconomic status, or personality characteristics (such as openness to experience), the age-related changes observed in studies involving college students may not be completely attributable to "pure ageing" processes. Therefore, we minimised age-extrinsic confounds, after which we found no age by decision type interaction. This might suggest that age-related cognitive change in extreme age-group designs is not necessarily attributable to intrinsic age effects. This should be investigated in future research by carefully screening and classifying participants in order to reduce age-extrinsic confounds.

Another possible explanation for the equal vulnerability to slowing in middle age for different levels of word processing may be sought in the slowing function representing age effects in sequential complexity conditions. Sequential complexity refers to any task manipulation that leads to a variation in the number of independent processing steps but that does not increase the amount of information exchange between single steps (Mayr & Kliegl, 1993). In particular, no simultaneous storage and processing demands should be involved in these tasks, which makes working memory load comparatively low. This contrasts with task manipulations on the coordinative complexity dimension in which simultaneous processing in working memory is varied. Age-related slowing is found to be larger if coordinative complexity is increased than if sequential complexity is increased (Mayr & Kliegl, 1993). The stability of age differences in RT across decision types in the current study suggests that the present task manipulation involves sequential rather than coordinative complexity. It should be investigated in future research whether there is disproportionate slowing in middle age with respect to tasks that increase in coordinative complexity.

We additionally investigated age-related differences in RT between stimulus types within decision tasks in order to provide insight into the use of search strategies. With respect to case decision, no difference in RT was found between responses on uppercase and lowercase words and there was no interaction with age. This was expected, because no search processes are involved. In the "e" detection task, an effect of response type was found, indicating that the RT for the words containing the letter "e" is shorter than for the words not containing an "e". Interestingly, this difference was larger in the middle-aged group. This pattern of results suggests that participants terminated the search of the letter string when the "e" was identified, and that middle-aged participants were slower in performing this search strategy than the younger ones. The suggestion that a terminating search strategy (Schneider & Shiffrin, 1977) was adopted in which each letter was assessed implies that the "e" detection task does not draw on orthographic or phonological processing of the whole word.

On the semantic decision task, an interaction between age and stimulus type was found: The age difference in RT was larger for nonliving than for living words. This suggests that middle-aged adults are more constrained by the reduced semantic accessibility of nonliving words than younger adults. In conclusion, although no overall age by level of processing interaction was found, the age by stimulus type interactions in the deeper processing tasks suggest that some vulnerability to cognitive decline already exists in middle age.

Concerning the role of education in visual word processing, higher educated persons had consistently shorter RTs than lower educated persons. Education did not interact with any of the other independent variables, however. This suggests that education is not a moderating factor of age-related changes in visual word processing, at least not over the age span investigated in the present study. It should be noted, however, that the level of education of the older cohorts is more often related to socioeconomic status than to true intellectual ability (Jolles, Houx, van Boxtel, & Ponds, 1995). As a consequence, there is a risk of underestimating the cognitive differences associated with age in lower educated people. By including a young and a middle-aged group and by adjusting the level of educational achievement, cohort differences were minimised in the current study. It is noteworthy that the precise mechanisms for the hypothesised protective effect of education remain unclear. One of the proposed mechanisms is that education serves as a marker for other socioeconomic conditions, including health status, which is also known to influence age-related cognitive decline (van Hooren et al., 2005). Thus, a protective effect of education might not have been demonstrated in the present study because all our participants were screened for health problems to exclude potential age-extrinsic confounds.

It is not clear yet on which cognitive domains education may have such a protective effect. Three large-scale studies examining the effects of education on age-related cognitive differences in a broad age range shed more light on this matter. First, Capitani, Barbarotto, and Laiacona (1996) studied 307 adults aged between 40 and 85 years. They found that age-related differences on tasks of visual attention and verbal memory were attenuated in higher educated individuals, but not on tasks of verbal fluency, spatial memory, and nonverbal intelligence. Similar results were found in a second study by Heaton, Grant, and Matthews (1986) on 553 individuals aged 15–81 years: The performance decrement with age was smaller for higher educated people on two WAIS subtests (Picture Arrangement and Block Design) but no effects were found on the other subtests. Also the third study, which involved 806 healthy people aged 16–85 (Ardila, Ostrosky-Solis, Rosselli, & Gomez, 2000), was consistent with the notion that higher educated subjects are characterised by less pronounced cognitive deterioration with age. A short neuropsychological battery was used in this study and effects were found on word recall (but not on word recognition), motor performance, verbal fluency, and digit span backwards. The general picture that emerges from these three studies is that the effect of education on age-related decrements in cognitive performance is indeed present, albeit not on all cognitive measures. These equivocal results may be due to the assessment of multiple cognitive domains by standard neuropsychological tasks. Because the responses generated in these tasks are often supposed to draw upon multiple cognitive processes, including visual scanning, working memory, mental flexibility, sustained attention, and psychomotor speed (Lezak, 1995),it is not clear which cognitive processes are particularly sensitive to the protective effects of education. Moreover, compensatory strategies may be more readily recruited in the execution of these tasks than when performing tasks that draw on a narrower range of cognitive processes, such as the decision tasks in the present study. The present findings are in accordance with a recent experimental study by van Gerven, Meijer, and Jolles (2007) in which the effects of age and education on switching focal attention in working memory, as measured with a numeric *n*-back task, were investigated among the same age groups as in the present study. The age-related decline of this process turned out to be independent of education. The present findings are also in accordance with the review by Anstey and Christensen (2000), in which none of the studies using measures of information processing speed found protective effects of education. Systematically testing a broad range of functions may further delineate the "protective reach" of education.

In conclusion, different levels of word processing appeared to be equally vulnerable to slowing in middle age. This may suggest that particular mechanisms of cognitive ageing, in which disproportional age-related slowing as a function of the number of processing steps is predicted, do not apply to middle age. Another possibility is that the decision tasks involve variations of sequential complexity, which do not interact with age. Although no overall age by level of processing interaction was found, the age by stimulus type interactions in the deeper processing tasks suggest that a vulnerability to age-related cognitive decline already exists in middle age. Finally, we conclude that high education has no protective effect on age-related changes in visual word processing.

REFERENCES

Allen, P. A., Madden, D. J., Weber, T. A., & Groth, K. E. (1993). Influence of age and processing stage on visual word recognition. *Psychology and Aging*, *8*, 274–282.

Anstey, K., & Christensen, H. (2000). Education, activity, health, blood pressure and apolipoprotein E as predictors of cognitive change in old age: A review. *Gerontology*, *46*(3), 163–177.

Ardila, A., Ostrosky-Solis, F., Rosselli, M., & Gomez, C. (2000). Age-related cognitive decline during normal aging: The complex effect of education. *Archives of Clinical Neuropsychology*, *15*(6), 495 513.

Baltes, P. B., Staudinger, U. M., & Lindenberger, U. (1999). Lifespan psychology: Theory and application to intellectual functioning. *Annual Review of Psychology*, *50*, 471–507.

Bentin, S., Mouchetant-Rostaing, Y., Giard, M. H., Echallier, J. F., & Pernier, J. (1999). ERP manifestations of processing printed words at different psycholinguistic levels: Time course and scalp distribution. *Journal of Cognitive Neuroscience*, *11*, 235–260.

Borowsky, R., & Besner, D. (1993). Visual word recognition: A multistage activation model *Journal of Experimental Psychology: Learning, Memory, and Cognition*, *19*, 813–840.

Bosma, H., van Boxtel, M. P., Ponds, R. W. H. M., Houx, P., & Jolles, J. (2003). Education and age-related cognitive decline: The contribution of mental workload. *Educational Gerontology*, *29*, 1–9.

Buchner, A., Faul, F., & Erdfelder, E. (1992). *GPOWER: A priori-, post hoc-, and compromise power analyses for the Macintosh (Version 2.1)*. Bonn, Germany: Bonn University.

Capitani, E., Barbarotto, R., & Laiacona, M. (1996). Does education influence the age-related cognitive decline? A further inquiry. *Developmental Neuropsychology*, *12*, 231–240.

Caramazza, A., & Shelton, J. R. (1998). Domain-specific knowledge systems in the brain the animate–inanimate distinction. *Journal of Cognitive Neuroscience*, *10*, 1–34.

Christensen, H., Anstey, K. J., Parslow, R. A., Maller, J., Mackinnin, A., & Sachdev, P. (2007). The brain reserve hypothesis, brain atrophy and aging. *Gerontology*, *53*, 82–95.

Christensen, H., Korten, A. E., Jorm, A. F., Henderson, A. S., Jacomb, P. A., Rodgers, B., & Mackinnon, A. J. (1997). Education and decline in cognitive performance: Compensatory but not protective. *International Journal of Geriatric Psychiatry*, *3*, 323–330.

Coffey, C. E., Saxton, J. A., Ratcliff, G., Bryan, R. N., & Lucke, J. F. (1999). Relation of education to brain size in normal aging: Implications for the reserve hypothesis. *Neurology*, *53*, 189–196.

Colsher, P. L., & Wallace, R. B. (1991). Longitudinal application of cognitive function measures in a defined population of community-dwelling elders. *Annals of Epidemiology*, *1*(3), 215–230.

Daselaar, S. M., Veltman, D. J., Rombouts, S. A., Raaijmakers, J. G., & Jonker, C. (2003). Deep processing activates the medial temporal lobe in young but not in old adults. *Neurobiology of Aging*, *24*, 1005–1011.

De Bie, S. E. (1987). *Standaardvragen 1987: Voorstellen voor uniformering van vraagstellingen naar achergrondkernmerken en interviews* [Standard questions 1987: Proposal for uniformisation of questions regarding background variables and interviews] (2nd ed.). Leiden, The Netherlands: Leiden University Press.

Dixon, R. A., de Frias, C. M., & Maitland, S. B. (2001). Memory in midlife. In M. E. Lachman (Ed.), *Handbook of midlife development* (pp. 248–279). New York: Wiley.

Ellis, A. W., & Young, A. W. (1996). *Human cognitive neuropsychology: A textbook with readings.* Hove, UK: Psychology Press.

Evans, D. A., Beckett, L. A., Albert, M. S., Hebert, L. E., Scherr, P. A., Funkenstein, H. H., & Taylor, J. O. (1993). Level of education and change in cognitive function in a community population of older persons. *Annals of Epidemiology, 3*, 71–77.

Farmer, M. E., Kittner, S. J., Rae, D. S., Bartko, J. J., & Regier, D. A. (1995). Education and change in cognitive function: The Epidemiologic Catchment Area Study. *Annals of Epidemiology, 5*(1), 1–7.

Gold, D. P., Andres, D., Etezadi, J., Arbuckle, T., Schwartzman, A., & Chaikelson, J. (1995). Structural equation model of intellectual change and continuity and predictors of intelligence in older men. *Psychology and Aging, 10*, 294–303.

Haug, H. (1985). Are neurons of the human cerebral cortex really lost during aging? A morphometric examination. In J. Traber & W. H. Gispen (Eds.), *Senile dementia of the Alzheimer type* (pp. 150–163). New York: Springer-Verlag.

Heaton, R. K., Grant, I., & Matthews, C. G. (1986). Differences in neuropsychological test performance associated with age, education, and sex. In I. Grant & K. M. Adams (Eds.), *Neuropsychological assessment of neuropsychiatric disorders* (pp. 100–120). New York: Oxford University Press.

Houx, P. J., & Jolles, J. (1993). Age-related decline of psychomotor speed: Effects of age, brain health, sex, and education. *Perceptual Motor Skills, 76*, 195–211.

Houx, P. J., Jolles, J., & Vreeling, F. W. (1993). Stroop interference: Aging effects assessed with the Stroop Color-Word Test. *Experimental Aging Research, 19*, 209–224.

Jolles, J., Houx, P., van Boxtel, M. P., & Ponds, R. W. (Eds.).(1995). *Maastricht Aging Study: Determinants of cognitive aging.* Maastricht: Neuropsych Publishers.

Lezak, M. D. (1995). *Neuropsychological assessment* (3rd ed.). New York: Oxford University Press.

Luteijn, F., & van der Ploeg, F. A. E. (1983). *Handleiding Groninger Intelligentietest (GIT)* [Manual Groningen Intelligence Test]. Lisse, The Netherlands: Swets & Zeitlinger.

Madden, D. J. (1985). Age-related slowing in the retrieval of information from long-term memory. *Journal of Gerontology, 40*, 208–210.

Madden, D. J. (1992). Four to ten milliseconds per year: Age-related slowing of visual word identification. *Journal of Gerontology, 47*(2), P59–P68.

Madden, D. J., Pierce, T. W., & Allen, P. A. (1993). Age-related slowing and the time course of semantic priming in visual word identification. *Psychology and Aging, 8*, 490–507.

Mahon, B. Z., & Caramazza, A. (2003). Constraining questions about the organisation and representation of conceptual knowledge. *Cognitive Neuropsychology, 20*, 433–450.

Mares, A. M. H. M. (Ed.). (2004). *Jaarboek onderwijs in cijfers* [Yearbook education in numbers]. Voorburg/Heerlen, the Netherlands: Centraal Bureau voor de Statistiek.

Mayr, U., & Kliegl, R. (1993). Sequential and coordinative complexity: Age-based processing limitations in figural transformations. *Journal of Experimental Psychology: Learning, Memory, and Cognition, 19*, 1297–1320.

Myerson, J., Hale, S., Wagstaff, D., Poon, L. W., & Smith, G. A. (1990). The information-loss model: A mathematical theory of age-related cognitive slowing. *Psychological Review, 97*, 475–487.

Petros, T. V., Zehr, D., & Chabot, R. (1983). Adult age differences in accessing and retrieving information from long-term memory. *Journal of Gerontology, 38*, 589–592.

Proverbio, A. M., Vecchi, L., & Zani, A. (2004). From orthography to phonetics: ERP measures of grapheme-to-phoneme conversion mechanisms in reading. *Journal of Cognitive Neuroscience, 16*, 301–317.

Rabbitt, P., Chetwynd, A., & McInnes, L. (2003). Do clever brains age more slowly? Further exploration of a nun result. *British Journal of Psychology, 94*, 63–71.

Salthouse, T. A. (1996). The processing-speed theory of adult age differences in cognition. *Psychological Review, 103*, 403–428.

Schaie, K. W. (Ed.).(1996). *Intellectual development in adulthood.* New York: Cambridge University Press.

Schmand, B., Smit, J. H., Geerlings, M. I., & Lindeboom, J. (1997). The effects of intelligence and education on the development of dementia: A test of the brain reserve hypothesis. *Psychological Medicine, 27*, 1337–1344.

Schneider, W.', Eschman, A., & Zuccolotto, A. (Eds.).(2002). *E-prime user's guide (Version 1.0).* Pittsburgh, PA: Psychology Software Tools.

Schneider, W., & Shiffrin, R. M. (1977). Controlled and automatic human processing: 1. Detection, search, and attention. *Psychological Review, 84*, 1–66.

Seidenberg, M. S., & McClelland, J. L. (1989). A distributed, developmental model of word recognition and naming. *Psychological Review, 96*, 523–568.

Shapiro, L. R., & Olson, A. C. (2005). Does normal processing provide evidence of specialized semantic subsystems? *Language and Cognitive Processes, 20*, 697–724.

Shichita, K., Hatano, S., Ohashi, Y., Shibata, H., & Matuzaki, T. (1986). Memory changes in the Benton Visual Retention Test between ages 70 and 75. *Journal of Gerontology, 41*, 385–386.

Stern, Y. (2002). What is cognitive reserve? Theory and research application of the reserve concept. *Journal of the International Neuropsychological Society, 8*, 448–460.

Sternberg, S., Grigorenko, E. L., & Oh, S. (2001). The development of intelligence at midlife. In M. E. Lachman (Ed.), *Handbook of midlife development* (pp. 217–248). New York: Wiley.

Tisserand, D. J., McIntosh, A. R., van der Veen, F. M., Backes, W. H., & Jolles, J. (2005). Age-related reorganization of encoding networks directly influences subsequent recognition memory. *Cognitive Brain Research, 25*, 8–18.

Tisserand, D. J., Pruessner, J. C., Sanz Arigita, E. J., van Boxtel, M. P., Evans, A. C., Jolles, J., & Uylings, H. B. M. (2002). Regional frontal cortical volumes decrease differentially in aging: An MRI study to compare volumetric approaches and voxel-based morphometry. *NeuroImage, 17*, 657–669.

Tombaugh, T. N., & McIntyre, N. J. (1992). The mini-mental state examination: A comprehensive review. *Journal of the American Geriatric Society, 40*, 922–935.

UNESCO. (1976). *International standard classification of education (ISCED).* Paris: Author.

Van der Elst, W., van Boxtel, M. P., van Breukelen, G. J., & Jolles, J. (2006a). Normative data for the Animal, Profession and Letter M Naming verbal fluency tests for Dutch speaking participants and the effects of age, education, and sex. *Journal of the International Neuropsychological Society, 12*, 80–89.

Van der Elst, W., van Boxtel, M. P., van Breukelen, G. J., & Jolles, J. (2006b). The Stroop color-word test: Influence of age, sex, and education, and normative data for a large sample across the adult age range. *Assessment, 13*, 62–79.

Van Dijk, K. R. A., van Gerven, P. W. M., van Boxtel, M. P. J., van der Elst, W., & Jolles, J. (2008). No protective effects of education in normal cognitive aging: Results from the 6-year follow-up of the Maastricht Aging Study (MAAS). *Psychology and Aging, 23*, 119–130.

Van Gerven, P. W. M., Meijer, W. A., & Jolles, J. (2007). Education does not protect against age-related decline of switching focal attention in working memory. *Brain and Cognition, 64*, 158–163.

Van Hooren, S. A., Valentijn, S. A., Bosma, H., Ponds, R. W., van Boxtel, M. P., & Jolles, J. (2005). Relation between health status and cognitive functioning: A 6-year follow-up of the Maastricht Aging Study. *Journal of Gerontology B: Psychological Sciences, 60*, 57–60.

Van Loon-Vervoorn, W. A. (1985). *Voorstelbaarheidswaarden van Nederlandse woorden: 4600 substantieven, 1000 verba en 500 adjectieven* [Imagery values of Dutch words: 400 nouns, 1000 verbs, and 500 adjectives]. Lisse, The Netherlands: Swets & Zeitlinger.

Willis, S. L., & Schaie, K. W. (2005). Cognitive trajectories in midlife and cognitive funcioning in old age. In S. L. Willis & M. Martin (Eds.), *Middle adulthood: A lifespan perspective* (pp. 243–277). Thousand Oaks, CA: Sage.

EUROPEAN JOURNAL OF COGNITIVE PSYCHOLOGY
2009, 21 (2/3), 235–254

Psychology Press
Taylor & Francis Group

Effects of ageing on associative memory for related and unrelated pictures

Angela H. Gutchess
Brandeis University, Waltham, MA, USA

Denise C. Park
University of Texas at Dallas, Dallas, TX, USA

Associative memory deficits are pervasive with age. Memory for complex pictures, however, also seems to require the association of several scene elements into one representation, but picture memory is often age-invariant. We speculated that the natural relationships contained in pictures may explain this distinction and that memory for scenes with unusual novel relationships would be affected with ageing. In three experiments, we found that, counter to our predictions, the relatedness of scene elements exerted little influence on picture memory and did not differentially affect older compared to younger adults. These data suggest that the semantically rich associations contained in pictures need not rely on prior knowledge and experiences in order to support age-invariant picture memory. Our results indicate that associative memory for complex pictures may differ from memory for interitem associations, which may be more affected by ageing.

Keywords: Ageing; Associative memory; Picture memory; Recognition; Relatedness.

Associative memory undergoes pronounced impairment with age. Older adults exhibit difficulty associating, or "binding", pieces of information together into a single memory trace (Chalfonte & Johnson, 1996; Navch-

Correspondence should be addressed to Angela Gutchess, Department of Psychology, Brandeis University, 415 South Street, MS 062, Waltham, MA 02454-9110, USA. E-mail: gutchess@brandeis.edu

Grant support from the National Institute on Aging (R01 AG006265 and P50 AG011715; awarded to DCP) and a seed grant from the Center on Aging and Cognition: Health, Education, and Training (awarded to AHG) supported this research, and funds from Brandeis University supported the preparation of this manuscript. We thank Julie Hautamaki, Siva Sethuraman, Laura Rallo, and Nora Goudsmit for experimental assistance. We also thank John Henderson's laboratory at Michigan State University for making some of their stimuli available on their website.

http://www.psypress.com/ecp DOI: 10.1080/09541440802257274

Benjamin, 2000). Naveh-Benjamin (2000) has proposed an associative deficit hypothesis of ageing, suggesting that older adults' intact ability to encode items is dissociated from their impaired ability to encode interitem relationships. Deficits in associative memory occur for items and contexts (Chalfonte & Johnson, 1996; Park & Puglisi, 1985; Park, Puglisi, & Lutz, 1982) as well as for pairs of distinct items, including word pairs, object picture pairs, and name–face pairs (Naveh-Benjamin, 2000; Naveh-Benjamin, Guez, Kilb, & Reedy, 2004; Naveh-Benjamin, Hussain, Guez, & Bar-On, 2003), even when item memory is intact. Memory for complex pictures also seemingly requires the ability to associate various components of scenes into a single representation in memory, but picture memory is largely invariant with age (e.g., Park, Puglisi, & Smith, 1986; Park, Smith, Morrell, Puglisi, & Dudley, 1990; Smith, Park, Cherry, & Berkovsky, 1990; Smith, Park, Earles, Shaw, & Whiting, 1998). In the present studies, we investigate the extent to which complex pictures place demands on associative memory under a variety of conditions.

One possible explanation for the age-invariance in picture memory is that complex pictures demand less associative processing than other types of items. There is some evidence that particular task conditions can reduce associative memory demands. For example, unitisation, that is, merging two distinct items into one single item such as the words "jail" and "bird" into "jailbird" or connecting two words in a sentence, reduces the extent of amnesic patients' associative memory impairments for word pairs (Giovanello, Keane, & Verfaellie, 2006; Quamme, Yonelinas, & Norman, 2007). With ageing, the effects of unitisation have been assessed by asking research participants to enact object-action phrases (e.g., "put the money in the wallet"), and this manipulation equivalently enhances young and older adults' memory for the object-action associations (Mangels & Heinberg, 2006). Age differences in associative memory also can be reduced with incidental encoding strategies that support associative memory (Naveh-Benjamin, Brav, & Levy, 2007).

Another important factor could be the inherent interrelatedness of picture elements. For complex pictures, the elements to be bound typically share a natural, meaningful relationship with each other. Information that is highly meaningful and interrelated, as is the case for the information contained in complex pictures, may reduce the binding demands and determine which medial temporal regions are implicated in associative processes. Memory for complex meaningful pictures can be astonishingly good (Standing, 1973), and memory for these types of pictures can be largely equivalent across young and older adults (Park et al., 1986, 1990; Smith et al., 1990, 1998). Age differences emerge in picture memory, however, when pictures are not meaningfully related or lack rich semantic or perceptual details (Park et al., 1990; Smith et al., 1990, 1998). One aspect of picture memory that has not been investigated is the importance of the relatedness of elements in complex scenes. Previous studies using related and unrelated picture pairs used simple drawings of related (e.g., ant-spider) and unrelated (e.g., spider-cherry) objects and noted that older adults exhibited poorer memory for the pairings than young (Naveh-Benjamin et al., 2003; Park et al., 1990). However, the associative demands and support provided by the interrelated picture information could differ for complex scenes.

We conducted three picture memory experiments in which we systematically manipulated intrapicture information, comparing the effects of ageing on recognition for scenes that contained related, predictable elements versus scenes that were composed of elements that would be unexpected and might not be automatically bound together. We expected that unrelated, low plausibility scenes would place large demands on binding processes and thus older adults' memory would be impaired relative to young adults' memory for unrelated scenes. We expected that scenes with related and predictable context would have reduced binding demands so that the previously mentioned pattern of age-equivalent picture memory (Park et al., 1986, 1990; Smith et al., 1990, 1998) would be replicated.

The inclusion of two additional factors, environmental support and encoding intentionality, allowed us to investigate the contribution of relatedness to binding under a variety of conditions. Environmental support, such as rich contextual information, can improve older adults' performance on memory tasks by reducing the demands on cognitive resources (Craik & Byrd, 1982; Craik & Jennings, 1992). Past research suggests that the encoding of rich, meaningful stimuli, particularly when tested in a recognition paradigm, can provide appropriate environmental support. As shown in Park, Puglisi, and Sovacool (1984), one way to manipulate environmental support is by removing seemingly extraneous picture backgrounds at recognition, and this impairs performance of both young and elderly adults. We incorporated this manipulation in the present study and predicted that an increase in environmental support would reduce binding demands and thus reduce age differences in memory (as in Park et al., 1984). Varying the amount of environmental support provides a measure of binding in that memory for tightly bound information may be disrupted when environmental support is reduced. This predicts that "unbinding" of information, through the removal of environmental support, will affect young more than elderly because young should have more successfully bound information together during the initial encoding phase. Likewise, the loss of environmental support should impact memory for related more than unrelated scenes because this type of scene should undergo greater binding when environmental support is present. Although we predict that older adults will be less affected by the removal of background information than young, it is possible that they will be more prone to misrecognition, on the basis that poorly bound representations are subject to distortion (Lyle & Johnson, 2006). We manipulated encoding intentionality by directing participants to associate the object and background together, as opposed to encoding the object alone. We expected that encoding intentionality would support greater association of object with background for the young, so that age differences would become larger under conditions of intentionality (as in Naveh-Benjamin et al., 2007).

The specifics of the three experiments are as follows. In the first two experiments, we assessed the effects of "unbinding" a scene. Subjects studied a complex picture with a central object presented against a background that was highly related or relatively unrelated. At recognition, we removed the backgrounds leaving only the central target object to be recognised. We expected that the loss of picture background context would impair performance of both young and elderly adults, due to a loss of environmental support at recognition (Park et al., 1984). Although this procedure relies upon correct recognition of picture elements rather than associations per se, we have used similar procedures successfully and found them to be sensitive to the effects of age on memory for backgrounds versus objects (Gutchess et al., 2007). Moreover, we also hypothesised that older adults would be relatively less affected than young by the removal of the backgrounds in the unrelated condition, because they were less effective at binding target to context than young. In contrast, removal of the related background would strongly impact target recognition, because the target should be more tightly bound to the background compared to the unrelated condition. In the third experiment, we examined the impact of intact and recombined target-background relationships on recognition for related and unrelated items.

EXPERIMENT 1

In the first experiment, participants intentionally encoded an object in relation to a background that was either related or unrelated. At recognition, the backgrounds were removed for half of the pictures, representing a loss of environmental support (Park et al., 1984). In this study, we hypothesised that young would be more effective than old at binding a target to a context in the unrelated condition, but that both age groups would be effective in the related condition. Thus, when subjects had to recognise items without backgrounds, the old would be less impaired than the young in the unrelated condition, due to the fragile binding for the target/background pair in the old.

Methods

Participants. Thirty-four young (ages 17–23; M age = 20.15, SD = 1.26; 17 females) and 34 elderly (ages 62–86; M age = 72.03, SD = 6.20; 17 females) participants took part in the study in exchange for payment or credit towards course requirements. Based on self-report, older adults were screened to have at least a 10th grade education, to be free from visual, auditory or cognitive impairments that would affect their participation, and to not have been hospitalised or had surgery in the previous 6 months. Older adults had more years of education (M = 14.94, SD = 2.06) than the young (M = 13.50, SD = 1.20), $t(66) = 3.53$, $p < .002$. The samples exhibited the expected pattern of age-related differences in measures of speed of processing (Hedden et al., 2002) and vocabulary (Shipley, 1986). Older adults had higher vocabulary scores (M = 34.65, SD = 3.28) than young adults (M = 31.47, SD = 3.18), $t(66) = 4.05$, $p < .001$, but completed fewer items on the digit comparison task (older adult M = 53.66, SD = 11.39 vs. young adult M = 74.61, SD = 11.58) on a speed of processing measure, $t(63) = 7.35$, $p < .001$. All participants provided written informed consent for a protocol approved by the Institutional Review Board.

Materials and procedure. In the study, we used 105 line-drawing pictures consisting of a target object and a supporting, related background (e.g., a squirrel eating a nut in a tree). The backgrounds were then swapped among pictures such that each target object was re-paired with an unrelated background to create an additional 105 pictures (e.g., a squirrel eating a nut on a kitchen counter). Finally, the background of each picture was removed to create a set of 105 pictures of the target-item only. See Figure 1 for examples of the three types of stimuli. This set of 315 pictures was counterbalanced such that, across subjects, each object was seen at recognition with a related background, an unrelated background, and without a background, as well as appearing as a studied target item and an unstudied lure item.

Participants viewed 60 line-drawings of a target item on a background. Many of the previous studies report age-equivalent memory for line-drawings of scenes (e.g., Park et al., 1986; Smith et al., 1990), which suggests that even these stimuli can impart sufficiently complex contextual information. Half of the encoded pictures consisted of a pairing of a background and target item that together constituted a familiar scene while the other half of the pictures consisted of pairings of a background with a target item that comprised an unusual or unrelated scene at encoding (see Figure 1). Participants were instructed to "study and try to remember the entire picture. Attempt to associate the target item with the background so that you can remember them together when you are tested later." Pictures

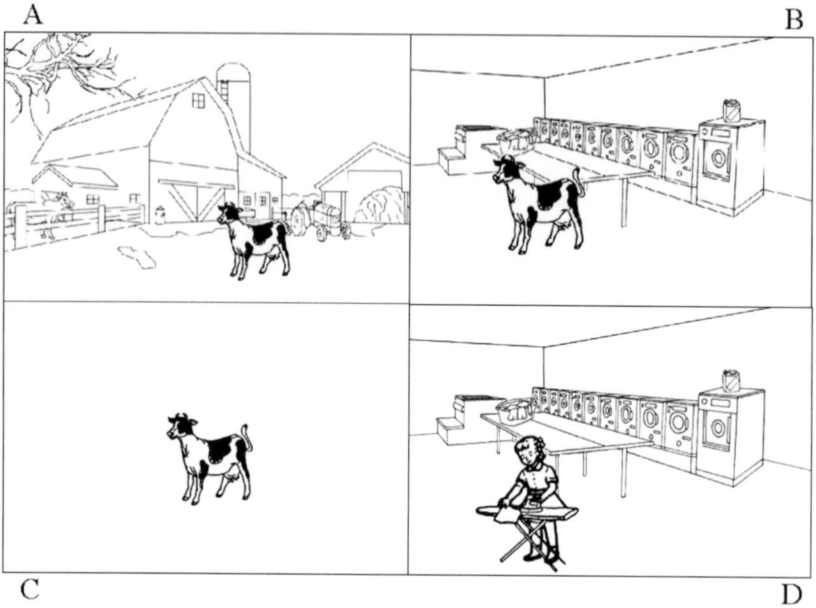

Figure 1. Examples of picture stimuli, consisting of a related picture (A), an unrelated picture (B), and a no-background picture (C). In Experiment 3, lure pictures consisted of recombinations of objects and backgrounds originally encoded in different picture pairings. Using these examples, a participant could have originally encoded the pictures displayed in Panels A and D (both in the related condition) and then encounter the same elements at recognition in the unrelated combination depicted in Panel B; this would constitute an RR-U trial (i.e., object and background were studied in separate Related pairings at encoding, but tested in a new Unrelated pairing at recognition).

were presented on a computer for 4 s each with a 1 s interstimulus interval. These pictures consisted of a central target item and a related or unrelated background (30 of each type). To reinforce the encoding instruction, we provided the participants with four practice encoding and recognition trials before studying the pictures on the computer. Participants were instructed, "remember that you are basing your decision on the entire picture you just studied. If you saw the target item before but it was not paired with the same background, you would respond NO because you did not study the entire identical picture previously." After the practice recognition test, the correct responses were explained to the participants.

After encoding, there was a 12 min retention interval, during which time participants completed the vocabulary subscale of the Shipley Institute of Living Scale (Shipley, 1986). Then, participants' picture memory was assessed. The recognition test consisted of 105 pictures: the 60 that were previously studied and 45 new lures. Half of the previously studied pictures (15 related and 15 unrelated) and one-third of the lures (i.e., 15) had the background removed while the other pictures had backgrounds intact (15 related and 15 unrelated targets; 15 related and 15 unrelated new lures). Participants were instructed to respond on the basis of the item only, ignoring the background information. Participants pressed a key labelled "yes" for pictures with target items they had studied previously and one labelled "no" for pictures they had not studied earlier. The backgrounds were removed from half of the previously studied pictures and a third of the lure items so that we could assess the contribution to memory of the environmental support provided by the presence of the background. Stimuli were presented in a random ordering for each subject with PsyScope software (Cohen, MacWhinney, Flatt, & Provost, 1993). Participants also completed the digit comparison task (Hedden et al., 2002; modelled after Salthouse & Babcock's, 1991, Letter Comparison Task) as a measure of speed of processing.

Results and discussion

To assess recognition performance, we calculated A' scores (Snodgrass & Corwin, 1988) as a measure of corrected recognition, using the hit rates to either the related or unrelated target pictures and the false alarm rates to related and unrelated lure pictures, with and without backgrounds. Results were tested using a mixed design ANOVA, with age (young/older) as a between-subjects variable and relatedness (related/unrelated) and background (present/absent at recognition) as within-subject variables. The only effect to reach significance was that of background, $F(1, 66) = 71.27$, $p < .001$, $\eta_p^2 = .52$), with pictures containing a background at recognition ($M = 0.92$) supporting more accurate recognition than pictures without a background ($M = 0.85$), consistent with the findings of Park et al. (1984). No other effects approached significance (Fs < 1). Results are shown in Figure 2. Contrary to our predictions, unrelated backgrounds did not disproportionately affect older adults compared to younger adults and, in fact, memory for objects presented on unrelated backgrounds was no worse than memory for objects presented on a related background. Even when the backgrounds were removed, pictures encoded in related and unrelated contexts were remembered equivalently, suggesting that the presence of an unrelated background did not inhibit recognition of object pictures. Consistent with prior studies, the age groups did not differ in picture recognition ability.

The results suggest that the different types of background contexts do not differ in their binding demands for younger or older adults. Both unrelated and related backgrounds enhance memory performance compared to pictures that lack background context.

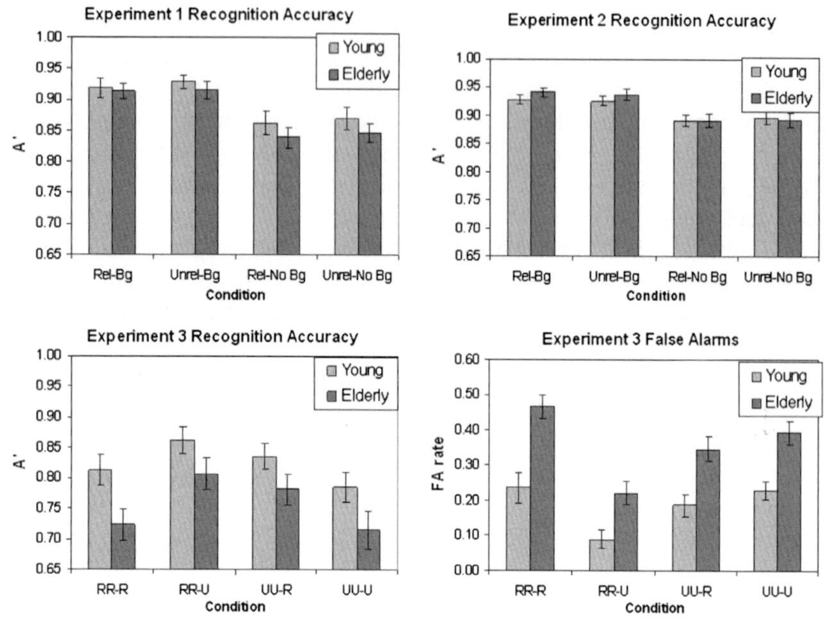

Figure 2. Memory performance for young and elderly adults in each of the three experiments.

EXPERIMENT 2

Although the complex scene context may engender semantic meaning that supports memory for both related and unrelated information, it is possible that our instructions contributed to the pattern of performance on this task. Our instructions emphasised encoding objects with their backgrounds, and this may have encouraged participants to place undue emphasis on the backgrounds. Even though prior studies have identified larger associative deficits with age under associative encoding instructions rather than item encoding instructions (Naveh-Benjamin, 2000), picture contexts could operate differently. In the case of unrelated backgrounds, participants may have focused on the bizarre nature of the unrelated pairings, which enhanced memory performance on these pictures (e.g., McDaniel & Einstein, 1986). Experiment 2 deemphasised the encoding of backgrounds; encoding instructions emphasised encoding of the items only and background information was incidental to the task.

Methods

Participants. Thirty-two young (ages 19–28; *M* age = 22.25, *SD* = 2.16; 16 females) and 33 elderly (ages 60–81; *M* age = 72.06, *SD* = 6.05; 16 females) participated in the study. Although participants were drawn from the same population as those in Experiment 1, the samples were non-overlapping (as also was the case for Experiment 3). Older adults had completed more years of education ($M = 15.73$, $SD = 2.27$) than young ($M = 14.73$, $SD = 1.03$), $t(63) = 2.26$, $p < .03$, and had higher Shipley vocabulary scores (older adult $M = 35.18$, $SD = 3.92$; young adult $M = 31.66$, $SD = 3.59$), $t(63) = 3.78$, $p < .001$. Young adults completed more items on the speed of processing task ($M = 72.53$, $SD = 10.12$) than older adults ($M = 56.71$, $SD = 13.89$), $t(61) = 5.18$, $p < .001$.

Materials and procedure. With the sole exception of the instructions and practice, the task was identical to that of Experiment 1. Whereas in Experiment 1 participants were instructed to associate the target item to the background during the encoding task, participants in Experiment 2 were instructed, "study and try to remember the target item only. … Try to remember the item regardless of the background so that you can recognise it when you are tested later." This instruction allowed us to assess the contribution of the background to recognition memory, even when the binding of related or unrelated information was incidental to the encoding task. The practice encoding and recognition trials were consistent with this instruction. Participants were instructed, "remember that you are basing your decision on only the target items you just studied. If you saw the target item before but now it is on a different (or blank) background, you would respond YES because you did study that target item previously."

Results and discussion

A' corrected recognition scores were calculated and subjected to a mixed design ANOVA. As was the case for Experiment 1, the effect of background was the only effect to reach significance, $F(1, 63) = 34.97$, $p < .001$, $\eta_p^2 = .36$. Pictures containing a background at recognition ($M = 0.93$) were more accurately recognised than pictures lacking a background ($M = 0.89$). No effects or interactions involving age emerged (Fs < 1.2), again illustrating the age-invariant nature of picture recognition ability. Results are displayed in Figure 2.

Experiment 2 replicates the pattern of results seen for Experiment 1, and suggests that the relatedness of background information has no effect on picture memory for both young and older adults even when the background information is not emphasised at encoding. Even when background information is incidentally encoded, young and elderly show equivalent support from backgrounds at recognition through superior memory when backgrounds are re-presented. This pattern suggests that backgrounds, whether relevant or irrelevant, are automatically bound to the target objects at the time of encoding. In contrast to the findings of age impairments in binding ability in a number of tasks (Naveh-Benjamin, 2000; Naveh-Benjamin et al., 2003, 2004), associative memory ability seems to be intact when the elements to be bound together are related in a semantically meaningful and perceptually rich environment, as is the case for complex pictures. Unrelated pictures do not differ from related pictures, regardless of whether the background is presented with the object at recognition. Our results replicate Smith et al.'s (1990) findings that young and elderly adults can exhibit equivalent picture memory when pictures are complex and semantically meaningful. Whereas the earlier study reports age differences in memory for abstract pictures that lack semantically meaningful content, we find that memory can be age-invariant for unrelated pictures. These data suggest that elements need not be schematically related based on familiar experiences, but need only lend themselves to rich interpretation.

EXPERIMENT 3

Although the previous two experiments are consistent in their findings that the relatedness of scene elements does not differentially affect picture recognition in young or older adults, the results do not present a pure test of binding ability. That is, accurate recognition could be achieved on the basis of recognising a previously studied object, regardless of the background. Even though we argue that "unbinding", or removing background information at the time of recognition, provides a test for how well item and background elements are bound together at the time of encoding, Experiment 3 adopts a more conventional associative memory task in which accurate recognition relies on the ability to correctly identify intact object–background associations from recombined object–background pairs. Based on the results of Experiments 1 and 2, we predict that both age groups will respond similarly to manipulations of the relatedness of object and background pairs.

Methods

Participants. Drawn from the same populations as the previous experiments, 28 young (*M* age $= 20.96$, $SD = 1.82$; 19 females) and 32 older adults (*M* age $= 69.66$, $SD = 4.22$; 18 females) participated in the study. Older adults tended to have more years of education ($M = 15.72$; $SD = 2.36$) than young adults ($M = 14.95$; $SD = 1.29$), but this difference was not significant, $t(58) = 1.54$, $p = .13$. As in the previous experiments, older adults ($M = 56.63$; $SD = 9.11$) completed fewer items on the digit comparison speed of processing task than young adults ($M = 78.71$; $SD = 12.60$), $t(58) = 7.85$, $p < .001$.

Materials and procedure. Participants intentionally encoded 96 line-drawing pictures, 48 consisting of objects placed in related backgrounds and 48 consisting of objects placed in unrelated backgrounds. Participants were instructed to "study and try to remember the entire picture. Attempt to associate the target object with the background so that you can remember them together when you are tested later." This instruction was reinforced with four practice study and test trials that contained intact pictures as well as some in which the background had been changed. Pictures were encoded for 4 s each. Following a 12 min retention interval, participants completed the recognition task, during which time participants judged whether the *exact* picture had been encoded previously and made a "yes" or "no" response with a keypress. Participants were reminded that "some pictures may have both a background and a target item that you studied previously but they were not paired together before. For those items you should respond NO. Only respond YES if you studied all of the parts in the SAME picture previously." Each participant was tested on 48 old target pictures (half related, half unrelated), and 48 lure pictures consisting entirely of previously studied elements. Lure pictures were recombinations of previously encoded object–background pairs, and object and the background always had the same encoding history (i.e., both studied in related pairs or both studied in unrelated pairs) but were drawn from two different encoded pictures. For the 48 lure pictures, 12 consisted of elements that were encoded in related pairings and were tested in a new related combination (RR-R), 12 consisted of elements that were encoded in related pairings and were tested in a new unrelated combination (RR-U), 12 consisted of elements that were encoded in unrelated pairings and were tested in a new related combination (UU-R), and 12 consisted of elements that were encoded in unrelated pairings and were tested in a new unrelated combination (UU-U). Using this naming convention, the first two letters indicate the relatedness of the encoding condition for the object and background elements (which always have the same encoding condition), and the last letter indicates the relatedness of the recognition condition, in which encoded elements from two separate studied pictures are combined into a single picture. See Figure 1 for an example of a recombination. Four counterbalanced orders were used to vary whether pictures were tested as targets or lures and for lures, to alternate which versions of the pictures were presented at encoding versus recognition. The encoding and recognition tasks were presented using E-Prime software (Psychology Software Tools, Pittsburgh, PA).

Results and discussion

In this study, there were two types of hit rate for previously studied pictures: one for related pictures and one for unrelated pictures. In contrast, there were four false alarm rates for the recombinations of old pictures: RR-R, RR-U, UU-R, UU-U. Corrected recognition A' scores were calculated for related and unrelated encoding items using the two hit rates and four different false alarm rates. We calculated the A' for RR-R by using hit rates for related items that had been presented at encoding along with the false alarm rates to RR-R pictures (i.e., both the object and background were originally presented in different related scenes but participants mistakenly claimed to recognise the lure picture that was a recombination of these elements into a new related scene) and the A' for UU-U by using hit rates for unrelated items that had been presented at encoding along with the false alarm rates to UU-U pictures (i.e., both the object and background were originally presented in different unrelated scenes but participants mistakenly claimed to recognise the lure picture that was a recombination of these elements into a new unrelated scene). For the pairings that changed their relatedness status, we chose to use the hit rate that matched the *recognition* condition.[1] Therefore, the A' score for RR-U was calculated by using the hit rates for unrelated items and the false alarm rates to RR-U pictures (i.e., both the object and background were originally presented in different related scenes but participants mistakenly claimed to recognise the lure picture that was a recombination of these elements into a new unrelated scene). The A' score for the UU-R condition was calculated by using the hit rates for related items and the false alarm rates to UU-R pictures (i.e., both the object and background were originally presented in different unrelated scenes but participants mistakenly claimed to recognise the lure picture that was a recombination of these elements into a new related scene).

In analyses of the corrected recognition scores (A'), the main effect of relatedness at encoding reached significance, with higher scores for related pictures ($M = 0.80$) than unrelated pictures ($M = 0.78$), $F(1, 58) = 4.76$, $p < .05$, $\eta_p^2 = .08$. The relatedness of the backgrounds and objects at encoding interacted with the relatedness of the scenes at recognition, $F(1, 58) = 36.87$, $p < .001$, $\eta_p^2 = .39$. As seen in Figure 2, corrected recognition scores tend to be higher when there is a mismatch between the relatedness of the pairing at encoding and recognition. We collapsed across the different conditions in order to compare average A' scores for pictures in which the relatedness at encoding and recognition matched versus mismatched. The results of a 2

[1] The other alternative would have been to calculate A' scores with the hit rate that matched the *encoding* condition (e.g., using the related hit rate for the RR-U condition). When A' scores are calculated with these hit rates, the pattern of significant main effects and interactions is unaffected.

(match/mismatch) × 2 (young/elderly) ANOVA supports the observation that recognition was more accurate for the mismatched ($M = 0.82$) compared to the matched relatedness ($M = 0.76$), $F(1, 58) = 36.87$, $p < .001$, $\eta_p^2 = .39$. It is hardest to reject novel repairings of objects and backgrounds when the elements share the same type of related or unrelated relationship as at encoding (i.e., RR-R and UU-U conditions, relative to RR-U and UU-R conditions). This difference is significant for both types of pairs, RR-R vs. RR-U, $F(1, 58) = 17.63$, $p < .001$, $\eta_p^2 = .23$, and UU-U vs. UU-R, $F(1, 58) = 10.70$, $p < .003$, $\eta_p^2 = .16$. Although the difference appears to be slightly larger for RR-U compared to RR-R pairings, in comparison to the difference between the UU-R and UU-U conditions, this was not borne out statistically ($F < 1$). There was also a main effect of age with higher corrected recognition scores for young than older adults, $F(1, 58) = 4.85$, $p < .05$, $\eta_p^2 = .08$. No other effects approached significance ($Fs < 2$).

Because the corrected recognition scores were affected by the relatedness of the objects and backgrounds and differed across the age groups, we conducted additional analyses on the hit and false alarm rates. Hit rates exhibited a main effect of relatedness, $F(1, 58) = 12.75$, $p < .001$, $\eta_p^2 = .18$, with higher hit rates for object presented in a related background ($M = 0.74$) compared to those presented in unrelated backgrounds ($M = 0.68$). Although older adults ($M = 0.74$) exhibited a trend for higher hit rates than young adults ($M = 0.68$), this effect did not reach significance, $F(1, 58) = 2.58$, $p = .11$, $\eta_p^2 = .04$. The Age × Relatedness interaction did not approach significance ($F < 1$).

For the false alarm rates (see Figure 2), the main effects of the relatedness at encoding, $F(1, 58) = 4.22$, $p < .05$, $\eta_p^2 = .07$, and the relatedness at recognition, $F(1, 58) = 16.54$, $p < .001$, $\eta_p^2 = .22$, reached significance. Participants committed more false alarms when encoding was unrelated ($M = 0.29$) as opposed to related ($M = 0.25$), but at recognition, committed more false alarms to related ($M = 0.31$) than unrelated ($M = 0.23$) pairs. Older adults committed significantly more false alarms than young adults, $F(1, 58) = 23.18$, $p < .001$, $\eta_p^2 = .29$, but none of the interactions involving age approached significance ($Fs < 2$). These main effects were qualified by an interaction of the relatedness at encoding and recognition, $F(1, 58) = 43.01$, $p < .001$, $\eta_p^2 = .43$. Note that the relative benefit for RR-U compared to RR-R trials on the corrected recognition A' measure seems to be driven by the substantially lower false alarm rate in the RR-U condition, compared to the heightened false alarm rate in the RR-R condition. This observation was supported by a follow-up 2 × 2 ANOVA comparing the false alarm rates to RR-U and RR-R lures for young and elderly, which revealed a significant main effect of relatedness, $F(1, 58) = 54.42$, $p < .001$, $\eta_p^2 = .48$. There was also a trend for difference between false alarms to RR-U and RR-R lures to be larger for young than older adults, $F(1, 58) = 3.42$, $p < .08$, $\eta_p^2 = .06$, and a significant main effect of age such that older adults committed more false alarms than young, $F(1, 58) = 19.70$, $p < .001$, $\eta_p^2 = .25$.

Unlike the previous experiments, we find that older adults perform less accurately than young adults in the binding of related and unrelated picture elements, and that this performance difference is due primarily to a heightened false alarm rate. Indeed, young and elderly exhibit rather high false recognition rates on some conditions of this task, a pattern that is in stark contrast to their highly accurate picture recognition ability demonstrated in Experiments 1 and 2. In this experiment, the relatedness of information affected recognition ability in young and elderly, in contrast to the findings from Experiments 1 and 2. As in the previous experiments, however, the relatedness of the objects and backgrounds does not *differentially* affect memory across the two age groups. Although older adults are less accurate than young, this age difference occurs across the board; the binding of both related and unrelated information is similar for young and elderly. Although binding unrelated information together at encoding seemed to be somewhat more difficult than binding related information together, changes in the relatedness condition at recognition substantially affected memory performance. Changing the type of relationship between scene elements (i.e., related to unrelated and vice versa; RR-U and UU-R conditions) from the time of encoding to the time of recognition generally benefited performance compared to memory for pictures tested with novel relationships of the same type (i.e., RR-R or UU-U). Although relatedness affects binding ability, it generally appears to be the case that relatedness facilitates encoding, although relatedness can backfire at recognition by leading to higher levels of memory errors when a lure pair shares a naturally occurring relationship (as in the RR-R pairs).

Even though older adults bind information together more poorly than young adults, the associative memory impairment is rather modest compared to previous studies (i.e., a .07 difference between the mean A' score for our young and elderly compared to a .15 age difference in A' scores in Naveh-Benjamin et al., 2003, Exp. 1). This seems to suggest that even under heavy binding demands, older adults benefit from rich pictorial information. Importantly, relatedness does not differentially impact memory binding across the age groups. Unrelated pairings are bound proportionately as well for older adults as for young adults. This finding suggests that in the case of pictures containing rich semantic information, contextual information can be used to support binding even if the contexts do not have longstanding associations with the objects through extensive prior experience. In contrast, relatedness severely impacts the ability of older adults to associate pairs of words, simple pictures of objects, or name–face pairs (Naveh-Benjamin, 2000; Naveh-Benjamin et al., 2003, 2004). Whereas age differences were modest in the ability to remember related word pairs on an associative memory test, older adults performed substantially worse on memory for unrelated word pairs. Taken together, the pattern of findings underscores the supportive nature of picture contexts for memory. Despite the preponderance of age-related impairments in associative memory for many types of information, both related and unrelated picture contexts are bound relatively well to objects with age.

GENERAL DISCUSSION

Across three experiments, we report evidence that ageing exerts little influence on associative memory for complex pictures. Counter to our predictions, our manipulation of relatedness does not affect older adults' associative memory performance any more than it affects young adults across all three experiments. In fact, the relatedness of object and background information had no effect on either group in Experiments 1 and 2; in Experiment 3, information that was related at encoding was remembered somewhat better than information that was unrelated at encoding, but there was no overall advantage for remembering information presented in a related pairing at recognition. The pattern of data reported in our studies differs from previous findings (e.g., Naveh-Benjamin et al., 2003), in which older adults' associative deficits are larger for unrelated information than related information.

Furthermore, our manipulations of environmental support and encoding intentionality did not interact with ageing or the relatedness of the scenes. Older adults recognise re-presented bound pictures just as well as young adults and the removal of previously bound background information affects older adults no differently than young (Experiments 1 and 2). We had predicted that the environmental support provided by backgrounds would be particularly important for related scenes, and that the removal of background information would disproportionately impair memory for related scenes. However, recognition of both related and unrelated scenes was similarly affected by the loss of environmental support, and this did not differ across the age groups. Unlike previous studies (e.g., Naveh-Benjamin, 2000), intentional associative encoding instructions, a factor varied across Experiments 1 and 2, do not magnify older adults' associative memory impairments. This provides further evidence that the relationships contained in complex pictures support associative memory for young and older adults, even if those relationships are of an unusual or unexpected nature.

Regarding the two candidate explanations for age-invariant picture memory that we put forth in the introduction, that complex pictures have relatively low associative processing demands and that the natural relationships contained in pictures support memory, our evidence tends to support the first, but not the second, hypothesis. Elderly remember pictures with novel and unusual relationships just as well as young adults. The divergence of our results from the previous findings suggests that complex scene associations are special and distinct from other types of associative memory. Related and unrelated components are bound together equally well by both younger and older adults, and associative and item-based encoding instructions support young and older adults' memory equally well. This finding is surprising, given the contribution of top-down contextual influences on the identification of objects in schema-consistent and schema-inconsistent scenes (Biederman, Mezzanotte, & Rabinowitz, 1982; see reviews by Bar, 2004; Henderson & Hollingworth, 1999). Our findings suggest that these top-down influences may be less important for memory and/or when there is a relatively lengthy encoding period. It is also surprising in terms of the ageing literature, which suggests that older adults have more difficulty integrating schema-inconsistent information into a script (Hess & Tate, 1992). We propose that the natural supporting relationship between a meaningful background and an object automatically engenders the formation of associations in memory. Even when the elements are combined in an unusual fashion, the rich semantic information contained in scenes supports a meaningful interpretation of the interacting components. A novel semantic association can be created easily to explain how the elements came to be combined in such a way; this interpretation is consistent with Smith et al.'s (1998) finding that semantically meaningful pictures can be remembered equivalently by young and elderly. Although we suggest that perceptual complexity is an important factor (as found by Smith et al., 1990), it is possible that the rich associations imparted by contexts, visual or not, are the critical component (see Bar, 2007) that supports older adults' memory. The high level of recognition for pictures containing unusual relationships does not seem to be explained simply as a bizarreness effect. In the present studies, we found no evidence that bizarreness enhanced item memory relative to typical scenes in Experiments 1 and 2, or that bizarreness improved binding, as assessed by Experiment 3. In addition, previous studies suggested that bizarreness enhances item, but not source, memory (Macklin & McDaniel, 2005), which would preclude an effect on memory for associations.

Another possibility, as suggested by Mayes, Montaldi, and Migo (2007), is that distinct regions of the medial temporal lobes contribute based on the properties of the information to be associated. The hippocampus plays a role in binding (Giovanello, Schnyer, & Verfaellie, 2004; Henke, Weber, Kneifel, Wieser, & Buck, 1999; Preston, Shrager, Dudukovic, & Gabrieli, 2004; Sperling, Chua, et al., 2003), and ageing is known to affect the function of the hippocampus, with several studies identifying decreased activation of the medial temporal lobes for older adults (e.g., Daselaar, Veltman, Rombouts,

Raaijmakers, & Jonker, 2003; Grady et al., 1995; Grady, McIntosh, Rajeh, Beig, & Craik, 1999; Park et al., 2003; Sperling, Bates, et al., 2003). However, ageing may not equivalently affect all regions of the medial temporal lobes. Perirhinal cortex does not lose volume with age, in contrast to the hippocampus and entorhinal and posterior parahippocampal cortices, which do lose volume with age (Dickerson et al., in press; Du et al., 2006; Raz, Rodrigue, Head, Kennedy, & Acker, 2004). These differences may be particularly important given recent evidence suggesting that subregions of the medial temporal lobes differ in their contributions to associative memory depending on the type of information. Across-domain associations (e.g., sound–picture) require the hippocampus to a greater extent than within-domain associations, which may be supported in part by the perirhinal cortex (Mayes et al., 2007). This explanation predicts that associative memory for complex scene elements should be governed by different regions than associative memory for other information. In contrast to other types of association (e.g., object–object; word–word) that are bound through hippocampally mediated mechanisms, it is possible that our complex scenes engaged the perirhinal cortex in an age-invariant manner (Dickerson et al., in press), possibly because the highly interrelated picture elements promoted unitisation (Mayes et al., 2007).

Although neuroimaging data are needed to evaluate potential differences in the neural regions that contribute to complex picture memory for related and unrelated elements, at present we favour an account that emphasises the supportive nature of the task conditions in picture memory. Even if complex pictures promote unitisation via the perirhinal cortex, one might expect that the novel relationships depicted in unrelated pictures would recruit the hippocampus (Köhler, Danckert, Gati, & Menon, 2005). Because the hippocampus is more sensitive to the effects of ageing, this would seem to predict poorer memory for older adults on unrelated picture pairs, which was not the case in our data. The semantically rich and meaningful associations that can be generated amongst even novel and unrelated picture elements engage the associative memory network in young and older adults. Recent functional neuroimaging data from our laboratory identified age-equivalent engagement of the hippocampus for unrelated and related pictures in an associative memory task, even though the stimuli were simple pictures of objects (Leshikar, Gutchess, Hebrank, Sutton, & Park, 2008). We suggest that the pattern of similar neural results reflected the supportive nature of the task conditions, in which young and elderly created a sentence to integrate the two depicted items. Complex pictures, as used in the present study, may engage integrative processes automatically.

In summary, our findings build on previous literature demonstrating that picture memory is relatively intact with age (e.g., Park et al., 1986, 1990; Smith et al., 1990, 1998) by extending the findings of relative invariance with age to associative memory. Importantly, our results suggest that associative deficits do not characterise all types of memory with age.

REFERENCES

Bar, M. (2004). Visual objects in context. *Nature Reviews Neuroscience, 5*, 617–629.

Bar, M. (2007). The proactive brain: Using analogies and associations to generate predictions. *Trends in Cognitive Sciences, 11*, 280–289.

Biederman, I., Mezzanotte, R. J., & Rabinowitz, J. C. (1982). Scene perception: Detecting and judging objects undergoing relational violations. *Cognitive Psychology, 14*, 143–177.

Chalfonte, B. L., & Johnson, M. K. (1996). Feature memory and binding in young and older adults. *Memory and Cognition, 24*, 403–416.

Cohen, J. D., MacWhinney, B., Flatt, M., & Provost, J. (1993). PsyScope: A new graphic interactive environment for designing psychology experiments. *Behavioral Research Methods, Instruments and Computers, 25*, 257–271.

Craik, F. I. M., & Byrd, M. (1982). Aging and cognitive deficits: The role of attentional resources. In F. I. M. Craik & S. Trehaub (Eds.), *Aging and cognitive processes* (pp. 191–211). New York: Plenum.

Craik, F. I. M., & Jennings, J. M. (1992). Human memory. In F. I. M. Craik & T. A. Salthouse (Eds.), *The handbook of aging and cognition* (pp. 51–110). Hillsdale, NJ: Lawrence Erlbaum Associates, Inc.

Daselaar, S. M., Veltman, D. J., Rombouts, S. A., Raaijmakers, J. G., & Jonker, C. (2003). Deep processing activates the medal temporal lobe in young but not elderly adults. *Neurobiology of Aging, 24*, 1005–1011.

Dickerson, B. C., Feczko, E., Augustinack, J. C., Pacheco, J., Morris, J. C., Fischl, B., & Buckner, R. L.(in press). Differential effects of aging and Alzheimer's disease on medial temporal lobe cortical thickness and surface area. *Neurobiology of Aging*.

Du, A.-T., Schuff, N., Chao, L. L., Kornak, J., Jagust, W. J., Kramer, J. H., et al. (2006). Age effects on atrophy rates of entorhinal cortex and hippocampus. *Neurobiology of Aging, 27*, 733–740.

Giovanello, K. S., Keane, M. M., & Verfaellie, M. (2006). The contribution of familiarity to associative memory in amnesia. *Neuropsychologia, 44*, 1859–1865.

Giovanello, K. S., Schnyer, D. M., & Verfaellie, M. (2004). A critical role for the anterior hippocampus in relational memory: Evidence from an fMRI study comparing associative and item recognition. *Hippocampus, 14*, 5–8.

Grady, C. L., McIntosh, A. R., Horwitz, B., Maisog, J. M., Ungerleider, L. G., Mentis, M. J., et al. (1995). Age-related reductions in human recognition memory due to impaired encoding. *Science, 269*, 218–221.

Grady, C. L., McIntosh, A. R., Rajah, M. N., Beig, S., & Craik, F. I. M. (1999). The effects of age on the neural correlates of episodic encoding. *Cerebral Cortex, 9*, 805–814.

Gutchess, A. H., Hebrank, A., Sutton, B., Leshikar, E., Chee, M. W. L., Tan, J. C., et al. (2007). Contextual interference in recognition memory with age. *NeuroImage, 35*, 1338–1347.

Hedden, T., Park, D. C., Nisbett, R., Ji, L.-J., Jing, Q., & Jiao, S. (2002). Cultural variation in verbal versus spatial neuropsychological function across the life span. *Neuropsychology, 16*, 65–73.

Henderson, J. M., & Hollingworth, A. (1999). High-level scene perception. *Annual Review of Psychology, 50*, 243–271.

Henke, K., Weber, B., Kneifel, S., Wieser, H. G., & Buck, A. (1999). Human hippocampus associates information in memory. *Proceedings of the National Academy of Sciences of the USA, 96*, 5884–5889.

Hess, T. M., & Tate, C. S. (1992). Direct and indirect assessments of memory for script-based narratives in young and older adults. *Cognitive Development*, *7*, 467–484.

Köhler, S., Danckert, S., Gati, J. S., & Menon, R. S. (2005). Novelty responses to relational and non-relational information in the hippocampus and the parahippocampal region: A comparison based on event-related fMRI. *Hippocampus*, *15*, 763–774.

Leshikar, E. D., Gutchess, A. H., Hebrank, A. C., Sutton, B. P., & Park, D. C. (2008). *The impact of increased relational encoding demands on frontal and hippocampal function in older adults.* Unpublished manuscript, University of Illinois at Urbana-Champaign, IL.

Lyle, K. B., & Johnson, M. K. (2006). Importing perceived features into false memories. *Memory*, *14*, 197–213.

Macklin, C. B., & McDaniel, M. A. (2005). The bizarreness effect: Dissociation between item and source memory. *Memory*, *13*, 682–689.

Mangels, J. A., & Heinberg, A. (2006). Improved episodic integration through enactment: Implications for aging. *Journal of General Psychology*, *133*, 37–65.

Mayes, A., Montaldi, D., & Migo, E. (2007). Associative memory and the medial temporal lobes. *Trends in Cognitive Sciences*, *11*, 126–135.

McDaniel, M. A., & Einstein, G. O. (1986). Bizarre imagery as an effective memory aid: The importance of distinctiveness. Journal of Experimental Psychology: Learning, Memory. *and Cognition*, *12*, 54–65.

Naveh-Benjamin, M. (2000). Adult age differences in memory performance: Tests of an associative deficit hypothesis. *Journal of Experimental Psychology: Learning, Memory and Cognition*, *26*, 1170 1187.

Naveh-Benjamin, M., Brav, T. K., & Levy, O. (2007). The associative memory deficit of older adults: The role of strategy utilization. *Psychology and Aging*, *22*, 202–208.

Naveh-Benjamin, M., Guez, J., Kilb, A., & Reedy, S. (2004). The associative memory deficit of older adults: Further support using face-name associations. *Psychology and Aging*, *19*, 541–546.

Naveh-Benjamin, M., Hussain, Z., Guez, J., & Bar-On, M. (2003). Adult age differences in episodic memory: Further support for an associative-deficit hypothesis. *Journal of Experimental Psychology: Learning, Memory and Cognition*, *29*, 826–837.

Park, D. C., & Puglisi, J. T. (1985). Older adults' memory for the color of matched pictures and words. *Journal of Gerontology*, *40*, 198–204.

Park, D. C., Puglisi, J. T., & Lutz, R. (1982). Spatial memory in older adults: Effects of intentionality. *Journal of Gerontology*, *37*, 330–335.

Park, D. C., Puglisi, J. T., & Smith, A. D. (1986). Memory for pictures: Does an age-related decline exist? *Psychology and Aging*, *1*, 11–17.

Park, D. C., Puglisi, J. T., & Sovacool, M. (1984). Picture memory in older adults: Effects of contextual detail at encoding and retrieval. *Journal of Gerontology*, *39*, 213–215.

Park, D. C., Smith, A. D., Morrell, R. W., Puglisi, J. T., & Dudley, W. N. (1990). Effects of contextual integration on recall of pictures by older adults. *Journal of Gerontology: Psychological Sciences*, *45*, 52–57.

Park, D. C., Welsh, R. C., Marshuetz, C., Gutchess, A. H., Mikels, J., Polk, T. A., et al. (2003). Age differences in frontal and medial temporal activations associated with the maintenance of complex pictures in working memory. *Journal of Cognitive Neuroscience*, *15*, 1122–1134.

Preston, A. R., Shrager, Y., Dudukovic, N. M., & Gabrieli, J. D. (2004). Hippocampal contribution to the novel use of relational information in declarative memory. *Hippocampus*, *14*, 148–152.

Quamme, J. R., Yonelinas, A. P., & Norman, K. A. (2007). Effect of unitization on associative recognition in amnesia. *Hippocampus*, *17*, 192–200

Raz, N., Rodrigue, K. M., Head, D., Kennedy, K. M., & Acker, J. D. (2004). Differential aging of the medial temporal lobe: A study of a five-year change. *Neurology*, *62*, 433–438.

Salthouse, T. A., & Babcock, R. L. (1991). Decomposing adult age differences in working memory. *Developmental Psychology*, *27*, 763–776.

Shipley, W. C. (1986). *Shipley Institute of Living Scale.* Los Angeles, CA: Western Psychological Services.

Smith, A. D., Park, D. C., Cherry, K., & Berkovsky, K (1990). Age differences in memory for concrete and abstract pictures. *Journal of Gerontology: Psychological Sciences, 45*, P205–P209.

Smith, A. D., Park, D. C., Earles, J. L. K., Shaw, R. J., & Whiting, W. L. (1998). Age differences in context integration in memory. *Psychology and Aging, 13*, 21–28.

Snodgrass, J. G., & Corwin, J. (1988). Pragmatics of measuring recognition memory: Applications to dementia and amnesia. *Journal of Experimental Psychology: General, 117*, 34–50.

Sperling, R. A., Bates, J. F., Chua, E. F., Cocchiarella, A. J., Rentz, D. M., Rosen, B. R., et al. (2003). fMRI studies of associative encoding in young and elderly controls and mild Alzheimer's disease. *Journal of Neurology, Neurosurgery and Psychiatry, 74*, 44–50.

Sperling, R. A., Chua, E., Cocchiarella, A., Rand-Giovannetti, E., Poldrack, R., Schacter, D. L., & Albert, M. (2003). Putting names to faces: Successful encoding of associative memories activates the anterior hippocampal formation. *NeuroImage, 20*, 1400–1410.

Standing, L. (1973). Learning 10000 pictures. *Quarterly Journal of Experimental Psychology, 25*, 207–222.

EUROPEAN JOURNAL OF COGNITIVE PSYCHOLOGY
2009, 21 (2/3), 255–282

Psychology Press
Taylor & Francis Group

Effects of age and practice in sequence learning: A graded account of ageing, learning, and control

Vinciane Gaillard
Université de Genève, Switzerland

Arnaud Destrebecqz, Sandrine Michiels, and Axel Cleeremans
Université Libre de Bruxelles, Belgium

The influence of age and practice level was investigated in sequence learning by testing young, middle-aged, and older participants, who first performed a serial reaction time (SRT) task, either after a short or a long training phase (15 vs. 30 training blocks). Unknown to them, successive stimuli followed a repeating pattern. After training, participants performed a sequence generation task under inclusion and exclusion instructions, and a recognition task. SRT and generation data indicate (1) preserved learning and generation abilities in ageing and (2) beneficial effects of extended practice. By contrast, recognition data suggest that ageing tends to impair discrimination performance. Implications of these findings for understanding the effects of age and practice on the ability to control sequential knowledge are discussed in terms of the involvement of gradual representations of sequence structure.

Keywords: Ageing; Sequence learning; Practice; Ironic effects hypothesis; Gradual hypothesis.

Correspondence should be addressed to Vinciane Gaillard, Université de Genève, Faculté de Psychologie et des Sciences de l'Education, 40, bld du Pont d'Arve bureau 5160, 1205 Geneva, Switzerland. E-mail: Vinciane.Gaillard@pse.unige.ch

Axel Cleeremans is a Research Director with the National Fund for Scientific Research (Belgium). The study was conducted while Vinciane Gaillard was a Research Assistant with the same institution. This work was supported by an institutional grant from the Université Libre de Bruxelles to AC, by Concerted Research Action 06/11-342 entitled "Culturally modified organisms: What it means to be human in the age of culture", financed by the Ministère de la Communauté Française-Direction Générale de l'enseignement non obligatoire et de la Recherche Scientifique (Belgium) and by FRFC (grant 2.4577.06).

We are grateful to Lynn Hasher, Valérie Camos, and Pierre Barrouillet for useful discussions of some aspects of our results and to Don E. Dulany and another anonymous reviewer for helpful comments and suggestions on an earlier draft.

http://www.psypress.com/ecp DOI: 10.1080/09541440802257423

The acquisition of new information without intending to do so, and in such a way that the resulting knowledge is difficult to express, referred to as implicit learning, has been extensively studied over the last decades (Cleeremans, Destrebecqz, & Boyer, 1998; Dienes & Berry, 1997). An emerging focus of interest in the study of implicit learning concerns its lifelong developmental course (Forkstam & Petersson, 2005). Does implicit learning occur in young children? Does it wane with age, or is it in contrast relatively robust (Reber, 1993)? Many recent studies have explored these issues in the context of cognitive development (Bremner, Mareschal, Destrebecqz, & Cleeremans, 2007; Maybery, Taylor, & O'Brien-Malone, 1995; Meulemans, van der Linden, & Perruchet, 1998; Pacton, Fayol, & Perruchet, 2005; Pacton, Perruchet, Fayol, & Cleeremans, 2001; Saffran, Aslin, & Newport, 1996; Saffran, Senghas, & Trueswell, 2001; Thomas et al., 2004; Thomas & Nelson, 2001; Vinter & Perruchet, 2000, 2002). Likewise, several recent studies have been dedicated to assess implicit learning at the other end of the lifespan (for recent reviews, see Light, Prull, La Voie, & Healy, 2000; Prull, Gabrieli, & Bunge, 2000).

Here, we focus on the influence of practice on the ability of participants from different age groups to learn about and to control the knowledge associated with sequential regularities. To assess performance, we used both an indirect task—a sequence learning situation—and two direct tasks—sequence recognition and sequence generation under inclusion and exclusion instructions. In the following sections, we first focus on the effects of age on learning by providing a brief overview of relevant studies. Next, we discuss the effects of age on cognitive control, focusing specifically on the ironic effects first described by Jacoby (1999).

IMPLICIT LEARNING AND AGEING: AN OVERVIEW

Based on the extant literature, two broad perspectives on the influence of ageing on learning can be distinguished. According to the first perspective, explicit, but not implicit learning is influenced by age (Cherry & Stadler, 1995; Frensch, Buchner, & Lin, 1994; Howard & Howard, 1989, 1992; Jennings & Jacoby, 1993; Reber, 1993). According to the second perspective, both implicit and explicit learning show age-related decreases (Curran, 1997; Jackson & Jackson, 1992; Squire & Frambach, 1990). This lack of consistent data may originate in the fact that experimental methods differ substantially across studies. Thus, in the current study, we chose to focus on a single, well-defined task which we believe to be particularly appropriate for the study of ageing, that is, sequence learning (Salthouse, McGuthry, & Hambrick, 1999).

In a typical sequence learning experiment, participants first perform a Serial Reaction Time (SRT) task (Nissen & Bullemer, 1987), in which they are asked to react to each element of a sequentially structured and typically visual sequence of events. On each trial, participants see a stimulus appear at one of several locations on a computer screen and are instructed to press on the corresponding key as fast and as accurately as possible. Unknown to them, the sequence of successive stimuli follows a repetitive pattern. The paradigm offers the advantage of placing participants in truly incidental learning conditions, as knowledge relative to the sequence is not necessary to perform the SRT task correctly. Reaction times (RTs) tend to decrease progressively during practice, but typically increase dramatically when the repetitive pattern is modified in any of several ways (Destrebecqz & Cleeremans, 2001; Reed & Johnson, 1994; Shanks & Johnstone, 1999). This RT cost indicates that participants have acquired some knowledge regarding the repeating pattern. Many authors (Dienes, 2008; Dulany, 1997; Frensch & Rünger, 2003; Kihlstrom, Dorfman, & Park, 2007) suggest that SRT performance reflects the joint influence of implicit and explicit processes—a point that most likely also holds for the tasks typically used to assess the extent to which knowledge acquired incidentally in the SRT can be subsequently expressed directly upon instruction, such as generation and recognition.[1]

Using the SRT task, Salthouse and colleagues (1999) found no qualitative differences between young (18–39 years old), middle-aged (40–59 years old), and older (60–87 years old) participants. Other studies, however, have yielded inconsistent data, showing a gradually detrimental effect of age, not only when participants aged 65 years and above ("older" group) are compared to younger participants ("young" group), but also when the performance of 65- to 75-year-olds ("young-older" group) is compared with the performance of participants older than 75 years ("old-older" group) (Howard & Howard, 1997, Exps. 2a and 2b). The detrimental effect of age is even observed when participants aged 34–45 ("young" group) are compared to participants aged 46–53 ("middle-aged" group) (Feeney, Howard, & Howard, 2002). Thus, gradually manipulating participants' age might be a valuable way to look at the ability to learn and to control sequential knowledge.

Practice also seems to play an important role, even though this factor has not been systematically studied yet. In many SRT studies, training is rather limited, consisting for instance of 30 (Howard & Howard, 1992, Exp. 1), 50 (Negash et al., 2007), or 70 pattern repetitions (Dennis, Howard, & Howard, 2006, Exps. 1 and 2). In one study, however, participants were exposed to as

[1] The authors thank one of the reviewers for highlighting this point.

many as 1260 pattern repetitions (Feeney et al., 2002). In yet another study, Howard and colleagues (2004) examined the effects of sequence structure and extended practice (2100 pattern repetitions) on sequence learning. Results of the latter study clearly show that, even after extended practice, older adults remain unable to learn a complex sequence, unlike younger participants and despite the fact that they exhibit good performance on a simpler sequence.[2] Accuracy measures indeed suggest that younger participants only need the sequential material to be repeated 50 times to acquire some knowledge about the sequence, whereas their older counterparts need at least 150 sequential repetitions to exhibit some learning of the underlying structure.

Thus, whereas increased practice typically improves performance in any domain, the interactions between practice and ageing have seldom been explored systematically and have sometimes yielded inconsistent results. In particular, some authors have reported highly counterintuitive negative effects of increased practice amongst older participants (e.g., Jacoby, 1999), whereby extended training actually diminishes performance rather than increases it. We briefly review these "ironic" effects in the next section.

IRONIC EFFECTS IN AGEING

It is now well established that healthy cognitive ageing disrupts control processes (Braver et al., 2001; Bugaiska et al., 2007; Hasher, Quig, & May, 1997; Hogan, Kelly, & Craik, 2006; Kray, Eber, & Lindenberger, 2004; Taconnat, Clarys, Vanneste, Bouazzaoui, & Isingrini, 2007; Vanderaspoilden, Adam, van der Linden, & Morais, 2007; Verhaeghen & Hoyer, 2007; West & Schwarb, 2006). Yet, some age-related effects on intentional control still surprise us, thus being dubbed "ironic effects". For instance, Howard and Howard (2001) found an interaction between orientation to learn and age: Direct instructions to learn about the material were beneficial to younger participants, but detrimental to older participants. According to the authors, this negative effect of trying to learn can be attributed to the reduced number of pattern events that can be activated simultaneously in working memory, a well-known hypothesis in the field of cognitive ageing (Craik & Bialystok, 2006; Craik & Salthouse, 2000; Park & Schwarz, 2000).

These detrimental effects of trying to learn in implicit learning echo another age-related dissociation, namely, ironic effects of repetition in implicit memory (Jacoby, 1999). In a nutshell, the more older participants had to read a word in the training phase, knowing they would have to exclude it afterwards, the less they were able to suppress this to-be-inhibited

[2] Even though older adults learned less than the young ones.

word in a subsequent test phase. This "ironic" effect of repetition was not observed with young adults, unless they had been performing the task under divided attention or under time pressure. How can we explain the results observed by Jacoby? On the one hand, because repetition enhances both recollection (controlled process) and familiarity (automatic process), young adults perform better under repetition conditions. On the other hand, time pressure to respond and ageing both weaken recollection, but familiarity is left intact (see Yonelinas, 2002, for a review). This suggests that healthy cognitive ageing diminishes control ability.

The irony, of course, lies in the fact that experimental conditions supposed to help participants in the so-called implicit tasks (i.e., intentional instructions or items repetition) actually impair older adults, with impoverished performance as a result. To summarise, for older adults, but not for younger ones, attempting to discover and learn subtle spatial/sequential regularities reduced the extent to which they exhibited sensitivity to these regularities. According to Howard and Howard (2001), this ironic effect can be interpreted as reflecting the additional load that such intentional instructions impose on older participants' already diminished working memory capacity.

An alternative hypothesis, however, comes from Cleeremans's gradual framework, which posits that (1) learning is mandatory, (2) learning results in higher quality representations, and (3) higher quality representations enjoy increased access to intentional control (Cleeremans, 2006; Cleeremans & Jiménez, 2002). Crucially, developing high-quality representations—of, say, the sequential structure of the presented material in a SRT task—takes time. The age-related effects of temporal factors in learning have already been investigated in the timescale of a single trial in our lab (Vandenberghe, Gaillard, Destrebecqz, Fery, & Cleeremans, 2008). We manipulated the delay between successive stimuli in the training phase. Consistent with the framework, results invalidate the idea that longer temporal intervals between elements impair older participants' learning. Rather, making more time available for processing appears to be just as beneficial to elderly participants as it is to younger people.

According to this gradual framework, giving more time to learn sequential material by repeating the sequence will yield higher quality traces of the sequence, regardless of participants' age. Thus, in contrast to Jacoby's perspective, increasing the number of pattern repetitions will benefit older adults just as their younger counterparts. In other words, extended practice during the training phase should be equally beneficial to both young and older participants, simply because all will benefit equally from the higher quality representations promoted by increased training.

AIMS AND HYPOTHESIS OF THE PRESENT STUDY

Because of age-related "chronic divided attention" (Craik & Byrd, 1982), it is of most interest to investigate the age-related effects of extended practice in the retrieval of an incidentally learned sequence. Will ironic effects of repetition emerge, as in implicit memory, i.e., will practice level have different effects on performance depending on participants' age? Conversely, will participants react in the same way, and take advantage of the sequence repetitions regardless of their age? Will we observe gradual effects of age and practice level? The present study is aimed at answering these questions by exploring the extent to which practice influences participants' ability to exert intentional control over knowledge acquired during training.

Thus, after performing the SRT task, participants are presented with a free generation task, under both inclusion and exclusion conditions (Jacoby, 1991). Under inclusion instructions, participants are asked to reproduce the sequence as best as they can. This is a facilitation task because both recollection and familiarity may help participants generate the sequence they have been trained on. Under exclusion instructions, in contrast, participants are instructed to generate a different sequence, that is, to avoid reproducing the training sequence. This is an interference task because recollection and familiarity of the repetitive pattern act in opposition: Only recollection (controlled processes) can help participants reproduce the repetitive pattern to improve their performance. If the repetitive pattern is nevertheless produced under exclusion instructions, such responses can only be interpreted as reflecting the automatic influence of learned sequential regularities.

To further assess the extent to which participants exhibit memory for the trained pattern, they had to perform a recognition task that involved (1) reacting to novel and trained short series of stimuli as in the SRT task, and (2) indicating whether the performed series were sequential or not.

According to the ironic effects hypothesis, under exclusion instructions and because of age-related control deficits, middle-aged and older adults are expected to be less able to withhold prepotent responses (i.e., generating the sequence) than their younger counterparts. Furthermore, we may also expect to observe ironic effects of repetition, i.e., an age-dependent modulation of generation performance by practice level, with increased practice resulting in better performance amongst young adults, but in worse performance amongst older participants.

According to the gradual hypothesis, however, offering more time to learn sequential material by repeating the sequence will yield higher quality traces of the sequence, regardless of participants' age. In other words, extended practice during the training phase should not yield dissociation effects on young and older participants, because, by assumption, all will benefit from the availability of the higher quality representations acquired through extended practice.

METHOD

Participants

One hundred and fourteen subjects took part to the experiment. All were unfamiliar with the SRT task. They were assigned to three different age groups: 40 young adults (mean = 22.7 years old; range = 18–29), 37 middle-aged adults (mean = 45.5 years old; range = 39–51) and 37 old adults (mean = 71.3 years old; range = 59–90). Young people were recruited via an advertisement and were paid 7 or 11 Euros for their participation, depending on whether they had been presented with the short or the long training condition, respectively. Middle-aged and older adults were all community-dwelling volunteers and were recruited via an advertisement. None of them was institutionalised, neurologically damaged, depressed (as attested by the Geriatric Depression Scale; Brink et al., 1982), or demented (as attested by the Mattis Dementia Rating Scale; Schmidt et al., 1994). All participants had normal or corrected sight. The only difference between groups was that younger adults had a higher educational level than the middle-aged, $t(64.362) = 3.6$, $p < .01$, two-tailed, equal variances not assumed, and older adults, $t(55.156) = 2.321$, $p < .05$, two-tailed, equal variances not assumed. The characteristics of the participants are summarised in Table 1.

TABLE 1
Participant characteristics (means with standard deviations in parentheses)

	Age groups		
Participant Characteristics	*Young*	*Middle-aged*	*Older*
Gender	20 F, 20 M	23 F, 14 M	27 F, 10 M
Age (years)	22.7 (2.69)	45.5 (3.37)	71.3 (7.04)
Education (years)	14.68 (1.81)	12.84 (2.53)	13.34 (2.94)
Mattis Dementia Rating Scale	–	141.27 (1.98)	141.33 (2.38)
Geriatric Depression Scale	–	3.35 (3.35)	4.74 (3.16)

Dashes indicate that the Mattis Dementia Rating Scale and the Geriatric Depression Scale were not administered to young adults.

Design

The general design was a 3 (age) × 2 (practice) mixed factorial design, with age (young vs. middle-aged vs. older) and practice level (short training vs. long training) as between-subjects variables. Each age-related group was again divided according to the number of blocks the participants were trained on. Participants were randomly exposed to either 15 (short learning condition) or 30 blocks of training (long training condition). The within-subjects variables depended on the relevant task (blocks in the SRT task, instructions in the generation task, and type of triplets in the recognition task).

Material

The experiment was run on a Macintosh iBook G4 laptop, with an additional keypad for comfort. The display consisted of four dots arranged in a horizontal line on the computer screen and separated by intervals of 2.70 cm. The stimulus was a small black circle 0.35 cm in diameter that appeared on a white background, centred 0.50 cm below one of the four dots. Each screen position corresponded to a key on the computer keyboard. The spatial configuration of the keys was fully compatible with the screen positions. Participants were asked to respond with the index and middle finger of each hand.

Procedure

All age groups performed the three experimental tasks (SRT, generation, and recognition) in one session. Middle-aged and older participants were screened during a previous session for possible depression, dementia, or health troubles.

The experiment consisted of either 15 or 30 training blocks, during which subjects were presented with a serial four-choice RT task. Each block consisted of 96 trials, for a total of 1440 or 2880 trials, for the 15 and 30 blocks conditions respectively. On each trial, a stimulus appeared at one of the four possible screen locations. Participants were instructed to respond as fast and as accurately as possible by pressing on the corresponding key. The target was removed as soon as a key had been pressed, and the next stimulus appeared after a 250 ms interval. Erroneous responses were signalled by means of a tone. Short rest breaks occurred between any two experimental blocks, and a longer break occurred in the 30 blocks condition, in between blocks 15 and 16. The very same sequence was repeated throughout the blocks, except in a transfer block.

Unknown to them, participants were presented with one of the following 12 elements sequences regarding the stimulus locations: 342312143241 (SOC1), 341243142132 (SOC2). Each experimental block consisted of eight repetitions of the sequence. These sequences consisted entirely of so-called "second order conditional" (SOC) transitions (Reed & Johnson, 1994). These sequences are identical to those used by Destrebecqz and Cleeremans (2001) and by Wilkinson and Shanks (2004). In each age group in the short training condition, half of the subjects were trained on SOC1 during the first 13 blocks and during Block 15; and on SOC2 during Block 14. This design was reversed for the other half of the subjects. In each age group in the long training condition, half of the subjects were trained on SOC1 during the first 28 blocks and during Block 30; and on SOC2 during Block 29. This design was again reversed for the other half of the subjects. Participants were thus presented with either 112 or 232 pattern repetitions, in the short and long training conditions, respectively.

After the SRT task, participants were informed that the dots had followed a repeating pattern. Objective measures of explicit knowledge were then obtained by means of a generation task and of a recognition task.

First, participants were told that the same sequence of movements had occurred throughout the entire experiment, and were asked to perform a *generation task* under inclusion and exclusion conditions (Destrebecqz & Cleeremans, 2001). They were presented with a single stimulus that appeared in a random location and asked to freely generate a series of 108 trials that "resembled the training sequence as much as possible" (*inclusion* instructions). They were told to rely on intuition when feeling unable to recollect the location of the next stimulus. After that, participants were asked to generate another sequence of 108 trials, this time avoiding the reproduction of the sequential regularities contained in the training sequence (*exclusion* instructions). In both generation tasks, participants were also told not to repeat responses. The stimulus moved whenever participants had pressed one of the keys, and appeared at the corresponding location after a delay of 250 ms, just as in the first task.

After completion of the two generation tasks, participants were asked to perform a triplets *recognition task*. Here, we used a procedure identical with that described in Shanks and Johnstone (1999). Participants were presented with 24 fragments of three trials. Twelve were part of SOC1 and twelve were part of SOC2. Participants were asked to respond to stimuli as in the SRT task, and then to provide a rating of how confident they were that the fragment was part of the training sequence. Ratings involved a 6-point scale where 1 = "I am certain that this fragment was part of the training sequence", 2 = "I am fairly certain that this fragment was part of the training sequence", 3 = "I believe that this fragment was part of the training sequence", 4 = "I believe that this fragment was not part of the training sequence", 5 = "I am fairly certain that this fragment was not part of the training sequence", and 6 = "I am certain that this fragment was not part of the training sequence". It was emphasised to participants that they had to respond as fast as possible to the dots. Both ratings and reaction times were recorded.

RESULTS

In all analyses, a significance criterion of $\alpha = .05$ was used. Prior to each analysis of variance (ANOVA), data were tested with Mauchly's test of sphericity. Where sphericity was of concern, the degrees of freedom were modified with the Greenhouse-Geisser epsilon, and effects are reported significant according to the adjusted alpha level. Effect size and power to detect effects (if less than 1) are reported.

Serial reaction time task

We calculated mean RTs by block, for each age group and for each condition. RTs associated with the first two stimuli of each block were excluded, because their locations could not be predicted. RTs associated with erroneous responses were also excluded, as were RTs beyond two standard deviations above each subject's mean per block. Because the two subgroups of subjects presented with either SOC1 or SOC2 in both conditions and in both age groups were trained identically, their RTs were combined for subsequent analyses. The data from two older participants were discarded because their reaction times were too slow (beyond two standard deviations of the RTs mean of their respective group). Mean errors rate was very low: for young participants, 3% ($SD = 2.7$) and 2.5% ($SD = 2.9$) in the short training condition and in long training condition, respectively; for middle-aged participants, 2.2% ($SD = 2.9$) and 1% ($SD = 1.9$) in the short training condition and in long training condition, respectively; and for older participants, 1.7% ($SD = 2.7$) and 1.9% ($SD = 2.4$) in the short training condition and in long training condition, respectively. They will not be further discussed.

Figure 1 shows the average RTs obtained over the entire experiment, plotted separately for age groups and for participants trained with 15 blocks of trials (short training condition, Figure 1a) or with 30 blocks of trials (long training condition, Figure 1b). To analyse data in the short training condition, we performed a first ANOVA with blocks (13 levels, the first 13 training blocks) as a within-subject variable and age (3 levels, young, middle-aged, and older) as a between-subject variable. This analysis revealed significant effects of blocks, $F(4.746, 251.562) = 19.472$, $MSE = 94132.995$, $\eta_p^2 = .27$ and of age, $F(1, 53) = 29.05$, $MSE = 4377573.52$, $\eta_p^2 = .52$. As can be seen in Figure 1a,

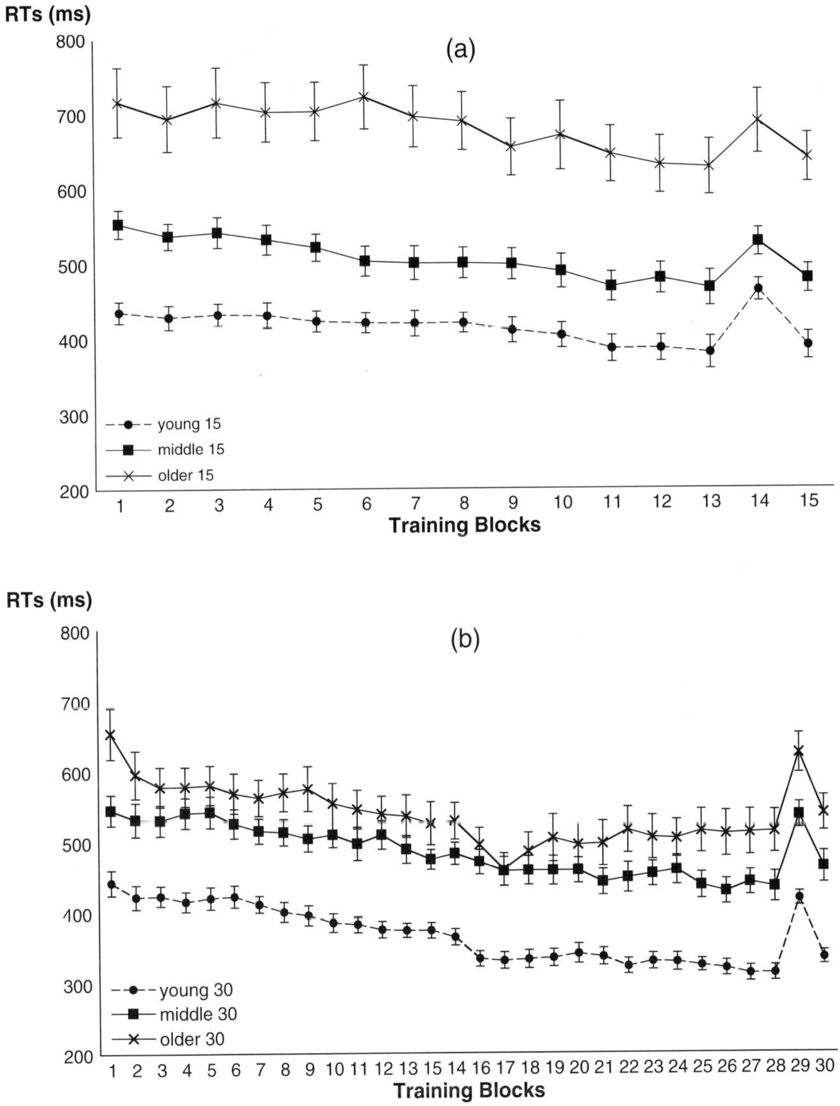

Figure 1. Mean reaction times for each training block, plotted separately for young, middle-aged, and older participants, and for participants trained with (a) 15 blocks of trials (short training condition) or (b) 30 blocks of trials (long training condition). Blocks 14 and 29 correspond to the transfer block of the short and the long training conditions, respectively. Error bars represent +/ −1 SE.

these main effects suggest that overall RTs decrease with practice (there is a mean overall decrease of 77.58 ms when comparing the first and the last sequential blocks). Moreover, overall RTs increased with age (young participants reacted faster than middle-aged ones, who also reacted faster than older participants). Importantly, the Blocks × Age interaction did not reach significance, $p > .17$, $\eta_p^2 = .05$, power = .92, which suggests that the decrease of RTs due to practice did not vary with age. Consistently, there is also evidence of significant learning when the groups are examined separately. The three analyses confirmed the significant effect of blocks, when performed only on young participants, $F(3.480, 66.127) = 5.364$, $MSE = 25597.189$, $\eta_p^2 = .22$, power = .95, on middle-aged participants, $F(4.791, 86.239) = 13.649$, $MSE = 38061.047$, $\eta_p^2 = .43$, and on older participants, $F(3.474, 55.578) = 5.562$, $MSE = 64398.296$, $\eta_p^2 = .26$, power = .95, respectively.

We then analysed the long training condition data with a second ANOVA with blocks (28 levels, the first 28 training blocks) as a within-subject variable and age (3 levels, young, middle-aged, and older) as a between-subject variable. Consistently with the analysis conducted on the short training condition, this analysis yielded both significant effects of blocks, $F(6.042, 320.217) = 55.971$, $MSE = 378153.454$, $\eta_p^2 = .51$ and of age, $F(2, 53) = 20.848$, $MSE = 4018463.71$, $\eta_p^2 = .44$. As can be observed in Figure 1b, these main effects suggest that overall RTs decrease with practice (there is an mean overall decrease of 127.16 ms when comparing the first and the last sequential blocks). Moreover, overall RTs increased with age (young participants reacted faster than middle-aged ones, who also reacted marginally faster than older participants).

In this case, the Blocks × Age interaction also reached significance, $F(12.084, 320.217) = 1.790$, $MSE = 12095.124$, $\eta_p^2 = .06$, power = .88. This result suggests that the decrease of RTs due to practice was modulated by age, perhaps because RTs in the older group change more between Blocks 15 and 19 than they do in the two other age groups. This can be explained by the longer break that takes place at the end of Block 15. Another ANOVA was again conducted on all training blocks, except Blocks 15–19. The analysis confirmed the significant effect of blocks, $F(5.192, 275.201) = 55.465$, $MSE = 374223.197$, $\eta_p^2 = .51$. However, in this case, the Blocks × Age interaction did not reach significance, $p > .14$, $\eta_p^2 = .05$, power = .75. This means that, except for the blocks surrounding the longer break, RTs decreased equally across age groups. Additionally, separate age-related analyses confirmed the significant effect of blocks, when performed only on young, $F(27, 513) = 34.080$, $MSE = 33996.577$, $\eta_p^2 = .64$, middle-aged, $F(27, 459) = 16.741$, $MSE = 25263.815$, $\eta_p^2 = .50$, and older participants, $F(27, 459) = 14.959$, $MSE = 31254.679$, $\eta_p^2 = .47$, respectively.

To sum up, in both the short and long training conditions, RTs decreased similarly over trials for the three age categories. More important is the negative transfer as assessed by the effects of switching from the training to the transfer sequence—an indirect measure of the extent to which participants have become sensitive to the regularities contained in the training sequence.

To assess negative transfer, another analysis of variance was carried out on the difference between RTs in the transfer blocks (Block 14 in the short training condition and Block 29 in the long training condition) and the average of RTs obtained for adjacent blocks (Blocks 13 and 15 in the short training condition, and Blocks 28 and 30 in the long training condition).[3] The ANOVA with transfer (2 levels, transfer block and mean of adjacent blocks) as a within-subjects variable and practice (2 levels, short vs. long training conditions) and age (3 levels, young, middle-aged, and older) as between-subjects variables showed significant effects of transfer, $F(1, 106) = 224.228$, $MSE = 337570.541$, $\eta_p^2 = .68$, age, $F(2, 106) = 51.068$, $MSE = 906589.166$, $\eta_p^2 = .49$, and practice, $F(1, 106) = 7.788$, $MSE = 138249.282$, $\eta_p^2 = .07$, power = .79.

This suggests that (1) RTs increased significantly in the three age-related groups when the sequence was modified; (2) RTs are overall faster when participants are younger; and (3) the overall RTs are faster for participants in the long training condition than for participants in the short training condition. Moreover, as can be seen in Figure 2, the Transfer × Practice interaction was also significant, $F(1, 106) = 8.509$, $MSE = 12809.703$, $\eta_p^2 = .07$, power = .82, whereas the Transfer × Age and the Transfer × Age × Practice interactions did not reach significance, $ps > .2$, $\eta_p^2 = .014$, power = .18, and $\eta_p^2 = .012$, power = .15, respectively. Importantly, this result demonstrates specific sequence learning and control of the acquired sequential knowledge in all age groups. However, sequence learning was influenced by the number of blocks participants had been trained on. Hence, regardless of their age, participants in the long training condition exhibited a larger transfer effect than participants in the short training condition (+ 92.93 ms vs. + 62.63 ms).

Taken together, SRT task results show that sequence learning was observed in the six groups of participants. Indeed, RTs decreased with practice when the same sequence was presented to the participants, increased when the sequence was modified and decreased again when the training sequence was presented anew. Our negative transfer results further suggest that all participants learned the sequential regularities to the same extent, regardless of their age. However,

[3] We also computed a proportional negative transfer effect, taking the age-related different RT baselines into account. In this case, we observed not only a significant Transfer × Practice interaction, but also a significant Transfer × Age interaction. However, this could be due to a general performance effect, because young adults reacted so quickly that their RTs show a ceiling effect. Moreover, as several authors argue against the use of proportional measures of performance, because they may exaggerate differences between groups (Cherry & Stadler, 1995; Howard & Howard, 1992; Schmitter-Edgecombe & Nissley, 2002), we will only consider the standard negative transfer measure.

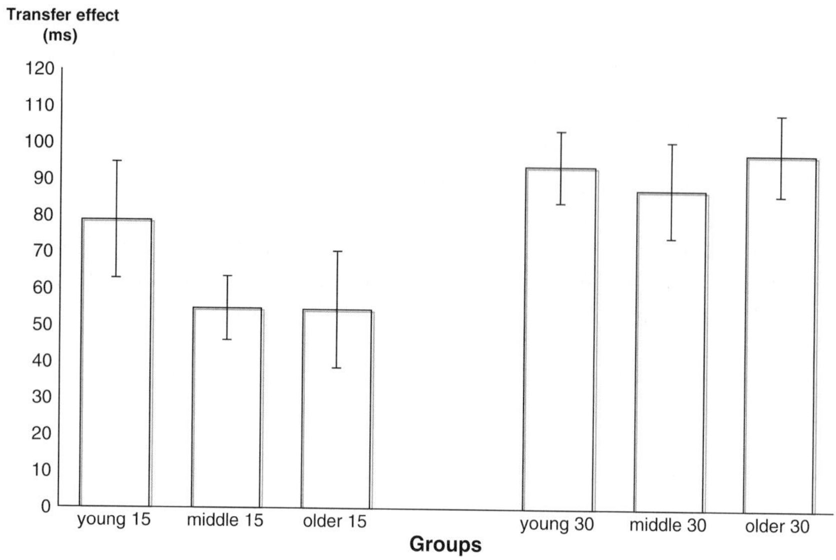

Figure 2. Mean transfer effects (in ms) for the six groups of participants. Error bars represent +/−1 SE.

because of the rather low power of the interactions involving age, the present data have to be interpreted with caution, even though the results clearly show that both young and older adults learn the sequence. More importantly, our data also indicate that increased practice results in better knowledge of the sequential regularities. This supports the gradual hypothesis across all age levels: Giving more time to learn yields higher quality traces of the sequence, regardless of participants' age.[4] We now examine whether participants differ in their ability to project their knowledge of the sequence in generation and recognition tasks.

Generation task

The first 12 trials served as practice trials and were removed from analysis both in inclusion and in exclusion. To measure generation performance, we computed the number of generated chunks of three elements (triplets) that were part of the training sequence. To obtain inclusion and exclusion scores for each subject, we divided the corresponding number of correct (e.g., sequential) triplets by the sum of the triplets that were part of the training sequence (correct triplets) and those that were part of the transfer sequence

[4] The authors thank one of the reviewers for highlighting this point.

(incorrect triplets). As training and transfer sequences share the same abstract structure, this comparison allows us to make sure that generation performance reflects learning of the sequential contingencies of the training sequence, and not merely basic frequency information (see Destrebecqz & Cleeremans, 2001; Shanks & Johnstone, 1999). Consequently, since only triplets from the training and from the transfer sequence were considered, chance level was .50.

Figure 3 shows average inclusion and exclusion scores, plotted separately for young, middle-aged, and older participants, and for both training groups. An ANOVA with instructions (2 levels, inclusion vs. exclusion) as within-subjects variable and age and practice as between-subjects variables revealed a significant effect of instructions, $F(1, 106) = 29.411$, $MSE = 0.556$, $\eta_p^2 = .22$. This effect showed that overall, participants produced more triplets from the training sequence in inclusion than in exclusion. More interesting was the Instructions × Practice interaction, which reached significance, $F(1, 106) = 6.067$, $MSE = 0.115$, $\eta_p^2 = .054$, power = .69, suggesting that the difference between inclusion and exclusion scores was larger in the long training condition than in the short training condition (.14 > .05). Interestingly, the analysis yielded neither and effect of age, $p > .9$, $\eta_p^2 = .002$, power = .07, nor any interaction involving age, all $ps > .4$, $\eta_p^2s < .014$, powers < .17. This suggests that middle-aged and older participants performed the generation task as well as younger participants, both under

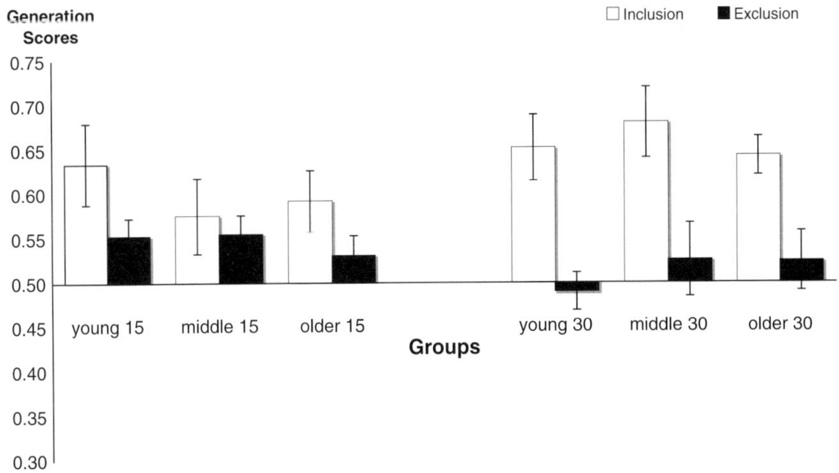

Figure 3. Mean proportions of generated second-order conditional transitions (SOCs) that were part of the training sequence, plotted separately for young, middle-aged, and older participants, and for participants trained with 15 blocks of trials (short training condition, left side of the figure) or with 30 blocks of trials (long training condition, right side of the figure). White bars represent inclusion scores and black bars represent exclusion scores. Error bars represent +/− 1 SE.

inclusion and exclusion instructions. In particular, the Instructions × Age × Practice interaction, which was of specific interest in this study, did not reach significance.

In order to determine whether practice had a similar influence on inclusion scores on the one hand, and on exclusion scores on the other, we also conducted two distinct one-way ANOVAs, with practice as a between-subjects variable. A marginal effect of practice was observed in inclusion scores only, $F(1, 110) = 3.478$, $MSE = 0.093$, $p = .065$, $\eta_p^2 = .03$, power = .46; $p > .1$, $\eta_p^2 = .02$, power = .32, for the exclusion scores. The absence of an effect of practice in the exclusion subtask might be due to a "floor" effect.

So far, the generation results are consistent with the SRT findings. Independently of age, learning produced knowledge that all participants could indeed control, because they were found to be successful in following instructions to either produce or avoid the reproduction of familiar fragments of the trained sequence. Moreover, increased practice resulted in better performance, with participants trained on 30 blocks expressing more sequential knowledge in inclusion than participants presented with 15 blocks only. No additional (especially "ironic") effects of age was evidenced. Admittedly, caution is again required when interpreting these null effects because of low power. In the next section, we will see that age differences can nevertheless be detected in the recognition task.

Recognition task

Subjects were asked to respond to sequences of three elements (triplets) and to rate from 1 to 6 the extent to which they felt these sequences were old or new. Sequences with erroneous responses were excluded. Mean recognition ratings for both structures of sequence (old vs. new) were plotted separately for age groups and for participants trained under short or long training. High ratings correspond to judgments of novelty and are expected for triplets from the transfer sequence, whereas low ratings correspond to judgements of oldness and are expected for training triplets. As can be seen in Figure 4, old and new triplets seem to be overall correctly discriminated, but this discrimination ability seems to be impaired as people get older.

An ANOVA with sequence (2 levels, old vs. new) as within-subjects variable and age and practice as between-subjects variables revealed a marginal effect of age, $F(2, 106) = 2.690$, $p = .072$, $MSE = 1.896$, $\eta_p^2 = .48$, power = .52. The analysis also yielded a main effect of sequence, $F(1, 106) = 32.461$, $MSE = 13.843$, $\eta_p^2 = .23$, and a marginal Sequence × Age interaction, $F(2, 106) = 2.758$, $p = .068$, $MSE = 1.176$, $\eta_p^2 = .05$, power = .53, probably due to the ratings attributed to new triplets. This latter finding is confirmed by two distinct one-way ANOVAs on "old" and "new" ratings,

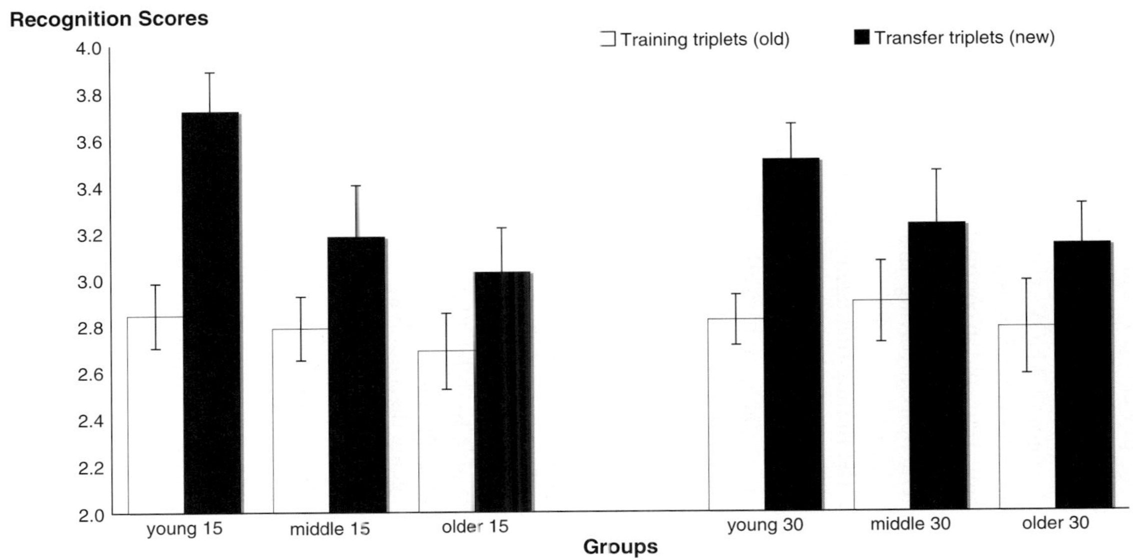

Figure 4. Mean recognition ratings given for the 24 test triplets, plotted separately for young, middle-aged, and older participants, and for participants trained with 15 blocks of trials (short training condition, left side of the figure) or with 30 blocks of trials (long training condition, right side of the figure). A high rating (between 4 and 6) is expected for a new sequence, and a low rating (between 1 and 3) is expected for an old sequence. Error bars represent +/ −1 SE.

with age and practice as between-subjects variables. A significant effect of age was observed for "new" ratings, $F(2, 106) = 4.327$, $MSE = 2.950$, $\eta_p^2 = .005$, power = .09, while this variable failed to reach significance for "old" ratings, $p > .7$, $\eta_p^2 = .08$, power = .74. Older participants may indeed have had a tendency to accept new triplets as old because they are very similar to each other as they only differ by the third element but share the same first two elements. In both one-way ANOVAs, neither the variable practice, nor the Age × Practice interaction reached significance, all $ps > .6$, $\eta_p^2\text{s} < .014$, powers < .01. In the same vein, and in contrast to what happened in SRT and generation tasks, the overall analysis of variance revealed neither an effect of practice, nor any interactions involving this factor, all $ps > .2$, $\eta_p^2\text{s} < .01$, powers < .08.

Let us now turn to the finding that ageing seems to reduce the difference between the scores attributed to old versus new triplets. As in the SRT task, we conducted separate age-related ANOVA's with sequence (2 levels, old vs. new) as within-subjects variable and practice as between-subjects variable. This analysis confirmed both the absence of any effect involving practice, all $ps > .2$, $\eta_p^2\text{s} < .03$, powers < .18, and the significant effect of sequence in the young, $F(1, 38) = 21.385$, $MSE = 12.270$, $\eta_p^2 = .36$, power = .99, middle-aged, $F(1, 35) = 5.360$, $MSE = 2.349$, $\eta_p^2 = .13$, power = .62, and older participants groups, $F(1, 33) = 9.333$, $MSE = 2.114$, $\eta_p^2 = .22$, power = .84, respectively. This suggests that, even though ageing overall seems to reduce the difference between the scores attributed to old versus new triplets, getting older does not totally suppress recognition abilities, since both middle-aged and older groups were able to differentiate between old and new triplets.

This finding is also supported by RTs analyses during the recognition task, evidencing that ageing does not bias the way stimuli are processed. One could indeed argue that middle-aged and older adults' above chance performance in recognition stems from a different process than younger adults' performance. In a nutshell, younger participants are assumed to respond based on recollection, whereas older participants might respond based primarily on familiarity. The assumption is that participants may tend to respond faster to familiar sequence fragments than to novel fragments. As a consequence, their ratings could reflect feelings of perceptual motor fluency rather than explicit recollection (see, e.g., Perruchet & Amorim, 1992).

To examine whether older participants are more likely to categorise triplets as old or new based on this perceptual motor fluency, we compared, for each group, the mean RTs associated to the third element of the 12 training triplets with the mean RTs associated to the third element of the 12 transfer triplets. As we know that two elements are necessary to predict the location of the third one, RT differences reflecting sequential knowledge can be observed only on the RT of the third element. If middle-aged and older

TABLE 2
Mean reaction times (in ms) in the recognition task, for old and new triplets, for the six groups of participants (standard deviations are in parentheses)

	Triplets	
Groups	*Training (old)*	*Transfer (new)*
Young 15	610.09 (467.55)	721.75 (541.59)
Middle 15	947.21 (457.76)	1076.91 (904.19)
Older 15	1397.47 (643.63)	1608.71 (976.63)
Young 30	507.14 (225.29)	589.25 (333.90)
Middle 30	877.55 (345.04)	1003.40 (433.33)
Older 30	1234.20 (683.45)	1738.03 (1743.90)

participants were to respond even more rapidly to familiar sequence fragments as compared to novel fragments than their younger counterparts, this would give support to the idea that getting older implies less recollection and more familiarity. On the other hand, if RTs to old and new triplets do not differ between age groups, this would indicate that participants process stimuli similarly, regardless of age. The latter assumption was supported by an ANOVA with sequence (2 levels, old vs. new) as within-subjects variable and age and practice as between-subjects variables (Table 2).

The main effect of sequence reached significance, $F(1, 106) = 9.869$, $MSE = 2101531.097$, $\eta_p^2 = .09$, power = .88, as was the effect of age, $F(2, 106) = 16.374$, $MSE = 14747674.13$, $\eta_p^2 = .24$. However, neither their interaction, nor the main effect of practice and all interactions involving this factor reached significance, all $ps > .18$, $\eta_p^2 s < .32$, powers < .17. This suggests that overall, participants tended to respond faster to old than to new triplets, regardless of their age and the number of training blocks they had previously been presented with. Thus, all participants' recognition performance may, at least partially, have been influenced by perceptual motor fluency. To summarise, recognition data indicate that recognition is preserved by ageing, even though middle-aged and older participants still exhibit reduced differences between old and new scores, as compared to their younger counterparts.

Finally, we examined whether SRT, generation, and recognition performances were associated to each other, and if so, to what extent these correlations would differ with age and practice. Therefore, we computed a performance index for each of the three tasks (Table 3). As already mentioned, the SRT index was computed as the RTs increase due to the sequence transfer. The generation and recognition indices were obtained by subtracting exclusion scores to inclusion scores, and by subtracting new triplets to old ones, respectively.

TABLE 3
Correlation coefficients between the direct and indirect tasks.

		SRT	*Generation*	*Recognition*
Young		SRT	0.46*	0.52**
	15 blocks	Generation		0.69**
		Recognition		
		SRT	.52*	.50*
	30 blocks	Generation		.71**
		Recognition		
Middle		SRT	−.09, ns	.31, ns
	15 blocks	Generation		.23, ns
		Recognition		
		SRT	.23, ns	.06, ns
	30 blocks	Generation		.26, ns
		Recognition		
Older		SRT	−.10, ns	−.37, ns
	15 blocks	Generation		.36, ns
		Recognition		
		SRT	.46, $p = .06$	.36, ns
	30 blocks	Generation		.12, ns
		Recognition		

*Correlations are significant at $\alpha = .05$, bilateral. **Correlations are significant at $\alpha = .01$, bilateral.

In young adults only (regardless of practice level), performance in the indirect SRT task was correlated with performance in both direct tasks. Moreover, generation and recognition tasks also correlated highly and significantly with each other in young adults. The older adults who were given long practice also showed a marginal positive correlation between SRT and generation tasks performance. All other correlations failed to reach significance.

DISCUSSION

The main goal of this study was to investigate the effects of age and practice in learning and in controlling sequential regularities. To achieve this, young, middle-aged, and older participants were exposed to either a 15 block or a 30 block SRT task. In order to assess participants' ability to use the acquired knowledge intentionally, they were required to perform two subsequent direct tasks (generation and recognition). In the following, we discuss our findings by focusing on each of the three tasks the participants had to perform.

Are there effects of age and practice on sequence learning?

Our main finding was that all six groups of participants (3 age levels × 2 practice levels) showed evidence of having become sensitive to the sequential regularities contained in the stimulus material. Participants in the long training condition exhibited a larger negative transfer effect than participants in the short training condition. This suggests that participants benefited from longer exposure to the sequence. Simply put, the more you are exposed to sequential structure, the more you will learn about the regularities of this sequence, and the more you will be able to react differentially to another sequence. In other words, longer training simply results in the increasing availability of high-quality representations of the trained material (Cleeremans, 2006; Cleeremans & Jiménez, 2002). When the training sequence is transferred to another one, middle-aged and older participants indeed showed a negative transfer effect as large as the one observed with younger participants. This result is congruent with previous data showing that, when a deterministic repeating sequence is used, ageing does not interfere with the ability to acquire new information implicitly, whereas explicit measures show an age-related deficit (Cherry & Stadler, 1995; Frensch et al., 1994; Howard & Howard, 1989, 1992). However, it differs from other sequence learning studies showing both implicit and explicit learning age-related decreases (Curran, 1997; Jackson & Jackson, 1992).

Did we observe any ironic effects of repetition in the generation task?

The generation task was designed to put familiarity and recollection processes in opposition, by using inclusion and exclusion instructions (e.g., see Jacoby, 1991; Yonelinas, 2002). Inclusion instructions required to reproduce the training sequence, whereas the exclusion subtask required not to generate the training sequence, i.e., to withhold a prepotent response. The ironic effects hypothesis (Jacoby, 1999) postulates that middle-aged and older adults would be less likely to be able to fit those requirements than their younger counterparts, because of age-related control deficits. Furthermore, ironic effects of repetition were expected, i.e., an age-related dissociative effect of practice level on the generation performance. According to the gradual hypothesis, however, extended practice during the training phase should not yield dissociative effects on young and older participants, because they would all benefit from higher quality representations. Nevertheless, a main effect of age was expected, since ageing is assumed to be associated with lower quality representations.

Interestingly, our results show no age-related differential effects on recollection and familiarity processes whatsoever. On the contrary, irrespective to age, generation performance suggests that participants were able to control their acquired sequential knowledge. Not only were they able to reproduce sequential regularities when needed, but they also were able to inhibit these regularities when required. This stands against all previous studies on implicit learning in the elderly, in which, even though preserved learning abilities were found in older participants, the expression of the acquired knowledge in subsequent direct tasks was found to be disrupted (Cherry & Stadler, 1995; Frensch et al., 1994; Howard & Howard, 1989, 1992; Jennings & Jacoby, 1993). Specifically, our data do not extend to sequence learning the ironic effects of repetition observed by Jacoby (1999) in an implicit memory task. One might argue that this test suffers from insufficient power to detect group differences. Effects related to age were indeed very small ($\eta^2 < .014$). Thus, even if we cannot totally reject the possibility of age differences in the generation task, these differences are certainly too small to be interpreted as confirming the ironic effects hypothesis.

However, as far as the practice effect is concerned, we unequivocally evidenced that sequence repetition actually enhances generation performance and particularly inclusion scores. That is, the more you have been presented with a sequential structure in the learning phase, the more you are subsequently able to express this acquired knowledge in the inclusion subtask.

How can we explain the discrepancy between our data and previous results? A first element might be the difference between, say, Jacoby's set-up and ours. In Jacoby's (1999) learning phase, young and older participants were exposed to words presented in visual or auditory modalities. They were instructed to read aloud written words and to repeat aloud heard words. The number of written words repetition was manipulated (i.e., from 1 to 3 presentations, in Experiment 1). In the subsequent classification phase, three lists of words were presented: words previously read, words previously heard, and novel words. In the inclusion task, participants were to differentiate between old and new words, that is, to *include* all previous words, irrespective of the modality of presentation. Conversely, in the exclusion task, participants had to classify as old previously heard words solely, thus *excluding* previously read words. In Jacoby's experiment, because of the age-related source monitoring deficit (Burke, 1997; Dehn & Engelkamp, 1997; Dehon & Bredart, 2004; Hashtroudi, Johnson, & Chrosniak, 1989; Johnson, Hashtroudi, & Lindsay, 1993; McElree, Dolan, & Jacoby, 1999; Siedlecki, Salthouse, & Berish, 2005), the read-words-list might have more interfered with the heard-words-list for older participants than for younger ones, especially with repeatedly read words. On the contrary, a single sequence is repeated in the present learning phase (the occurrence of a transfer sequence during a single block, at the end of training, is indeed unlikely to interfere with the training sequence). Hence, in our exclusion task, participants know exactly what to do with the acquired information, that is, to inhibit it. They do not have to select in between two different sequences, i.e., between two different sources. This might explain why middle-aged and older adults performed at the same level as younger adults, even after a longer training phase.

A second tentative explanation of the absence of any ironic effects of repetition in our experiment stems from the distinction between procedural and declarative memory systems (Tulving, 1995). The declarative system consists of the "know what", whereas the procedural system is the "know how". This latter system develops earlier (Homberg, Bickmann, & Muller, 1993), is preserved in amnesia (Squire & Zola, 1998; Warrington & Weiskrantz, 1974), and benefits from extensive training (Cleeremans & McClelland, 1991; Willingham, Nissen, & Bullemer, 1989). Jacoby's (1999) task is a declarative task, with words as stimuli, whereas ours is a procedural one, using a visuospatial setting. Therefore, it might be the case that repeating the training sequence either 112 times in the short training condition (15 blocks) or 232 times in the long training condition (30 blocks) was not even close to the number of repetitions that would be necessary to try to produce ironic effects of repetitions in sequence learning. Previous data indeed show that learning measures come to a floor level only after about 20,000 trials (Jiménez, Méndez, & Cleeremans, 1996). In this respect, it would worth replicating and extending the present findings by gradually manipulating practice level, up to 200 sequential blocks.

Age-related differences in the recognition task

The recognition task yielded a pattern of findings that is in sharp contrast with what has just been discussed in the generation task. First, practice level did not bias recognition performance, that is, participants in the long training condition did not perform better in the subsequent recognition task than participants in the short training condition. Second, age-related effects were observed, contrary to the SRT and generation tasks. Actually, middle-aged and older adults were still able to distinguish between old and new fragments, but younger participants outperformed them. Third, the same level of automatic fluency was observed in all experimental conditions, regardless of participants' age. However, one cannot rule out the possibility that older participants relied more on fluency than their younger counterparts in order to perform the recognition task.

Finally, the observed correlations between direct and indirect measures of learning show an highly coherent pattern of results in younger participants in which good learners are also able to follow generation and recognition instructions. In older participants, however, we did not find such a coherent pattern, suggesting maybe that the different measures of performance are differentially sensitive to factors such as forgetting or the similarity between test items. Such an interpretation might also explain why we found that older participants tend to produce more false alarms than younger subjects and to accept more often as "old" sequence triplets that have not been presented before in the recognition task.

As a conclusion, our results open a promising "third way" in the domain of sequence learning in older adults. Middle-aged and older adults indeed not only exhibited preserved learning abilities, but were also just as able to control the acquired knowledge in a generation task as younger participants. Conversely, an age-related deficit in recognition was evidenced, even though middle-aged and older adults were able to differentiate between old and new sequential fragments. Two kinds of conclusion can be drawn from these results: (1) The generation task and recognition tasks may not tap the same processes and can be dissociated based on them, and (2) sequence learning tasks and implicit memory tasks, beyond their similarities, do differ from each other in significant ways. Further research is necessary to fully explore these differences.

REFERENCES

Braver, T. S., Barch, D. M., Keys, B. A., Carter, C. S., Cohen, J. D., Kaye, J. A., et al. (2001). Context processing in older adults: Evidence for a theory relating cognitive control to neurobiology in healthy aging. *Journal of Experimental Psychology: General*, *130*(4), 746–763.

Bremner, A., Mareschal, D., Destrebecqz, A., & Cleeremans, A. (2007). Cognitive control of sequential knowledge at 2 years of age: Evidence from an incidental sequence learning and generation task. *Psychological Science*, *18*(3), 261–266.

Brink, T. L., Yesavage, J. A., Lum, O., Heersema, P. H., Adey, M., & Rose, T. L. (1982). Screening tests for geriatric depression. *The Clinical Gerontologist*, *1*, 37–43.

Bugaiska, A., Clarys, D., Jarry, C., Taconnat, L., Tapia, G., Vanneste, S., et al. (2007). The effect of aging in recollective experience: The processing speed and executive functioning hypothesis. *Consciousness and Cognition*, *16*(4), 797–808.

Burke, D. M. (1997). Language, aging, and inhibitory deficits: Evaluation of a theory *Journal of Gerontology. B: Psychological Sciences*, *52*, 254–264.

Cherry, K. E., & Stadler, M. A. (1995). Implicit learning of a nonverbal sequence in younger and older adults. *Psychology and Aging*, *10*(3), 379–394.

Cleeremans, A. (2006). Conscious and unconscious cognition: A graded, dynamic, perspective. In Q. Jing, M. R. Rosenzweig, G. d'Ydewalle, H. Zhang, H.-C. Chen, & K. Zhan (Eds.), *Progress in psychological science around the world: Neural, cognitive and developmental issues* (Vol. 1 (pp. 401–418)). Hove, UK: Psychology Press.

Cleeremans, A., Destrebecqz, A., & Boyer, M. (1998). Implicit learning: News from the front. *Trends in Cognitive Sciences*, *2*(10), 406–414.

Cleeremans, A., & Jiménez, L. (2002). Implicit learning and consciousness: A graded, dynamical perspective. In R. M. French & A. Cleeremans (Eds.), *Implicit learning and consciousness* (pp. 1–40). Hove, UK: Psychology Press.

Cleeremans, A., & McClelland, J. L. (1991). Learning the structure of event sequences. *Journal of Experimental Psychology: General, 120*(3), 235–253.

Craik, F. I. M., & Byrd, M. (1982). Aging and cognitive deficits: The role of attentional resources. In F. I. M. Craik & S. E. Trehub (Eds.), *Aging and cognitive processes* (pp. 191–211). New York: Plenum.

Craik, F. I. M., & Bialystok, E. (2006). Cognition through the lifespan: Mechanisms of change. *Trends in Cognitive Sciences, 10*(3), 131–138.

Craik, F. I. M., & Salthouse, T. A. (2000). *The handbook of aging and cognition* (2nd ed.). Hove, UK: Lawrence Erlbaum Associates Ltd.

Curran, T. (1997). Effects of aging on implicit sequence learning: Accounting for sequence structure and explicit knowledge. *Psychological Research, 60*, 24–41.

Dehn, D. M., & Engelkamp, J. (1997). Process dissociation procedure: Double dissociations following divided attention and speeded responding. *Quarterly Journal of Experimental Psychology, 50A*(2), 318–336.

Dehon, H., & Bredart, S. (2004). False memories: Young and older adults think of semantic associates at the same rate, but young adults are more successful at source monitoring. *Psychology and Aging, 19*(1), 191–197.

Dennis, N. A., Howard, J. H., Jr., & Howard, D. V. (2006). Implicit sequence learning without motor sequencing in young and old adults. *Experimental Brain Research, 175*(1), 153–164.

Destrebecqz, A., & Cleeremans, A. (2001). Can sequence learning be implicit? New evidence with the process dissociation procedure. *Psychonomic Bulletin and Review, 8*(2), 343–350.

Dienes, Z. (2008). Subjective measures of unconscious knowledge. Progress in Brain Research. *Models of Brain and Mind: Physical, Computational and Psychological Approaches, 168*, 49–64.

Dienes, Z., & Berry, D. (1997). Implicit learning: Below the subjective threshold. *Psychonomic Bulletin and Review, 4*, 3–23.

Dulany, D. E. (1997). Consciousness in the explicit (deliberative) and implicit (evocative). In J. Cohen & J. Schooler (Eds.), *Scientific approaches to consciousness* (pp. 179–212). Mahwah, NJ: Lawrence Erlbaum Associates, Inc.

Feeney, J. J., Howard, J. H., Jr., & Howard, D. V. (2002). Implicit learning of higher order sequences in middle age. *Psychology and Aging, 17*(2), 351–355.

Forkstam, C., & Petersson, K. M. (2005). Towards an explicit account of implicit learning. *Current Opinion in Neurology, 18*(4), 435–441.

Frensch, P., & Rünger, D. (2003). Implicit learning. *Current Directions in Psychological Science, 12*(1), 13–18.

Frensch, P. A., Buchner, A., & Lin, J. (1994). Implicit learning of unique and ambiguous serial transitions in the presence and absence of a distractor task. *Journal of Experimental Psychology: Learning, Memory, and Cognition, 20*(3), 567–584.

Hasher, L., Quig, M. B., & May, C. P. (1997). Inhibitory control over no-longer-relevant information: Adult age differences. *Memory and Cognition, 25*(3), 286–295.

Hashtroudi, S., Johnson, M. K., & Chrosniak, L. D. (1989). Aging and source monitoring. *Psychology and Aging, 4*(1), 106–112.

Hogan, M. J., Kelly, C. A., & Craik, F. I. (2006). The effects of attention switching on encoding and retrieval of words in younger and older adults. *Experimental Aging Research, 32*(2), 153–183.

Homberg, V., Bickmann, U., & Muller, K. (1993). Ontogeny is different for explicit and implicit memory in humans. *Neuroscience Letters, 150*(2), 187–190.

Howard, D. V., & Howard, J. H. (1989). Ages differences in learning serial patterns: Direct versus indirect measures. *Psychology and Aging, 4*, 357–364.

Howard, D. V., & Howard, J. H. (1992). Adult age differences in the rate of learning serial patterns: Evidence from direct and indirect tests. *Psychology and Aging*, *7*, 232–241.

Howard, D. V., & Howard, J. H., Jr. (2001). When it does hurt to try: Adult age differences in the effects of instructions on implicit pattern learning. *Psychonomic Bulletin and Review*, *8*(4), 798–805.

Howard, D. V., Howard, J. H., Jr., Japikse, K., DiYanni, C., Thompson, A., & Somberg, R. (2004). Implicit sequence learning: Effects of level of structure, adult age, and extended practice. *Psychology and Aging*, *19*(1), 79–92.

Howard, J. H., Jr., & Howard, D. V. (1997). Age differences in implicit learning of higher order dependencies in serial patterns. *Psychology and Aging*, *12*(4), 634–656.

Jackson, G. M., & Jackson, S. R. (1992). *Sequence structure and sequential learning: The evidence from ageing reconsidered*. Eugene, OR: Institute of Cognitive and Decision Sciences, University of Oregon.

Jacoby, L. L. (1991). A process dissociation framework: Separating automatic from intentional uses of memory. *Journal of Memory and Language*, *30*, 513–541.

Jacoby, L. L. (1999). Ironic effects of repetition: Measuring age-related differences in memory. *Journal of Experimental Psychology: Learning, Memory, and Cognition*, *25*(1), 3–22.

Jennings, J. M., & Jacoby, L. L. (1993). Automatic versus intentional uses of memory: Aging, attention and control. *Psychology and Aging*, *8*, 283–293.

Jiménez, L., Méndez, C., & Cleeremans, A. (1996). Comparing direct and indirect measures of sequence learning. *Journal of Experimental Psychology: Learning, Memory, and Cognition*, *22*(4), 948–969.

Johnson, M. K., Hashtroudi, S., & Lindsay, D. S. (1993). Source monitoring. *Psychological Bulletin*, *114*(1), 3–28.

Kihlstrom, J. F., Dorfman, J., & Park, L. (2007). Implicit and explicit memory and learning. In M. Velmans & S. Schneider (Eds.), *The Blackwell companion to consciousness* (pp. 525–539). Malden, MA: Blackwell Publishing.

Kray, J., Eber, J., & Lindenberger, U. (2004). Age differences in executive functioning across the lifespan: The role of verbalization in task preparation. *Acta Psychologica*, *115*(2–3), 143–165.

Light, L. L., Prull, M. W., La Voie, D. J., & Healy, M. R. (2000). Dual-process theories of memory in old age. In T. J. Perfect & E. A. Maylor (Eds.), *Models of cognitive aging* (pp. 238–300). New York: Oxford University Press.

Maybery, M. T., Taylor, M., & O'Brien-Malone, A. (1995). Implicit learning: Sensitive to age but not to IQ. *Australian Journal of Psychology*, *47*, 8–17.

McElree, B., Dolan, P. O., & Jacoby, L. L. (1999). Isolating the contributions of familiarity and source information to item recognition: A time course analysis. *Journal of Experimental Psychology: Learning, Memory, and Cognition*, *25*(3), 563–582.

Meulemans, T., van der Linden, M., & Perruchet, P. (1998). Implicit sequence learning in children. *Journal of Experimental Child Psychology*, *69*, 199–221.

Negash, S., Petersen, L. E., Geda, Y. E., Knopman, D. S., Boeve, B. F., Smith, G. E., et al. (2007). Effects of ApoE genotype and mild cognitive impairment on implicit learning. *Neurobiology of Aging*, *28*, 885–893.

Nissen, M. J., & Bullemer, P. (1987). Attentional requirement of learning: Evidence from performance measures. *Cognitive Psychology*, *19*, 1–32.

Pacton, S., Fayol, M., & Perruchet, P. (2005). Children's implicit learning of graphotactic and morphological regularities. *Child Development*, *76*(2), 324–339.

Pacton, S., Perruchet, P., Fayol, M., & Cleeremans, A. (2001). Implicit learning out of the lab: The case of orthographic regularities. *Journal of Experimental Psychology: General*, *130*(3), 401–426.

Park, D., & Schwarz, N. (2000). *Cognitive aging: A primer*. Philadelphia: Psychology Press.

Perruchet, P., & Amorim, M. A. (1992). Conscious knowledge and changes in performance in sequence learning: Evidence against dissociation. *Journal of Experimental Psychology: Learning, Memory, and Cognition, 18*(4), 785–800.

Prull, M. W., Gabrieli, J. D., & Bunge, S. A. (2000). Age-related changes in memory: A cognitive neuroscience perspective. In F. I. Craik & T. A. Salthouse (Eds.), *The handbook of cognitive aging and cognition* (2nd ed) (pp. 91–153). Mahwah, NJ: Lawrence Erlbaum Associates, Inc.

Reber, A. S. (1993). *Implicit learning and tacit knowledge: An essay on the cognitive unconsicous.* New York: Oxford University Press.

Reed, J., & Johnson, P. (1994). Assessing implicit learning with indirect tests: Determining what is learned about sequence structure. *Journal of Experimental Psychology: Learning, Memory, and Cognition, 20*(3), 585–594.

Saffran, J. R., Aslin, R. N., & Newport, E. L. (1996). Statistical learning by 8-month-old infants. *Science, 274*(5294), 1926–1928.

Saffran, J. R., Senghas, A., & Trueswell, J. C. (2001). The acquisition of language by children. *Proceedings of the National Academy of Sciences of the USA, 98*(23), 12874–12875.

Salthouse, T. A., McGuthry, K. E., & Hambrick, D. Z. (1999). A framework for analyzing and interpreting differential aging patterns: Application to three measures of implicit learning. *Aging, Neuropsychology, and Cognition, 6*(1), 1–18.

Schmidt, R., Freidl, W., Fazekas, F., Reinhart, B., Grieshofer, P., Kock, M., et al. (1994). The Mattis Dementia Rating Scale: Normative data from 1,001 healthy volunteers. *Neurology, 44*, 964–966.

Schmitter-Edgecombe, M., & Nissley, H. M. (2002). Effects of aging on implicit covariation learning. *Aging, Neuropsychology, and Cognition, 9*(1), 61–75.

Shanks, D. R., & Johnstone, T. (1999). Evaluating the relationship between explicit and implicit knowledge in a serial reaction time task. *Journal of Experimental Psychology: Learning, Memory, and Cognition, 26*(6), 1435–1451.

Siedlecki, K. L., Salthouse, T. A., & Berish, D. E. (2005). Is there anything special about the aging of source memory? *Psychology and Aging, 20*(1), 19–32.

Squire, L. R., & Frambach, M. (1990). Cognitive skill learning in amnesia. *Psychobiology, 18*, 109–117.

Squire, L. R., & Zola, S. M. (1998). Episodic memory, semantic memory, and amnesia. *Hippocampus, 8*(3), 205–211.

Taconnat, L., Clarys, D., Vanneste, S., Bouazzaoui, B., & Isingrini, M. (2007). Aging and strategic retrieval in a cued-recall test: The role of executive functions and fluid intelligence. *Brain and Cognition, 64*(1), 1–6.

Thomas, K. M., Hunt, R. H., Vizueta, N., Sommer, T., Durston, S., Yang, Y., et al. (2004). Evidence of developmental differences in implicit sequence learning: An fMRI study of children and adults. *Journal of Cognitive Neuroscience, 16*(8), 1339–1351.

Thomas, K. M., & Nelson, C. A. (2001). Serial reaction time learning in preschool- and school-age children. *Journal of Experimental Child Psychology, 79*(4), 364–387.

Tulving, E. (1995). Organization of memory: Quo vadis? In M. S. Gazzaniga (Ed.), *The cognitive neurosciences* (pp. 839–847). Cambridge, MA: MIT Press.

Vandenberghe, M., Gaillard, V., Destrebecqz, A., Fery, P., & Cleeremans, A. (2008). Is slowing down better than speeding up? Exploring the effects of temporal factors on adult age differences in sequence learning. *Manuscript in preparation.*

Vanderaspoilden, V., Adam, S., van der Linden, M., & Morais, J. (2007). Controlled processes account for age-related decrease in episodic memory. *Acta Psychologica, 125*(1), 20–36.

Verhaeghen, P., & Hoyer, W. J. (2007). Aging, focus switching, and task switching in a continuous calculation task: Evidence toward a new working memory control process. *Aging, Neuropsychology, and Cognition, 14*(1), 22–39.

Vinter, A., & Perruchet, P. (2000). Implicit learning in children is not related to age: Evidence from drawing behavior. *Child Development*, *71*(5), 1223–1240.

Vinter, A., & Perruchet, P. (2002). Implicit motor learning through observational training in adults and children. *Memory and Cognition*, *30*(2), 256–261.

Warrington, E. K., & Weiskrantz, L. (1974). The effect of prior learning on subsequent retention in amnesic patients. *Neuropsychologia*, *12*(4), 419–428.

West, R., & Schwarb, H. (2006). The influence of aging and frontal function on the neural correlates of regulative and evaluative aspects of cognitive control. *Neuropsychology*, *20*(4), 468–481.

Wilkinson, L., & Shanks, D. R. (2004). Intentional control and implicit sequence learning. *Journal of Experimental Psychology: Learning, Memory, and Cognition*, *30*(2), 354–369.

Willingham, D. B., Nissen, M. J., & Bullemer, P. (1989). On the development of procedural knowledge. *Journal of Experimental Psychology: Learning, Memory, and Cognition*, *15*(6), 1047–1060.

Yonelinas, A. P. (2002). The nature of recollection and familiarity: A review of 30 years of research. *Journal of Memory and Language*, *46*, 441–517.

EUROPEAN JOURNAL OF COGNITIVE PSYCHOLOGY
2009, 21 (2/3), 283–302

Psychology Press
Taylor & Francis Group

Constituent priming effects: Evidence for preserved morphological processing in healthy old readers

Jon Andoni Duñabeitia, Alejandro Marín, and Alberto Avilés
Universidad de La Laguna, Tenerife, Spain

Manuel Perea
Universitat de València, València, Spain

Manuel Carreiras
Universidad de La Laguna, Tenerife, Spain

How elderly adults process morphologically complex words is still a matter of controversy. The present study explored whether compound word recognition is affected by ageing. A group of young adults and a group of older healthy adults were tested on a lexical decision task. Compound words were presented primed by their first constituent (*book-BOOKSHOP*), their second constituent (*shop-BOOKSHOP*), or by an unrelated word (*house-BOOKSHOP*). Results revealed that morphological processing is fully preserved in advanced age and that the magnitude of the constituent priming effect was similar for young and older adults.

Keywords: Compound words; Morphological priming; Ageing.

How readers understand the meaning of morphologically complex words is a fundamental question for models of visual-word recognition (see Diependaele, Sandra, & Grainger, 2005). Words vary largely in terms of their morphological structure, ranging from monomorphemic words (i.e., words composed of a single meaningful unit, like *walk*) to polymorphemic words (i.e., words composed of more than a single morpheme, like *walker*).

Correspondence should be addressed to Jon Andoni Duñabeitia, Departamento de Psicología Cognitiva, Universidad de La Laguna, 38205, Tenerife, Spain. E-mail: jaduna@ull.es

The research reported in this article has been partially supported by Grants SEJ2004-07680-C02-02/PSIC, SEJ2006-09238/PSIC, and SEJ2005-05205/EDU from the Spanish Government, and by Grant BFI05.310 from the Basque Government. The authors thank Lars-Göran Nilsson and three anonymous reviewers for their helpful comments on an earlier draft. Thanks are also due to Margaret Gillon-Dowens for her support and priceless patience.

http://www.psypress.com/ecp DOI: 10.1080/09541440802281142

Empirical evidence from healthy young adults suggests that these polymorphemic words are decomposed early in the visual word recognition process (see Frost, Grainger, & Rastle, 2005a, for review). However, there is less evidence regarding other populations, such as children and older adults. In the present study we explore how older adults recognise morphologically complex words, and more specifically, how they recognise compound words.

COMPOUND WORDS AND CONSTITUENT PRIMING EFFECTS

Compound words are created from the union of two or more lexemes (e.g., *foot* + *ball* = *football*). These compound word forms are not necessarily written as a single unit (closed or "solid" compounds, as in *football*), but can also be scripted in a hyphenated fashion (e.g., *editor-in-chief*) or even in an unlinked way (e.g., *science fiction*). Furthermore, compound words can vary largely in degree of transparency, that is, in how the meaning of the compound word is tied to the meaning of each of the constituents. Hence, one can easily come across compound words in which the meaning of both constituents is directly related to the whole-word meaning (e.g., a transparent compound, such as *bedroom*), compound words in which only the meaning of the first or second lexeme fits the general meaning of the word (e.g., semiopaque compounds such as *jailbird* or *strawberry*), and compound words in which none of the constituent meanings coincide with the whole-word meaning (e.g., opaque compounds such as *deadline*; see Libben, 1998; see also Libben, Gibson, Yoon, & Sandra, 2003). In the present study, we focus on how transparent, solid compounds are processed and decomposed when presented visually—bear in mind that these compounds are critical to test morpho-orthographic versus morphosemantic decomposition effects (see Diependaele et al., 2005).

There is a large body of evidence consistently showing that young adult readers decompose compound words into their constituents at early stages of lexical access (e.g., Duñabeitia, Perea, & Carreiras, 2007b; Fiorentino & Poeppel, 2007; Hyönä & Pollatsek, 1998; Juhasz, Starr, Inhoff, & Placke, 2003; Koester, Gunter, & Wagner, 2007; Pollatsek, Hyönä, & Bertram, 2000). The most robust evidence on morphological processing has been obtained in priming experiments. For instance, a number of studies have shown a robust priming effect of the whole compound when primed by one of the constituent lexemes. Furthermore, it seems that the magnitude of the priming effect produced by the first constituent (e.g., *milk*-*MILKMAN*) and by the second constituent (e.g., *man*-*MILKMAN*) is approximately the same (Jarema, Busson, Nikolova, Tsapkini, & Libben, 1999; Libben et al., 2003; Monsell, 1985; Sandra, 1990; Zwitserlood, 1994). For instance,

Zwitserlood (1994) used immediate partial repetition priming, presenting the compound word for 300 ms followed by one of its constituents (e.g., *milkman-MILK* and *milkman-MAN*). She found similar priming effects for the first and second constituents. Importantly, these constituent priming effects have also been replicated using very brief prime exposures and briefly presented primes (i.e., the masked priming paradigm; Forster & Davis, 1984). Shoolman and Andrews (2003) presented the participants with compound target words (e.g., *BOOKSHOP*) that could be preceded by the brief presentation (57 ms) of either the first constituent (e.g., *book*), the second constituent (e.g., *shop*), or an unrelated word. For transparent compound words, they observed similar priming for the first and for the second constituents relative to the unrelated priming condition. Very recently, and with a more extreme manipulation, Duñabeitia, Laka, Perea, and Carreiras (in press-b) replicated these findings using a masked priming paradigm. Duñabeitia and colleagues presented compound target words which were briefly preceded by different compound words that shared either the first constituent (e.g., *milkshake-MILKMAN*), the second constituent (e.g., *postman-MILKMAN*), or by noncompound words that did not share any of the lexemes. Their results confirmed those from previous studies revealing a similar constituent priming effect that does not depend on the position of the shared lexeme (Monsell, 1985; Sandra, 1990; Shoolman & Andrews, 2003; Zwitserlood, 1994). In sum, constituent priming is a well-established phenomenon that can be interpreted in terms of a parallel activation of separate representations of the morphemic constituents (in line with Rastle, Davis, & New, 2004; Rastle, Davis, Tyler, & Marslen-Wilson, 2000; see also Duñabeitia, Perea, & Carreiras, 2007a, in press-c).

VISUAL WORD RECOGNITION IN YOUNG AND ELDERLY READERS: EVIDENCE FROM PRIMING

In priming experiments, the effect of a related prime on target performance is compared to the effect of an unrelated prime on the same target. That is, participants do not make explicit judgement on the link between the prime and the target, and hence this processing facilitation (i.e., a "priming" effect) is usually thought to reflect an automatic access to activation –at least when the stimulus-onset asynchrony between the prime and the target is brief. There are different types of possible relationships between prime and target words, based either on a pure orthographic/form overlap (e.g., *house-HORSE*; see Carreiras, Perea, & Grainger, 1997; Spieler & Balota, 2000), on a similarity at morpheme level (e.g., *reaction-REFORM*; see Giraudo & Grainger, 2003; Marslen-Wilson, Ford, Older & Zhou, 1996), or on semantic relationship between concepts (e.g., *nurse-DOCTOR*; see Duñabeitia, Carreiras, & Perea, in press-a; Meyer & Schvaneveldt, 1971; Perea, Duñabeitia, & Carreiras, 2008; Perea & Gotor, 1997; Perea & Rosa, 2002). Although the priming paradigm has been largely used in young adult samples, elderly readers have not been so extensively tested under priming conditions. Some of the priming studies that have tested elderly participants on semantic relationships between concepts have shown an interesting priming pattern, revealing that senior readers exhibit a greater semantic priming effect than younger readers (the so-called *hyperpriming*; Laver, 2000; Laver & Burke 1993; see Giffard, Desgranges, Piolino, Eustache, & Kerrouche, 2003, for a review). As indicated by Giffard and colleagues, this hyperpriming effect may be reflecting a storage deficit for specific details of the concepts (i.e., semantic priming could be an instance of repetition priming in those individuals), a mere artefact of a general slowing hypothesis (i.e., larger priming effects for the slower individuals), or some differing attentional processing (i.e., different strategies of processing for the elderly individuals). However, the presence of hyperpriming in semantic priming experiments is not entirely consistent, and a number of studies have reported that the magnitude of the semantic priming effects does not interact with age (Balota, Black, & Cheney, 1992; Balota & Duchek, 1988; Howard, McAndrews, & Lasaga, 1981; Ober, Shenaut, Jagust, & Stillman, 1991). With respect to sublexical manipulations, Carreiras, Baquero, and Rodríguez (in press) recently conducted a syllable priming experiment (e.g., does *ca****-CASINO* differ from *cas***-CASINO*?; see Carreiras & Perea, 2002) with senior readers. Carreiras and colleagues found that not only subword unit processing is preserved with age (i.e., there was a significant syllable priming effect for the elderly), but the magnitude of the priming effect was greater for senior readers than for young adults. In fact, the syllable congruency effect was approximately 10 times larger for older readers than for younger readers who were tested in a previous experiment with the same materials (Carreiras & Perea, 2002), revealing that the size of the orthographic/phonological priming effect is enlarged as a function of ageing. Hence, these results from sublexical priming together with those from previous semantic priming studies showing greater magnitudes of the effects for the elderly participants support the existence of a hyperpriming effect that emerges as a function of age.

The very few studies that have tackled morphological priming in the elderly have reached the conclusion that morpheme processing is preserved in advanced age. Kavé and Levy (2004) tested Hebrew participants with Alzheimer's disease and aged control participants in a cross-modal priming experiment. They found that healthy older readers produced strong morphological priming in the absence of phonological priming (similarly to Bentin & Feldman, 1990; see also Frost, Deutsch, Gilboa, Tannenbaum,

& Marslen-Wilson, 2000). These results led them to conclude that the morphological relationships that exist among lexical items are preserved (see also Stamatakis & Tyler, 2006, for an fMRI study). However, several points should be highlighted regarding these findings. First, Kavé and Levy did not include a group of young adults in their experiment—note that their interest was to compare healthy aged participants with patients with Alzheimer's disease, and hence nothing could be said about dissimilarities in morphological priming effects due to age differences. This comparison is highly interesting in order to explore the existence of a *morphological hyperpriming* effect. Second, their experiments were conducted in Hebrew, and the morphological properties of Semitic languages are very different to those of Indo-European languages (see Frost, Kugler, Deutsch, & Forster, 2005b). For instance, words in Hebrew are composed of a consonantal root that represents an independent morphological unit, embedded within other letters (e.g., *RGL* in *meRaGeL*, the Hebrew for *a spy*), and in many cases, shared roots imply shared meaning (e.g., *RGL* in *RiGuL*, translated as *spying*). Thus, considering that root extraction is a necessary process for Hebrew readers but not for non-Semitic language users, it is not a simple task to generalise their results to other languages.

THE PRESENT STUDY: GOALS AND PREDICTIONS

The present study is aimed at exploring morphological decomposition of transparent compound words in aged readers. A group of healthy elderly adults was tested in a constituent priming experiment: Compound words served as targets (e.g., *BOOKSHOP*) and could be briefly preceded by their first constituent lexeme (e.g., *book*), their second constituent lexeme (e.g., *shop*), or by an unrelated word (e.g., *house*). To test whether or not the elderly readers showed a morphological hyperpriming effect, a group of younger readers was also tested with the same materials. Considering previous research, several main predictions can be made. Prior research has shown that reading latencies (reaction times) tend to increase with age (Allen, Madden, & Crozier, 1991; Allen, Sliwinski, & Bowie, 2002; Lima, Hale, & Myerson, 1991; Ratcliff, Thapar, Gómez, & McKoon, 2004b). However, although reading times are generally longer for older adults, language processing is thought to be minimally affected by ageing (Davidson, Zacks, & Ferreira, 2003; Waters & Caplan, 2005)—that is, the longer reaction times may just be a consequence of a general slowing (the general slowing hypothesis; see Birren, 1965; Cerella, 1985, 1990; Lima et al., 1991; Myerson, Hale, Chen, & Lawrence, 1997). Hence, according to this hypothesis, a first straightforward prediction is that elderly readers should produce longer reaction times than younger adults. Second, according to recent findings in subword unit processing (at a syllable level), robust priming effects can be expected for the morphologically related primes with respect to the unrelated condition (Carreiras et al., in press). Indeed, if the results obtained in Hebrew (Kavé & Levy, 2004) can be generalised to Indo-European languages, and if morphological relationships are indeed preserved in aged readers, a robust constituent priming effect should be observed for the elderly participants. But importantly, there is a key aspect of this study that could shed some light on the way in which connections at the orthographic, morphological, and semantic levels are affected by age. The compound words employed in the experiment were always transparent; that is, the meaning of the whole-words were directly derived from its constituents (i.e., there was a shared orthographic and semantic component between primes and targets). Thus, this manipulation allows us to test whether, similarly to previous findings with semantic priming, the observed effects are of greater magnitude for elderly than for younger readers (a hyperpriming effect; Laver, 2000; Laver & Burke, 1993) or, alternatively, whether they are of the same magnitude for both groups (as reported, among others, by Balota et al., 1992, and Balota & Duchek, 1988). To our knowledge, this critical test with transparent compounds has not been conducted in previous research.

METHOD

Participants

A total of 48 Spanish speakers took part in the data collection. Twenty-four of them were undergraduate students from the University of La Laguna (the young adult readers group). They all had normal or corrected-to-normal vision. Another group of 24 elderly participants was also selected for the current experiment (the elderly readers group; mean age 65.6 ± 7.5, range: 60–81). They were all healthy, active, community-dwelling individuals, and none of them reported having suffered medical or neurological diseases causing cognitive impairment or psychiatric disorder. All of the seniors had corrected vision for reading, and they wore their glasses in the experiment. These participants had attended regular scholar education for an average of 8.5 years (± 3.1).

Neuropsychological study

All the 24 elderly readers underwent a neuropsychological testing session that lasted for approximately 1 hour. This protocol included a Spanish and Latin-American standardised set of neuropsychological tests (Peña-Casanova, 2005), in which general cognitive status, functional-emotional status, memory, language, attention, and executive abilities were assessed. Special attention was paid to screening for dementia, and four standardised tests were applied for this: the Mini-Mental State Exam (MMSE; Folstein, Folstein, & McHugh, 1975), the short version of the Geriatric Depression Scale (Yesavage, 1988), the Lawton Geriatric Functionality Scale (Lawton, 1971), and a self-perception memory loss test based on a questionnaire about memory complaint (Cano, Ruiz, & Plata, 2002). The 24 participants obtained scores similar to or above those expected in all the tests and questionnaires. Scores from these participants are presented in Table 1.

Materials

Before creating the final list of materials for this experiment, a total of 24 workers and undergraduate students from the University of La Laguna voluntarily completed a questionnaire that served as a norming survey of the

TABLE 1
Neuropsychological scores for participants in the elderly group

Test	*Average*	*Standard deviation*	*ES***
Education (years)	8.45	3.12	
MMSE*	27.6	1.90	24
QSM	7.91	6.04	19
Lawton	8	0	6
Yesavage	2.3	3.2	5
FVS	14.9	2.7	13
FVF	11.7	3.2	11
DEN	57	4.1	50
RAVLT (learning)	39.9	6.5	39
RAVLT (short term)	9	2.1	6
LISTA B	7	2.35	4
RAVLT (long term)	9	1.9	8
REC	12.7	4.2	10
CFCR	32	18.1	29
TMT (time)	50.4	11.9	60
TMT	23.86	1.12	20
D-S	34.4	1.5	27
Refrains	8.6	2.7	7
Resemblances	16.3	0	13
Grafo-Motor Series	3	0	3

*MMSE: Mini-Mental State Examination. QSM: Subjective Memory Complain. FVS: Semantic Verbal Fluency. FVF: Phonologic Verbal Fluency. DEN: Naming. RAVLT: Rey Auditory Verbal Learning Test. REC: Recall. CFCR: Rey Figure (Copy). TMT: Trail Making Test. D-S: Digit-Symbol. **ES: Expected Scores (fit by age and scholar education in each participant and to all groups).

transparency of the compound words. None of these participants took part in the data collection for the experiment. These participants were presented with a selected list of 82 Spanish compound words that were previously chosen from the Spanish lexical database (LEXESP; Sebastián-Gallés, Martí, Carreiras & Cuetos, 2000). These words were at first selected by two independent external judges who classified them as transparent compound words. In order to directly asses the transparency degree of these words, the 24 participants had to rate them following a 1–7 scale, 1 being completely opaque and 7 completely transparent. They were told to consider a compound word as transparent whenever the two constituents were directly related to the whole-word meaning (e.g., *blackboard*), and to rate the compound word as opaque when the meaning of the two constituents was not related to the general meaning of the word (e.g., *deadline*). They were instructed to give a medium rating when the meaning of only one of the two constituent lexemes was linked to the whole-word meaning (e.g., *strawberry, jailbird*). The results showed that 13 of the 82 compound words were rated with a mean score less than 4 (mean: 3.2 ± 0.7), indicating that the degree of transparency was low. Therefore, these 13 words were discarded for the experiments. The other 69 compound words were rated with a mean score of 5.7 (± 0.9), indicating that the meaning of both constituent lexemes was highly related to the general meaning of the whole compound word.

The 69 compound words rated as transparent in the norming study were used as target words for the present experiment. These words were analysed with the B-Pal software that provides the most relevant indexes influencing visual word recognition (Davis & Perea, 2005). These compound words were low frequency words (mean frequency: 3.23 ± 7.75 appearances per million words), and had a mean length of 9.9 ± 1.4 characters. They had a mean number of 0.3 ± 0.5 orthographic neighbours according to the index N (Coltheart, Davelaar, Jonasson, & Besner, 1977). The first constituent lexemes of these compound words had a mean frequency of 162.39 ± 331.91, a mean length of 4.7 ± 0.8 letters, and a mean number of 11.5 ± 7.7 orthographic neighbours. The second constituent lexemes closely matched these statistics, with a mean frequency of 145.88 ± 240.44, a mean length of 5.2 ± 1.2 characters, and a mean number of 9.1 ± 7.2 orthographic neighbours. An extra set of 69 different words was selected as unrelated prime words for the compound words. These words were matched as closely as possible to the constituent lexemes in frequency (157.29 ± 177.89), number of letters (5.3 ± 1.1), and number of orthographic neighbours (6.6 ± 6.0). The 69 compound words were used as targets (e.g., *PASATIEMPO*, meaning *pastime*, composed of *pasa*[*pass*] + *tiempo*[*time*]), and could be preceded by (1) the first constituent lexeme (e.g., *pasa-PASATIEMPO*), (2) the second constituent lexeme (e.g., *tiempo-PASATIEMPO*), or (3) a completely unrelated word (e.g., *mujer-PASATIEMPO*; *mujer* is the Spanish for *woman*). Another set of 207 Spanish noncompound words of approximately the same length and frequency as the target compounds was also selected as target words, so that the relatedness proportion of compound words in the experiment was kept constant at 25%. These noncompound words were preceded by a set of prime words composed by 207 different words. An extra set of 276 nonwords was created in order to make the lexical decision possible. These nonwords were created by replacing three or four letters from the target words (e.g., *PUFAMIESPO* from *PASATIEMPO*), and were preceded by nonword primes created by replacing two or three letters from the prime words (e.g., *pufa*, *miespo*, *rufer*). Three different lists were created with the stimuli, so that each critical target appeared only once in each list, but each time in a different priming condition. Different participants were assigned to each of the lists.

Procedure

The young readers group was tested in a well-lit, soundproofed room of the Cognitive Neuroscience and Psycholinguistics Group's installations at the University of La Laguna, while the elderly readers group was tested individually in a well-lit, quiet room at the senior centres where they were recruited. The presentation of the stimuli and recording of the responses was carried out using DMDX software (Forster & Forster, 2003) on a PC-compatible computer associated to a CRT monitor. Each trial consisted in the presentation of a fixation point (|) for 500 ms, followed by the displaying of the lowercase prime for 250 ms, and immediately followed by the presentation of the uppercase target. Primes and targets were presented in 12 point Courier New font. For the young readers group, target items remained on the screen for 2500 ms or until a response was given. For the elderly readers group, target items remained for 3500 ms or until a response was given. This was in order to provide aged participants with enough time for their responses, bearing in mind that older participants' response times tend to be much higher than those of younger participants. All participants were instructed to press the "M" button on the keyboard when the item displayed was a real Spanish word, and the "Z" button when it was not. They were told to do so as fast and as accurately as possible. All participants completed practice trials before the experiment for warm-up purposes. All the items were randomly presented to avoid order repetition effects across participants.

TABLE 2
Mean lexical decision times (ms) and percentage of errors (in parentheses) for word targets in the experiment

	Priming condition			*Priming effect*	
	First lexeme	*Second lexeme*	*Unrelated word*	*First lexeme*	*Second lexeme*
Young group	759 (5.98%)	757 (4.71%)	842 (8.33%)	83 (2.35)	85 (3.62)
Elderly group	1550 (8.70%)	1541 (7.97%)	1662 (7.79%)	112 (–0.91)	120 (–0.18)

Mean reaction times for nonwords and percentage of errors were 858 and 2.05% for the young adult group and 1976 and 13.59% for the elderly group.

RESULTS

Response latencies beyond or above three standard deviations from the mean values of each experimental condition and reaction times associated to incorrect responses (4.2% of the data) were excluded from the response time analyses.[1] Mean response times and percentages of errors are presented in Table 2. Planned comparisons were conducted to assess the effect of constituent priming (i.e., the difference between the unrelated condition and each constituent). We report only *F* analyses over participants, since there is evidence showing that *F*1 is the appropriate analysis for testing the significance of the effects in counterbalanced designs (see Raaijmakers, 2003; Raaijmakers, Schrijnemakers, & Gremmen, 1999). Group (young readers, elderly readers) was included as a between-subject variable. List (List 1, List 2, List 3) was also included in the analyses as a dummy variable to extract the variance due to the counterbalanced lists (see Pollatsek & Well, 1995).

First constituent priming

The results from the reaction time analyses revealed a significant effect of the first constituent priming relative to the unrelated condition, $F(1, 42) = 40.09$, $p < .001$, $MSE = 56740$, $1–\beta = 1$: Participants recognised much faster (97 ms faster) compound words when preceded by their first constituent. The main effect of group was also significant (young readers being faster than elderly readers), $F(1, 42) = 58.80$, $p < .001$, $MSE = 264763$, $1–\beta = 1$. But the key

[1] Even though on a priori grounds one could argue that the three standard deviation cutoff might leave a high number of outlier values in the data (e.g., see Ratcliff, 1993), it should be noted that the data trimming procedure did not have any significant impact on the results. An analysis of the same data with a two standard deviation cutoff produced exactly the same results, with almost identical *p*-values for the observed effects.

finding here is that there were no signs of an interaction between these two factors, $F(1, 42) = 0.35$, $p > .91$, $MSE = 5674$, $1–\beta = .15$.

Analyses on the percentages of errors did not show any significant effects. There were no statistical differences between the error rates for compound words preceded by their first constituent or by unrelated words, $F(1, 42) = 0.41$, $p > .50$, $MSE = 31$, $1–\beta = .10$. The effect of group was not significant, $F(1, 42) = 0.55$, $p > .45$, $MSE = 52$, $1–\beta = .11$. The interaction between the two factors was not significant either, $F(1, 42) = 2.06$, $p > .15$, $MSE = 31$, $1–\beta = .29$.

Second constituent priming

Compound words preceded by their second constituent were recognised significantly faster (102 ms faster) than those preceded by an unrelated word, $F(1, 42) = 37.04$, $p < .001$, $MSE = 6802$, $1–\beta = 1$. The effect of group was also significant, showing that the group of elderly readers made longer response times than the group of young readers, $F(1, 42) = 61.71$, $p < .001$, $MSE = 250290$, $1–\beta = 1$. Importantly, the interaction between the two factors was not significant, $F(1, 42) = 1.12$, $p > .25$, $MSE = 6802$, $1–\beta = .18$.

The percentage of error analyses showed no reliable effects. Compound words preceded by their second constituent were read equally accurately than compound words preceded by an unrelated word, $F(1, 42) = 2.39$, $p > .13$, $MSE = 30$, $1–\beta = .33$. The effect of group was not significant, $F(1, 42) = 0.74$, $p > .35$, $MSE = 60$, $1–\beta = .13$. The interaction between the two factors only approached significance, $F(1, 42) = 2.91$, $p = .09$, $MSE = 30$, $1–\beta = .38$.

First constituent priming versus second constituent priming

The priming effects for compound words preceded by their first or their second constituent lexemes did not show any significant difference, $F(1, 42) = 0.11$, $p > .70$, $MSE = 5638$, $1–\beta = .06$. The effect of group was significant, $F(1, 42) = 56.93$, $p < .001$, $MSE = 261505$, $1–\beta = 1$, but the interaction between the two factors was not, $F(1, 42) = 0.04$, $p > .80$, $MSE = 5638$, $1–\beta = .05$.

The analyses on the error rates showed that compound words preceded by their first constituent were recognised with similar accuracy to compound words preceded by their second constituent, $F(1, 42) = 1.07$, $p > .30$, $MSE = 22$, $1–\beta = .17$. The effect of group was significant, revealing that the group of elderly readers made more errors than the group of young readers, $F(1, 42) = 4.57$, $p < .05$, $MSE = 47$, $1–\beta = .55$. The interaction between the two factors was not significant, $F(1, 42) = 0.08$, $p = .78$, $MSE = 22$, $1–\beta = .06$.

There is a caveat, however: Response times for older individuals were longer than response times for younger individuals, and hence one could argue that this may complicate a straightforward interpretation of the present findings. To minimise the proportional increase in the response times between groups, we performed the same analysis with a logarithmic transformation of the response times. The ANOVAs on the transformed data confirmed the results obtained with the nontransformed data. Compound words preceded by their first constituent were recognised significantly faster than in the unrelated condition, $F(1, 42) = 51.21$, $p < .001$, $MSE = 0.004$, $1–\beta = 1$. The priming effect for the second constituent was also significant, $F(1, 42) = 52.27$, $p < .001$, $MSE = 0.004$, $1–\beta = 1$. No differences were found between the priming effects for the first and second constituents, $F < 1$ and $p > .90$; and finally, none of the interactions with group resulted significant, all $Fs < 1.4$ and all $ps > .25$.

DISCUSSION

The present results can be summarised as follows: (1) Young adult readers show robust constituent priming effects, which are independent of the position of the lexeme (initial, final); (2) older adults also show sizeable constituent priming effects for both the first and second lexemes; and (3) the magnitude of the constituent priming effects is similar for the young and the older adults, despite the fact that reaction times were longer for older than for younger adults.

As stated in the introduction, constituent priming effects have been consistently found at different ranges of stimulus–onset asynchronies (ranging from 50 to 300 ms; see Isel, Gunter, & Friederici, 2003, for a review). Importantly, the benefit of previewing the first constituent (e.g., *book-BOOKSHOP*) and the second constituent (e.g., *shop-BOOKSHOP*) is similar. That is, the two lexemes seem to exert a similar influence on compound word recognition (e.g., Shoolman & Andrews, 2003). The present results converge with previous studies that have explored the same issue in young adult populations, obtaining constituent priming effects of the same magnitude for the first and second lexeme. Importantly, this is the first time that a constituent priming experiment has been conducted with an elderly population, bearing in mind that research on morphological processing has been scarce in seniors. As indicated in the introduction, Kavé and Levy (2004) tested a group of healthy old Hebrew-speaking participants, and a group of Hebrew patients with Alzheimer's disease, in a cross-modal (auditory prime and visual target) morphological priming experiment. Their results confirmed that both patients and healthy aged participants showed morphological and morphosemantic priming effects (see also Bentin & Feldman, 1990, or Frost et al., 2000). However, the Kavé and Levy results are difficult to generalise because of the very different morphological properties of Hebrew and Indo-European languages (e.g., English, French, Spanish, etc; see Frost et al., 2005b, for extensive discussion) and because Kavé and Levy did not include a control group of young adults. Therefore, the present examination of how age-related changes influence the way in which compound words are recognised and decomposed at the initial stages of lexical access represents a step forward in the literature on morphological priming. Interestingly, the effects obtained were of the same magnitude for both initial and ending position for the young and the elderly. This finding reinforces the view of preserved morphological decomposition and processing in healthy aged individuals, generalising the findings of Kavé and Levy (2004) and Stamatakis and Tyler (2006), at least for transparent compound words.[2]

Not surprisingly, we found longer latencies for the older readers than for the young readers. The general slowing hypothesis (Birren, 1965; Cerella, 1985, 1990) has usually been applied to account for the increase in reading latencies as a function of advanced age. In spite of this increase in reaction times, language processing is thought to be only minimally affected by ageing (e.g., Davidson et al., 2003; Rayner, Reichle, Stroud, Williams, & Pollatsek, 2006; Waters & Caplan, 2005). In the present experiment, we obtained a main effect of group, revealing that reaction times for older adults were longer than for younger adults. Thus, the present results support this view of a general slowing in a direct comparison between young and elder readers. But more importantly, none of the interactions of group with the constituent priming effects resulted significant, revealing that the observed effects did not differ significantly between groups. That is, morphological processing of compound words seems to be fully preserved in aged participants, and hence it is reasonable to conclude that the process of segmentation of a compound word into its constituent lexemes is similar for both groups of readers.

As indicated in the introduction, because of their perceptual and/or cognitive deficits, older adults may be expected to benefit more from

[2] Interestingly, all the previous studies on constituent priming effects in healthy young adults have stated that their results confirmed early morphological decomposition of the compound words (e.g., the lexeme *book* is rapidly identified and processed when a reader encounters the word *BOOKSHOP*). However, it could be thought that the difference in the priming effect obtained from *book-BOOKSHOP* and the unrelated pair *house-BOOKSHOP* may reflect a mere form-based orthographic priming effect. Evidence against this assumption has recently been provided by Duñabeitia, Laka, Perea, and Carreiras (in press-b). Duñabeitia and colleagues showed that constituent priming effects like those from *book-BOOKSHOP* are largely different from orthographic priming effects such as those in pairs like *resta-RESTAURANT*. Further research is needed to test the same subjects with orthographically, morphologically, and semantically related prime-target pairs to test this issue.

contextual support (i.e., from a semantically related prime) than young adults (i.e., a *hyperpriming* effect, as explained by the interactive-compensatory hypothesis; see Laver & Burke, 1993). However, the present findings do not support the idea of hyperpriming in the elderly, at least in the context of morphological priming. In the present experiment, materials were composed of transparent compound words (e.g., *BOOKSHOP*) and all the related primes were not only morphologically linked to the target, but also orthographically and semantically linked (e.g., *book*, *shop*). Hence, because of the high semantic overlap between primes and targets in this experiment, and considering the interactive-compensatory hypothesis and previous results from orthophonological and semantic priming experiments (e.g., Carreiras et al., in press), one might have expected a hyperpriming effect for the elderly group. However, we failed to obtain any signs of an interaction between the magnitude of the effects and the age of the participants (young vs. elderly). Therefore, the present findings cannot be accounted for by the interactive-compensatory hypothesis. Instead, they are better understood in terms of a total preservation of morphological priming effects in healthy aged participants. This pattern of results is consistent with proposals that assume that morphological relationships are much more than a compendium of orthographic and semantic relationships, and that morphemes may have an autonomous representation in the lexicon, (e.g., Aronoff, 1994; Di Sciullo & Williams, 1987; Duñabeitia et al., in press-c; Roelofs & Baayen, 2002; Zwitserlood, Bölte, & Dohmes, 2000, 2002). Of course, we acknowledge that the lack of an interaction between morphological priming and age is a new finding that requires replication—note that a number of prior studies have obtained an additive pattern of semantic priming effects and age (e.g., Balota et al., 1992; Balota & Duchek, 1988; Howard et al., 1981; Ober et al., 1991). What we should note here is that the presence of slow latencies for older adults does not imply that the underlying central cognitive effects are affected, but instead the slow response times may be due to nondecision parameters ("boundary separation" or "nondecision time" rather than "drift rates" in a diffusion model; e.g., see Ratcliff et al., 2004b; Ratcliff, Perea, Colangelo, & Buchanan, 2004a). Thus, the conditions under which hyperpriming can be obtained with elderly readers is a question for further research.

Even though the present results provide the first unambiguous evidence in favour of a preservation of morphological priming effects in the elderly, there are some possible shortcomings of the experiment that should be addressed. First, the neuropsychological performance of only the elderly participants was assessed, since this is the population with higher risk of neuropsychological disorders. However, it could have been of interest to have a psychological assessment for the younger adults (a group of healthy college students). In any case, we conducted a correlation analysis to explore whether the performance across some of the critical neuropsychological tests of the elderly group was related to the constituent priming effects. To this end, net priming effects for the first and second constituents were obtained for each of the elderly participants, and the correlation between these effects and the performance in four critical tests was assessed. These tests were the MMSE test (Folstein et al., 1975), the semantic fluency test (Benito-Cuadrado, Estaba-Castillo, S., Böhm, P., Cejudo-Bolívar, J., & Peña-Casanova, 2002; Spreen & Strauss, 1991), the naming test (based on Snodgrass & Vanderwart, 1980), and the memory test of the RALVT (Rey, 1958). The reason behind this selection is to have a representative test for the screening for dementia (MMSE), and to employ three tests that directly or indirectly measure the linguistic skills of the participants (note that these are the ones most related to the task). As can be seen in Table 3, this analysis did not show any significant correlation between the first/second constituent priming effects and the results in the four tests for the elderly (all $ps > .14$). Therefore, despite some (small) differences in the performance of the elderly participants in the tests that examined their language skills and dementia, these variations did not have a relevant influence on their performance in the experiment. Second, while the use of only transparent compound words as materials has provided a clear picture of morphological processing and ageing, we acknowledge that studying other types of compound may help to complete this picture. Future work should be aimed at exploring how ageing might modulate morphological decomposition effects with opaque, semi-opaque and pseudocompound words (e.g., *deadline*, *strawberry*, and *mayhem*, respectively). For instance, using opaque compounds (i.e., compound words in which the meaning of the constituents is not clearly linked to the whole-word meaning) may shed some light on the morpho-orthographic level of processing, since the semantics of the elements do not completely match, whereas the orthographic representations do.

TABLE 3
Correlation analysis between the net constituent priming effects of the elderly participants and their performance in four critical tests: MMSE, semantic fluency, naming, and the memory test of the RALVT

	MMSE	*Semantic fluency*	*Naming*	*RALVT*
First constituent priming effect	$r = -.12$ $p = .56$	$r = .09$ $p = .67$	$r = .17$ $p = .41$	$r = .18$ $p = .39$
Second constituent priming effect	$r = .15$ $p = .48$	$r = -.05$ $p = .80$	$r = .30$ $p = .15$	$r = .21$ $p = .32$

In summary, the present study has extended previous findings in compound word processing to healthy elderly adults, revealing that morphological processing is unaffected by age as the magnitude of the priming effects was similar for young and old adults. Therefore, meaningful subword units seem to be processed normally by aged participants, at least in the case of transparent, solid compound words.

REFERENCES

Allen, P. A., Madden, D. J., & Crozier, L. C. (1991). Adult age differences in letter-level and word-level processing. *Psychology and Aging, 6*, 261–271.

Allen, P. A., Sliwinski, M., & Bowie, T. (2002). Differential age effects in semantic and episodic memory: Part II. Slope and intercept analyses. *Experimental Aging Research, 28*, 111–142.

Aronoff, M. (1994). *Morphology by itself.* Cambridge, MA: MIT Press.

Balota, D. A., Black, S., & Cheney, M. (1992). Automatic and attentional processes in young and older adults: A reevaluation of the two-process model of semantic priming. *Journal of Experimental Psychology: Human Perception and Performance, 18*, 485–502.

Balota, D. A., & Duchek, J. M. (1988). Age related differences in lexical access, spreading activation, and simple pronunciation. *Psychology and Aging, 3*, 84–93.

Benito-Cuadrado, M. M., Estaba-Castillo, S., Böhm, P., Cejudo-Bolívar, J., & Peña-Casanova, J. (2002). Semantic verbal fluency of animals: A normative and predictive study in a Spanish population. *Journal of Clinical Experimental Neuropsychology, 24*, 1117–1122.

Bentin, S., & Feldman, L. B. (1990). The contribution of morphological and semantic relatedness to repetition priming at short and long lags: Evidence from Hebrew. *Quarterly Journal of Experimental Psychology, 42A*, 693–711.

Birren, J. E. (1965). Age changes in speeded behavior: Its central nature and physiological correlates. In A. T. Welford & J. E. Birren (Eds.), *Behavior, aging and the nervous system* (pp. 191–216). Springfield, IL: Charles C. Thomas.

Cano, C., Ruiz, A., & Plata, S. (2002). Capacidad operativa de una prueba de tamizado en el diagnóstico temprano de la enfermedad de Alzheimer. *Revista Asociación Colombiana Gerontología Geriatrica, 16*, 428–429.

Carreiras, M., Baquero, S., & Rodríguez, E. (in press). Syllabic processing in visual word recognition in Alzheimer patients, the elderly and young adults. *Aphasiology.* Epub ahead of print. DOI: 10.1080/02687030701820337.

Carreiras, M., & Perea, M. (2002). Masked priming effects with syllabic neighbors in the lexical decision task. *Journal of Experimental Psychology: Human Perception and Performance, 28*, 1228–1242.

Carreiras, M., Perea, M., & Grainger, J. (1997). Effects of orthographic neighborhood in visual word recognition: Cross-task comparisons. *Journal of Experimental Psychology: Learning, Memory, and Cognition, 23*, 857–871.

Cerella, J. (1985). Information processing rates in the elderly. *Psychological Bulletin, 98*, 67–83.

Cerella, J. (1990). Aging and information-processing rate. In J. E. Birren & K. W. Schaie (Eds.), *Handbook of the psychology of aging* (3rd ed., pp. 201–221). San Diego, CA: Academic Press.

Coltheart, M., Davelaar, E., Jonasson, J. T., & Besner, D. (1977). Access to the internal lexicon. In S. Dornič (Ed.), *Attention and performance VI.* Hillsdale, NJ: Lawrence Erlbaum Associates, Inc.

Davidson, D. J., Zacks, R. T., & Ferreira, F. (2003). Age preservation of the syntactic processor in production. *Journal of Psycholinguistic Research, 32*, 541–566.

Davis, C. J., & Perea, M. (2005). BuscaPalabras: A program for deriving orthographic and phonological neighborhood statistics and other psycholinguistic indices in Spanish. *Behavior Research Methods, 37*, 665–671.

Diependaele, K., Sandra, D., & Grainger, J. (2005). Masked cross-modal morphological priming: Unravelling morpho-orthographic and morpho-semantic influences in early word recognition. *Language and Cognitive Processes, 20*, 75–114.

Di Sciullo, M., & Williams, E. (1987). *On the definition of word.* Linguistic Inquiry Monographs 14. Cambridge, MA: MIT Press.

Duñabeitia, J. A., Carreiras, M., & Perea, M. (in press-a). Are *coffee* and *toffee* served in a *cup*? Ortho-phonologically mediated associative priming. *Quarterly Journal of Experimental Psychology.* Epub ahead of print. DOI: 10.1080/17470210701774283.

Duñabeitia, J.A., Laka, I., Perea, M., & Carreiras, M. (in press-b). Is *Milkman* a superhero like *Batman*? Constituent morphological priming in compound words. *European Journal of Cognitive Psychology.* Epub ahead of print. DOI: 10.1080/09541440802079835.

Duñabeitia, J. A., Perea, M., & Carreiras, M. (2007a). Do transposed-letter similarity effects occur at a morpheme level? Evidence for morpho-orthographic decomposition. *Cognition, 105*, 691–703.

Duñabeitia, J. A., Perea, M., & Carreiras, M. (2007b). The role of the frequency of constituents in compound words: Evidence from Basque and Spanish. *Psychonomic Bulletin and Review, 14*, 1171–1176.

Duñabeitia, J. A., Perea, M., & Carreiras, M. (in press-c). Does *darkness* lead to *happiness*? Masked suffix priming effects. *Language and Cognitive Processes.* Epub ahead of print. DOI: 10.1080/01690960802164242.

Fiorentino, R., & Poeppel, D. (2007). Compound words and structure in the lexicon. *Language and Cognitive Processes, 22*, 953–1000.

Folstein, M. F., Folstein, S. E., & McHugh, P. R. (1975). Mini-Mental State: A practical method for grading the cognitive state of patients for the clinician. *Journal of Psychiatric Research, 12*, 189–198.

Forster, K. I., & Davis, C. (1984). Repetition priming and frequency attenuation in lexical access. *Journal of Experimental Psychology: Learning, Memory and Cognition, 10*, 680–698.

Forster, K. I., & Forster, J. C. (2003). DMDX: A Windows display program with millisecond accuracy. *Behavior Research Methods, Instruments and Computers, 35*, 116–124.

Frost, R., Deutsch, A., Gilboa, O., Tannenbaum, M., & Marslen-Wilson, W. (2000). Morphological priming: Dissociation of phonological, semantic, and morphological factors. *Memory and Cognition, 28*, 1277–1288.

Frost, R., Grainger, J., & Rastle, K. (2005a). Current issues in morphological processing: An introduction. *Language and Cognitive Processes, 20*, 1–5.

Frost, R., Kugler, T., Deutsch, A., & Forster, K. I. (2005b). Orthographic structure versus morphological structure: Principles of lexical organization in a given language. *Journal of Experimental Psychology: Learning, Memory and Cognition, 31*, 1293–1326.

Giffard, B., Desgranges, B., Piolino, P., Eustache, F., & Kerrouche, N. (2003). The hyperpriming phenomenon in normal aging: A consequence of cognitive slowing? *Neuropsychology, 17*, 594–601.

Giraudo, H., & Grainger, J. (2003). On the role of derivational affixes in recognizing complex words: Evidence from masked priming. In R. H. Baayen & R. Schreuder (Eds.), *Morphological structure in language processing* (pp. 209–232). Berlin: Mouton de Gruyter.

Howard, D. V., McAndrews, M. P., & Lasaga, M. I. (1981). Semantic priming of lexical decisions in young and old adults. *Journal of Gerontology, 36*, 707–714.

Hyönä, J., & Pollatsek, A. (1998). Reading Finnish compound words: Eye fixations are affected by component morphemes. *Journal of Experimental Psychology: Human Perception and Performance, 24*, 1612–1627.

Isel, F., Gunter, T. C., & Friederici, A. D. (2003). Prosody-assisted head-driven access to spoken German compounds. *Journal of Experimental Psychology: Learning, Memory and Cognition, 29*, 277–288.

Jarema, G., Busson, C., Nikolova, R., Tsapkini, K., & Libben, G. (1999). Processing compounds: A cross-linguistic study. *Brain and Language, 68*, 362–369.

Juhasz, B., Starr, M., Inhoff, A. W., & Placke, L. (2003). The effects of morphology on the processing of compound words: Evidence from naming, lexical decisions, and eye fixations. *British Journal of Psychology, 94*, 223–244.

Kavé, G., & Levy, Y. (2004). Preserved morphological decomposition in persons with Alzheimer's disease. *Journal of Speech, Language and Hearing Research, 47*, 835–847.

Koester, D., Gunter, T. C., & Wagner, S. (2007). The morphosyntactic decomposition and semantic composition of German compound words investigated by ERPs. *Brain and Language, 102*(1), 64–79.

Laver, G. D. (2000). A speed-accuracy analysis of word recognition in young and older adults. *Psychology and Aging, 15*, 705–709.

Laver, G. D., & Burke, D. M. (1993). Why do semantic priming effects increase in old age? A meta-analysis. *Psychology and Aging, 8*, 34–43.

Lawton, M. P. (1971). The functional assessment of elderly people. *Journal of American Geriatric Society, 19*, 465–481.

Libben, G. (1998). Semantic transparency in the processing of compounds: Consequences for representation, processing, and impairment. *Brain and Language, 61*, 30–44.

Libben, G., Gibson, M., Yoon, Y.-B., & Sandra, D. (2003). Compound fracture: The role of semantic transparency and morphological headedness. *Brain and Language, 84*, 26–43.

Lima, S. D., Hale, S., & Myerson, J. (1991). How general is general slowing? Evidence from the lexical domain. *Psychology and Aging, 6*, 416–425.

Marslen-Wilson, W. D., Ford, M., Older, L., & Zhou, X. (1996). The combinatorial lexicon: Priming derivational affixes. In G. Cottrell (Ed.), *Proceedings of the 18th annual conference of the Cognitive Science Society* (pp. 223–227). Mahwah, NJ: Lawrence Erlbaum Associates, Inc.

Meyer, D. E., & Schvaneveldt, R. W. (1971). Facilitation in recognizing pairs of words: Evidence of a dependence between retrieval operations. *Journal of Experimental Psychology, 90*, 227–234.

Monsell, S. (1985). Repetition and the lexicon. In A. Ellis (Ed.), *Progress in the psychology of language* (pp. 147–195). Hove, UK: Lawrence Erlbaum Associates Ltd.

Myerson, J., Hale, S., Chen, J., & Lawrence, B. (1997). General lexical slowing and the semantic priming effect: The roles of age and ability. *Acta Psychologica, 96*, 83–101.

Ober, B. A., Shenaut, K., Jagust, W. J., & Stillman, R. C. (1991). Automatic semantic priming with various category relations in Alzheimer's disease and normal aging. *Psychology and Aging, 6*, 647–660.

Peña-Casanova, J. (2005). *Test neuropsicológicos: fundamentos para una neuropsicología clínica basada en evidencias*. Barcelona: Masson.

Perea, M., Duñabeitia, J.A., & Carreiras, M. (2008). Masked associative/semantic priming effects across languages with highly proficient bilinguals. *Journal of Memory and Language, 58*, 916–930.

Perea, M., & Gotor, A. (1997). Associative and semantic priming effects occur at very short SOAs in lexical decision and naming. *Cognition, 62*, 223–240.

Perea, M., & Rosa, E. (2002). The effects of associative and semantic priming in the lexical decision task. *Psychological Research, 66*, 180–194.

Pollatsek, A., Hyönä, J., & Bertram, R. (2000). The role of morphological constituents in reading Finnish compound words. *Journal of Experimental Psychology: Human Perception and Performance, 26*, 820–833.

Pollatsek, A., & Well, A. (1995). On the use of counterbalanced designs in cognitive research: A suggestion for a better and more powerful analysis. *Journal of Experimental Psychology: Learning, Memory and Cognition, 21*, 785–794.

Raaijmakers, J. G. W. (2003). A further look at the "language-as-fixed-effect fallacy". *Canadian Journal of Experimental Psychology, 57*, 141–151.

Raaijmakers, J. G. W., Schrijnemakers, J. M. C., & Gremmen, F. (1999). How to deal with "the language as a fixed effect fallacy:" Common misconceptions and alternative solutions. *Journal of Memory and Language, 41*, 416–426.

Rastle, K., Davis, M. H., & New, B. (2004). The broth in my brother's brothel: Morpho-orthographic segmentation in visual word recognition. *Psychonomic Bulletin and Review, 11*, 1090–1098.

Rastle, K., Davis, M. H., Tyler, L. K., & Marslen-Wilson, W. D. (2000). Morphological and semantic effects in visual word recognition: A time-course study. *Language and Cognitive Processes, 15*, 507–537.

Ratcliff, R. (1993). Methods for dealing with reaction time outliers. *Psychological Bulletin, 114*, 510–532.

Ratcliff, R., Perea, M., Colangelo, A., & Buchanan, L. (2004a). A diffusion model account of normal and impaired readers. *Brain and Cognition, 55*, 374–382.

Ratcliff, R., Thapar, A., Gómez, P., & McKoon, G. (2004b). A diffusion model analysis of the effects of aging in the lexical-decision task. *Psychology and Aging, 19*, 278–289.

Rayner, K., Reichle, E. D., Stroud, M. J., Williams, C. C., & Pollatsek, A. (2006). The effects of word frequency, word predictability, and font difficulty on the eye movements of young and elderly readers. *Psychology and Aging, 21*(3), 448–465.

Rey, A. (1958). *L'examen clinique en psychologie.* Paris: Press Universitaires de France.

Roelofs, A. P. A., & Baayen, R. H. (2002). Morphology by itself in planning the production of spoken words. *Psychonomic Bulletin and Review, 9*(1), 132–138.

Sandra, D. (1990). On the representation and processing of compound words: Automatic access to constituent morphemes does not occur. *Quarterly Journal of Experimental Psychology, 42A*, 529–567.

Sebastián-Gallés, N., Martí, M. A., Carreiras, M., & Cuetos, F. (2000). *LEXESP: Léxico informatizado del español.* Barcelona, Spain: Edicions Universitat de Barcelona.

Shoolman, N., & Andrews, S. (2003). Racehorses, reindeers and sparrows: Using masked priming to investigate morphological influences on word identification. In S. Kinoshita & S. Lupker (Eds.), *Masked priming: The state of the art* (pp. 241–278). Hove, UK: Psychology Press.

Snodgrass, J. G., & Vanderwart, M. (1980). A standardized set of 260 pictures: Norms for name agreement, image agreement, familiarity, and visual complexity. *Journal of Experimental Psychology: Human Learning and Memory, 6*, 174–215.

Spieler, D. H., & Balota, D. A. (2000). Factors influencing word naming in younger and older adults. *Psychology and Aging, 15*, 225–231.

Spreen, O., & Strauss, E. (1991). *A compendium of neuropsychological tests.* New York: Oxford University Press.

Stamatakis, E. A., & Tyler, L. K. (2006). Language lateralisation as a function of age. *Journal of Cognitive Neuroscience, 18*(Suppl.), A128.

Waters, G., & Caplan, D. (2005). The relationship between age, processing speed, working memory capacity, and language comprehension. *Memory, 13*, 403–413.

Yesavage, J. A. (1983). Development and validation of a geriatrics depression scale. *Journal of Psychiatric Research*, *17*, 31–49.

Zwitserlood, P. (1994). The role of semantic transparency in the processing and representation of Dutch compounds. *Language and Cognitive Processes*, *9*, 341–368.

Zwitserlood, P., Bölte, J., & Dohmes, P. (2000). Morphological effects on speech production: Evidence from picture naming. *Language and Cognitive Processes*, *15*, 563–591.

Zwitserlood, P., Bölte, J., & Dohmes, P. (2002). Where and how morphologically complex words interplay with naming pictures. *Brain and Language*, *81*, 358–367.

EUROPEAN JOURNAL OF COGNITIVE PSYCHOLOGY
2009, 21 (2/3), 303–329

Psychology Press
Taylor & Francis Group

Memory accuracy in old age: Cognitive, metacognitive, and neurocognitive determinants

Ainat Pansky, Morris Goldsmith, and Asher Koriat
Department of Psychology, University of Haifa, Haifa, Israel

Shiri Pearlman-Avnion
Department of Education, Tel-Hai Academic College, Tel Hai, Israel

Age differences in memory accuracy were examined within a conceptual framework specifying the mediating role of metacognitive monitoring and control processes (Koriat & Goldsmith, 1996b). Replicating previous results, older adults showed poorer memory quantity and accuracy performance compared to young adults. Even when memory quantity performance was equated, by dividing the young adults' attention during encoding, the difference in memory accuracy was not eliminated. Examination of the underlying metacognitive processes revealed that the age-related reduction in memory accuracy stemmed partly from less effective memory monitoring, apparently the result of poorer encoding, and also from differences in two aspects of metacognitive control: (1) a more liberal report criterion—greater tendency to volunteer incorrect (and correct) answers, and (2) reduced control sensitivity—less reliance on subjective monitoring as a basis for responding. This latter control reduction was associated with lower neuropsychological measures of executive functioning, suggesting a decline in frontal-lobe efficiency.

Keywords: Memory accuracy; Metamemory; Ageing; Executive processes; Memory control.

Memory decline in old age is both ubiquitous and multifaceted. Much of the work on this topic has focused on the amount of information that can be recalled or recognised. In the last few years, however, accumulating evidence indicates an age-related decline in memory accuracy as well. Older adults have been found to be particularly vulnerable to memory slips and errors that can have serious consequences, such as taking the same medicine twice

Correspondence should be addressed to Ainat Pansky, Department of Psychology, University of Haifa, Haifa 31905, Israel. E-mail: pansky@research.haifa.ac.il

This research was supported by the Charles E. Smith Extended Grant on the Subject of Memory, awarded by the National Institute for Psychobiology in Israel to AK, MG, and AP.

http://www.psypress.com/ecp DOI: 10.1080/09541440802281183

(Koriat, Ben-Zur, & Sheffer, 1988) or being taken in by scams and frauds (Jacoby & Rhodes, 2006).

There are numerous references in the literature to possible links between the memory impairments associated with ageing and neuropsychological deficits in frontal-lobe functioning. Thus, the age-related pattern of memory errors that is characteristic of old age resembles the pattern found in patients suffering frontal lobe lesions (see Moscovitch & Winocur, 1992, 1995; Perfect, 1997, for reviews). This similarity suggests that one source of age-related deficits in memory accuracy may be a decline in frontal lobe efficiency. This idea is supported further by converging anatomical, physiological, and neurological evidence indicating pronounced frontal lobe deficits in old age (see Raz, 2000; Stuss, Craik, Sayer, Franchi, & Alexander, 1996; West, 1996; but see Greenwood, 2000).

Frontal-lobe functioning, in turn, has been broadly associated with so-called "executive functions". These functions are generally assumed to include the monitoring and control of one's own behaviour, the ability to suppress irrelevant information and to inhibit prepotent responses, the ability to shift between mental sets or tasks and to control attention, and the monitoring of working memory contents (see, e.g., Miyake et al., 2000; Shimamura, 2000). Executive functions are also assumed to include higher cognitive processes such as reasoning and planning (Waltz et al., 1999; West, 1996). Focusing specifically on memory processes, converging evidence suggests the frontal lobe is involved in strategic processes that support memory encoding, recovery, monitoring, and verification (see Moscovitch & Winocur, 2002).

Finally, some of the age-related impairments in memory functioning appear to be linked to executive functions. Thus, recent behavioural studies employing a wide range of memory paradigms have found superior memory performance for older adults achieving high scores on neuropsychological tests of executive functioning compared to older adults scoring poorly on such tests (e.g., Butler, McDaniel, Dornburg, Price, & Roediger, 2004; Chan & McDermott, 2007; Davidson & Glisky, 2002; Glisky, Polster, & Routhieaux, 1995; Glisky, Rubin, & Davidson, 2001; McDaniel, Glisky, Rubin, Guynn, & Routhieaux, 1999; Roediger & Geraci, 2007).

In this study, we aimed to shed further light on the links between memory accuracy deficits, neuropsychological deficits, and ageing, within a general theoretical model specifying the mediating role of metacognitive processes. That model was developed in previous work with young adults (Koriat & Goldsmith, 1996b) with the goal of clarifying the role of metacognitive processes in the strategic regulation of both memory quantity and memory accuracy performance.

Traditionally, memory research has focused on *memory quantity*—the amount of information that can be recalled or recognised after a retention interval. Hence, measures of memory performance have typically been calculated conditional on the input, by expressing the number of items recalled or recognised as the proportion or percentage of the total number of items presented. Such measures reflect the amount of presented or studied information that has been retained and is currently accessible. More recently, however increasing interest has been directed to *memory accuracy*—the extent to which the person's memory report accords with what has been presented. A very common and simple measure of memory accuracy is *output-bound proportion correct*: The number of correct items recalled or recognised is expressed as a proportion or percentage of the total number of items reported. Unlike the input-bound quantity measures, this type of accuracy measure is conditional on the output, reflecting the probability that a reported item is correct. Consider, for example, a participant who is presented with 30 words (items of information), and in a recall test reports 15 words (provides answers to 15 questions), 12 of which are correct and 3 are commission errors (wrong answers). Input-bound memory quantity performance in this case is 0.40 (12/30), that is, 40% of the input-studied items (questions) have been successfully recalled (answered). In contrast, output-bound memory accuracy is 0.80 (12/15). That is, 80% of the output-reported items (answers) are, in fact, correct. This latter measure uniquely reflects the *dependability* of the information that is reported—the degree to which each reported item can be trusted to be correct. Essentially, then, whereas the input-bound quantity measure holds the rememberer responsible for what he or she fails to report, the output-bound accuracy measure holds the person accountable only for what he or she does report.

Importantly, output-bound accuracy and input-bound quantity measures can be distinguished operationally only under conditions of *free report*, that is, only when the rememberer has the option of deciding which items of information to report and which to withhold. This condition is typical of most real-life memory situations. In contrast, under forced-report conditions, in which people are required to answer each and every question (as in standard forced-choice recognition tests), the input-bound (quantity) and output-bound (accuracy) memory measures are operationally equivalent. This is because the number of output items is the same as the number of input items (see Koriat & Goldsmith, 1994, 1996a).

The option of free report is essential when the focus is on output-bound memory accuracy. Just as an eyewitness cannot be expected to uphold the oath to tell "nothing but the truth" under forced-report conditions, neither does it make sense to hold participants accountable for the errors that they make under such conditions. Indeed, only under free-report conditions, when rememberers have the option to respond "don't know", can we assume that they are actually committed to the accuracy of their memory output.

THE STRATEGIC REGULATION OF MEMORY REPORTING: A METACOGNITIVE FRAMEWORK

The focus on memory accuracy in addition to memory quantity has led researchers to incorporate a wider range of phenomena and processes into the study of memory than has been done in traditional memory research (e.g., Koriat, Goldsmith, & Pansky, 2000). For example, a great deal of research in the area of metacognition has examined the processes by which people monitor the validity of their memories, as well as the accuracy of this monitoring (e.g., Koriat, 1993; Koriat, Lichtenstein, & Fischhoff, 1980; Schwartz, 1994). Other studies have examined the manner in which monitoring processes are actually used in controlling the process of remembering, and in regulating memory performance (e.g., Barnes, Nelson, Dunlosky, Mazzoni, & Narens, 1999; Goldsmith & Koriat, 1999, 2008; Higham, 2002, 2007; Koriat & Goldsmith, 1994, 1996b; Koriat, Goldsmith, & Halamish, 2008; Nelson & Narens, 1990). Most relevant to present purposes, the examination of monitoring and control processes operating during memory retrieval has provided important insights regarding memory deficits in old age (e.g., Henkel, Johnson, & de Leonardis, 1998; Jacoby, Bishara, Hessels, & Toth, 2005; Kelley & Sahakyan, 2003; Koutstaal, 2006; Rhodes & Kelley, 2005).

We now outline the conceptual framework proposed by Koriat and Goldsmith (1996b), which guided the present investigation. Their model of the strategic regulation of memory reporting allows the examination of memory quantity and memory accuracy performance within a common framework, focusing on the manner in which performance is mediated by metacognitive processes that operate during memory reporting. As shown in Figure 1, in addition to an unspecified retrieval (or ecphory, reconstruction, etc.) mechanism, the model includes a *monitoring* mechanism that is used to subjectively assess the correctness of potential memory responses, and a *control* mechanism that determines whether or not to volunteer the best available candidate answer (for similar models, see Barnes et al., 1999; Higham, 2002). The control mechanism operates by setting a report criterion on the monitoring output: The answer is volunteered if its assessed probability of being correct passes the criterion, but is withheld otherwise. The criterion is set on the basis of implicit or explicit payoffs, that is, the perceived gain for providing correct information relative to the cost of providing incorrect information.

Based on this simple model, the overall quality of free-report memory performance (quantity and accuracy) may be seen to depend on four components: (1) *overall retention*—the amount of correct information (i.e., the number of correct candidate answers) that can be retrieved; (2) *monitoring effectiveness*—the extent to which the subjective confidence

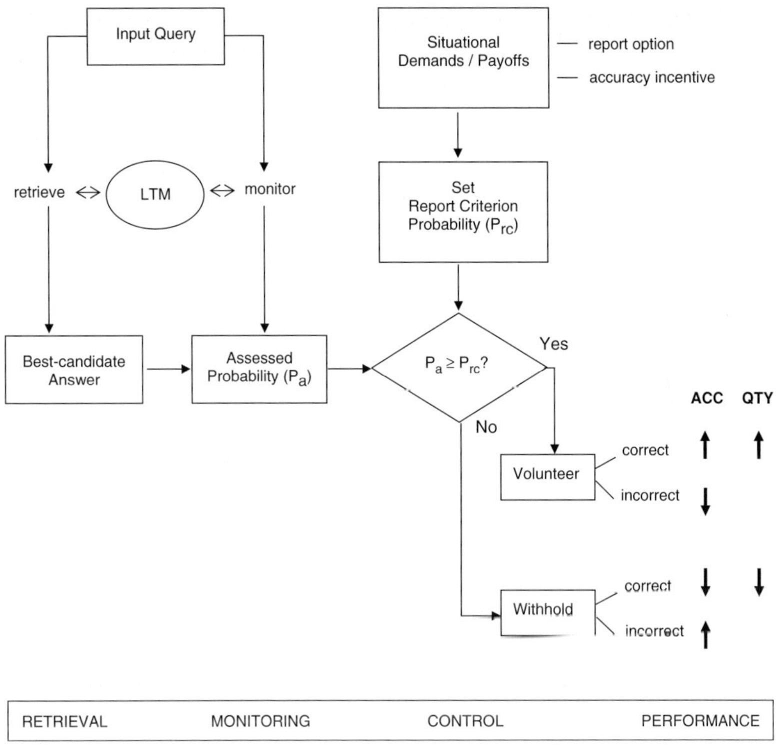

Figure 1. A schematic model of the strategic regulation of memory accuracy and memory quantity performance, utilising the option of free report. The upward and downward pointing arrows on the right of the figure signify positive and negative performance outcomes. LTM = long-term memory; ACC = accuracy; QTY = quantity; P_a = assessed probability; P_{rc} = response criterion probability (adapted from Koriat & Goldsmith, 1996b).

judgements successfully differentiate correct from incorrect candidate answers; (3) *control sensitivity*—the extent to which the volunteering or withholding of answers is in fact based on the monitoring output; (4) *report criterion setting*—the report criterion above which answers are volunteered, below which they are withheld.

Results from various studies have provided strong support for the model, revealing the manner in which monitoring and control processes mediate between memory retrieval on the one hand and memory performance on the other (Danion, Gokalsing, Robert, Massin-Krauss, & Bacon, 2001; Goldsmith, Koriat, & Pansky, 2005; Goldsmith, Koriat, & Weinberg-Eliezer, 2002; Higham, 2002; Higham & Tam, 2005; Kelley & Sahakyan, 2003; Koren et al., 2004; Koriat & Goldsmith, 1996b; Payne, Lambert, & Jacoby, 2002; Rhodes & Kelley, 2005; for a review see Goldsmith & Koriat, 2008).

Most important for the present study is the methodology that was developed to assess the contribution of each component to free-report memory performance (Koriat & Goldsmith, 1996b). This methodology, which was adapted here to the study of age-related deficits, will be described briefly. It is based on a two-phase, free-forced paradigm. Participants are exposed to a memory input stimulus and later given either a recall or recognition test using the following procedure:

1. *Forced-report phase*: A cue is presented for each studied item, and participants are required to provide an answer even if they have to guess. In addition, the participant also indicates his/her confidence regarding the correctness of each answer.
2. *Free-report phase*: The participant is presented with the same cues again (either the cues alone or the cue-answer pairs from the previous phase) under free-report instructions: He/she must indicate whether he/she would like to "volunteer" the answer or "withhold" it. Monetary or point incentives for accurate volunteering are offered, for example, a 1-point bonus for each correct volunteered answer but a 2-point penalty for each incorrect volunteered answer (withheld answers receive no bonus but also no penalty).

The measures that can be derived are as follows:

1. *Free-report accuracy* and *quantity* performance (output-bound and input-bound proportions correct, respectively), based only on the Phase-2 answers. These can be treated as measure of "actual" memory performance.
2. *Forced-report quantity correct*, based only on Phase-1 answers. This can be used as an estimate of how much information is accessible in memory ("retention" or "ecphory").
3. *Monitoring effectiveness*, based on the relationship between confidence judgements and the forced-report answers (Phase 1). Within-subject gamma correlations (Nelson, 1984) are generally used to measure *monitoring resolution*—the extent to which the confidence judgements distinguish between correct and incorrect answers. Calibration bias scores, reflecting over/underconfidence (i.e., the extent to which the confidence judgements are higher or lower than the actual proportions correct; see Lichtenstein, Fischhoff, & Phillips, 1982) may sometimes also be calculated.
4. *Control sensitivity*, the extent to which the free-report volunteering and withholding decisions in Phase 2 are based on the monitoring output (confidence ratings in Phase 1). This can be indexed by within-

participant gamma correlations between confidence (Phase 1) and volunteering-withholding decisions (Phase 2).

5. *Control policy (report criterion)*, the minimum level of confidence that is required by the participant before he/she is willing to volunteer an answer. This can be estimated by finding a cutoff on the confidence ratings that best separates the items that were volunteered and those that were withheld in Phase 2. Alternatively, Phase-2 volunteering or withholding ratios can be compared, while partialling out differences in forced-report quantity correct and/or differences in mean confidence ratings (cf. B''_D in Higham, 2002).

Neuropsychological evidence suggests that frontal lobes are at least partially involved in metamemory judgements (e.g., Janowsky, Shimamura, & Squire, 1989; Vilkki, Servo, & Surma-aho, 1998; see also Fernandez-Duque, Baird, & Posner, 2000). Assuming that old age is associated with a decline in frontal lobe functioning, then we may expect age-related declines in metamemory processes, but the evidence so far has been mixed and inconclusive (see Hertzog & Dunlosky, 2004; Hertzog & Hultsch, 2000; Souchay &Isingrini, 2004; Souchay, Isingrini, & Espagnet, 2000).

Recently, Kelley and colleagues (Kelley & Sahakyan, 2003; Rhodes & Kelley, 2005) utilised Koriat and Goldsmith's (1996b) model and methodology in conjunction with Kato's (1985) associative interference paradigm to compare the strategic regulatory processes of younger and older adults. Kelley and Sahakyan (2003, Exp. 1) found that for control word-pairs (not expected to elicit associative interference), forced-report performance was superior for younger than for older participants. However, the older participants were successful in taking advantage of the option to withhold answers to narrow the gap between their level of free report accuracy performance and that of the younger participants. In contrast, for "deceptive" word-pairs (in which the retrieval cues evoke a highly accessible associate that competes with the target, thereby presenting a difficult challenge to memory monitoring), the age difference in accuracy performance became, if anything, somewhat larger under free-report than under forced report. This interactive pattern was accounted for in terms of age-related differences in monitoring effectiveness. Indeed, although both older and younger participants were highly overconfident in the correctness of their responses to the deceptive items, the degree of overconfidence was more pronounced for the older participants. Furthermore, the older participants exhibited lower levels of monitoring resolution for both deceptive and control items.

Additional experiments suggested that the impaired monitoring of the older participants derived from impoverished encoding: When the encoding of the younger participants was disrupted by having them study the word list under divided attention, they exhibited a pattern of performance that was very similar to that of the older participants in terms of both memory accuracy and memory monitoring. Kelley and Sahakyan (2003) suggested that the poorer memory monitoring of older adults derives primarily from their greater reliance on the familiarity of candidate responses rather than on recollection of details of the study experience (Jacoby, 1999; Jacoby, Debner, & Hay, 2001), which in turn stems, at least in part, from poor encoding. A similar conclusion was reached by Rhodes and Kelley (2005), who used the same approach to investigate age differences in memory performance, but now tying these to neuropsychological measures of executive functioning. In their study, path analyses supported a model in which ageing impairs executive functioning, which in turn impairs retention (forced-report performance—a product of both encoding quality and retrieval), which in turn impairs free-report memory accuracy, both directly, and also indirectly by way of impaired monitoring. No age-related differences in control processes were found in either of these studies.

THE CURRENT STUDY

The current study also examined age-related differences in metacognitive and neurocognitive functioning that contribute to accurate memory performance. However, in contrast to Kelley and Sahakyan (2003) and Rhodes and Kelley (2005), we were primarily interested in potential age-related differences in metacognitive control. This focus was motivated by several results indicating systematic population differences in measures of control (see Goldsmith & Koriat, 2008; and see later). Consequently, rather than use a list-learning task with deceptive pairs, which placed a large burden on monitoring, we used a more naturalistic memory task, testing the memory for a simple slide show, without making any special attempt to mislead or hamper memory monitoring.

We followed the recommendation of previous researchers to facilitate the interpretation of age-related metamemory comparisons by equating the baseline quantity performance of the older and younger participants (see Perfect & Stollery, 1993). Because of the well-documented age-related decline in episodic memory quantity (Craik & Anderson, 1999), we included in our study a group of young participants who were presented with the stimulus materials under divided attention at study (e.g., Jennings & Jacoby, 1993; Kelley & Sahakyan, 2003). Thus, the experiment included three groups: young full-attention control, young divided-attention, and older adults. All participants were presented with a computerised slide show and accompanying narration describing an event in the life of a family. The young divided-attention pariticipants performed a concurrent auditory task while watching the show. Thirty questions about the show were then presented in multiple-choice recognition format. Report option was manipulated as follows: In the first phase, the participants were required to answer all 30 questions, and to indicate their confidence in the correctness of each answer. In the second phase, the participants were asked to take the same test again under free-report instructions, deciding which answers to volunteer and which to withhold, with a monetary incentive for accurate reporting. Note that, in contrast to Kelley and Sahakyan (2003) and Rhodes and Kelley (2005), who implemented the two phases on an item-by-item basis, we followed Koriat and Goldsmith's (1996b) procedure in which the confidence judgements and volunteering decisions are elicited in two separate phases of the experiment. Although the item-by-item method has its advantages (see Goldsmith & Koriat, 2008), we thought that the two-phase method might reduce possible demand characteristics, by which the expectation that one's volunteering decisions should be based on one's confidence judgements might be conveyed implicitly in the procedure itself, making it more difficult to find differences in control sensitivity.

In order to assess the role of executive functioning as a potential mediator of the age-related decline in memory accuracy, the older participants were administered two tests that are commonly used in neuropsychological research to evaluate executive functioning (see, e.g., Rhodes, 2004; Salthouse, Atkinson, & Berish, 2003).[1] The older adults were sampled across a wide range of ages, with the goal of achieving adequate variation on measures of executive functioning, metacognitive functioning, and free-report performance within this age group.

METHOD

Participants

The experiment included three groups of participants: (1) 20 older adults (aged 62 to 87, mean = 73, *SD* = 7.11) (2) 20 young adults (aged 17 to 26, mean = 23), assigned to the full-attention group, and (3) 20 young adults assigned to the divided-attention group (aged 20 to 28, mean = 22). These groups will be designated as older, Young-FA, and Young-DA, respectively. All the participants were healthy and had normal hearing and normal or corrected vision.

[1] We did not administer these neuropsychological tests to the young adults because, based on previous research (see Rhodes, 2004), we did not expect to find much meaningful variance for this population.

Materials

The participants were presented with a computerised slide show lasting about 4 min. It consisted of 27 colour photographs presented on a high-resolution (super VGA) screen controlled by an IBM-PC compatible computer. The pictures were presented at a rate of 8 s per picture, with about 0.5 s between pictures. Each picture was accompanied by a recorded narration spoken in Hebrew by a professional radio broadcaster, which was produced through speakers attached to the computer.

The show ("On the Way to the Picnic") depicts a staged incident in the life of a family preparing to go out on a picnic, in which the family cat climbed up an electricity pole and had to be enticed by various means to come down. The story begins with an introduction to each family member, which is followed by a sequence of events culminating in the successful rescue of the cat. For the Young-DA group, a pseudorandom sequence of 300 Hz and 600 Hz tones was presented concurrently with the slide show. The participants were asked to count how many tones of each type (low frequency, high frequency) were sounded.

A 30-item memory questionnaire concerning the slide show was developed in a five-alternative recognition format. The questions related both to aspects that were central to the story and to peripheral details (e.g., Why did the cat . . .? What was the colour of the mother's dress?). Most of the answers consisted of a single word or name. In the forced-report phase, each question was accompanied by a 5-point "thermometer" scale, ranging from "very cold" to "very hot", on which the participants were asked to indicate their confidence that their chosen answer was correct. Higher confidence was indicated by "hotter" ratings. We chose to use this rating scale, rather than subjective probability assessments of correctness used Koriat and Goldsmith's (1996b) study with young adults, because we wanted to obtain a "gut feeling" rather than an analytic judgement, and because we suspected that some of the older adults might encounter difficulties in assigning such probabilities. This decision precluded some of the standard measures associated with the Koriat and Goldsmith framework (e.g. calibration bias), and required a few modifications in the data analyses which will be described in the Results section.[2]

Two tests of executive function were used. The first test was a Hebrew version of the Verbal Fluency (FAS) test, including three speeded tasks (60 s each) requiring the listing of as many words as possible: (1) in the ANIMAL category, (2) in either the fruit or vegetable category, and (3) starting with the

[2] In light of the findings of two studies that were published after the current study was conducted (Kelley & Sahakyan, 2003; Rhodes & Kelley, 2005), perhaps we were overcautious regarding these considerations.

Hebrew letters SHIN or MEM. The total number of unique words produced served as the dependent measure. The second test was the Wisconsin Card Sorting Task (WCST; Hart, Kwentus, Wade, & Taylor, 1988). The two most commonly used scores—number of categories achieved and number of perseverative errors committed—served as dependent measures.

Procedure

After viewing the slide show, the participants' memory was tested in two phases. The first was a forced-report five-alternative multiple choice recognition test in which the participants were asked to answer each item (guessing if necessary) and to indicate their level of confidence in the correctness of their answer on the 5-point "thermometer" scale.

In the second, free-report phase, participants went over the answers they had provided in the previous phase, now without the associated confidence judgements (which were cut away), and were given the option to either volunteer or withhold each of the answers. This phase included a payoff schedule according to which participants were told that they would gain 10 bonus points for each correct answer volunteered, but would lose 10 points for each incorrect answer volunteered. However, they need not volunteer all the answers; for those answers withheld they would not gain any points but neither would they lose any points. The participants were told that when the study was over, they would receive a monetary prize proportional to the number of points each of them earned.

Finally, the older participants (only) were tested on the FAS and WCST.

RESULTS

Based on Koriat and Goldsmith's (1996b) model, we compared the three groups of participants on free-report memory performance, both accuracy and quantity, and on four component measures: (1) memory retention (the amount of remembered information), (2) monitoring effectiveness (the ability to discriminate between correct and incorrect answers), (3) control sensitivity (the extent to which the decision to volunteer a particular answer is based on the monitoring output), and (4) free-report volunteering rate (after equating mean confidence) as an indirect measure of control policy. Post hoc paired comparisons were performed using Scheffe's test (.05 criterion value).

As expected, memory retention, measured in terms of forced-report memory performance (quantity or accuracy), was superior for the Young-FA participants (.84) than for both the older participants (.69) and the Young-DA participants (.68), $F(2,\ 57) = 10.32$, $MSE = 139.43$, $p < .001$, $\eta^2 = .27$.

The latter two groups did not differ, indicating our success in equating baseline quantity performance.

As shown in Figure 2, the option of free report allowed all three groups of participants to enhance the accuracy of their reports considerably. However, a one-way analysis of variance (ANOVA) indicated that there were still substantial differences between the groups in free-report memory accuracy, $F(2, 57) = 5.72$, $MSE = 108.51$, $p < .01$, $\eta^2 = .17$. The older adults showed inferior accuracy performance (.87) than both the Young-DA (.94) and the Young-FA adults (.98). In comparing memory accuracy under free and

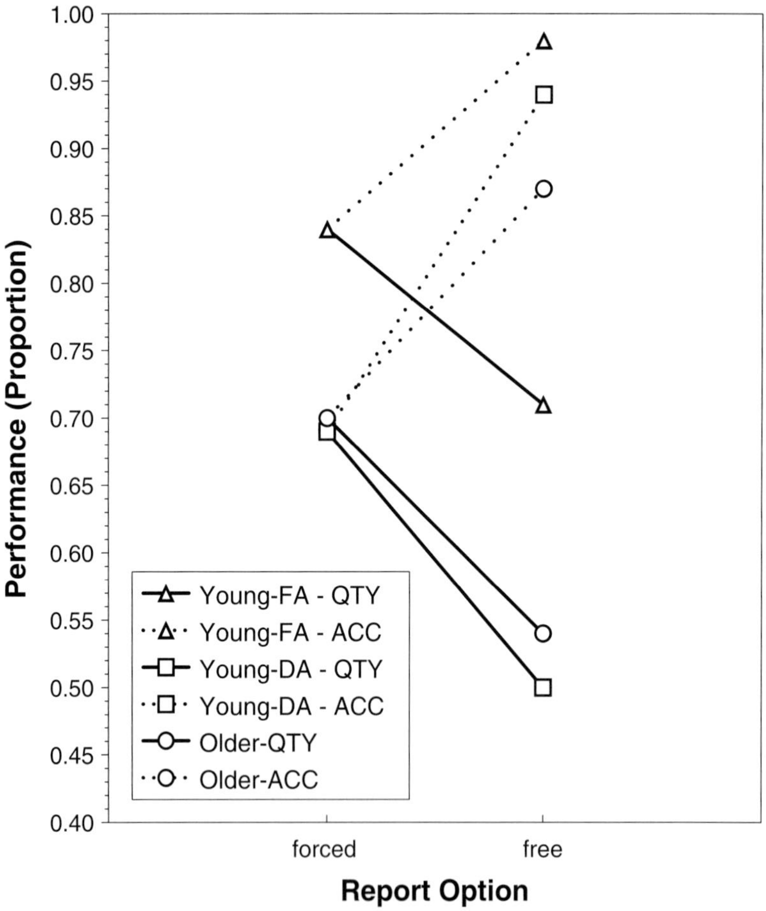

Figure 2. Quantity (QTY) and accuracy (ACC) performance, under free versus forced memory reporting, for the three groups of participants: (1) young adults in the full attention condition (Young-FA), (2) young adults in the divided attention condition (Young-DA), and (3) older adults (Older).

forced instructions, it appears that although the older participants' memory performance was practically identical to that of the Young-DA group under forced-report conditions, the older group did not gain as much as the Young-DA group did from the opportunity to screen out wrong answers, with free-forced accuracy improvements of .17 and .25, respectively, $F(1, 38) = 4.25$, $MSE = 147.03$, $p < .05$, $\eta^2 = .10$. Note that by exercising the option to withhold answers, the Young-DA group was able to close the gap with the Young-FA group, achieving comparable free-report accuracy. The increase in memory accuracy due to the exercise of free-report option, however, came at the cost of a reduction in memory quantity performance. This cost was more pronounced for the Young-DA group (.19) than for the older group (.13), $F(1, 38) = 6.48$, $MSE = 58.70$, $p < .05$, $\eta^2 = .15$. Thus, it appears that the two groups chose different strategies in trading quantity for accuracy, with the older group putting more emphasis on quantity and the Young-DA group putting more emphasis on accuracy. In fact, given the particular incentive matrix used in the current experiment, these two different tradeoffs yielded equivalent payoffs: The average number of points earned in the free-report stage did not significantly differ for the older group (143) and for the Young-DA group (138.5), but both groups earned significantly less bonus points than the Young-FA group (209), $F(2, 57) = 10.88$, $MSE = 2864.12$, $p < .001$, $\eta^2 = .28$.

What are the mechanisms underlying age-related changes in memory performance? Our paradigm allowed us to trace the observed age differences in free-report accuracy and quantity performance to differences in metacognitive monitoring and control. Regarding monitoring, one can use the option of free report to enhance accuracy only to the extent that one is able to discriminate correct from incorrect answers. *Monitoring effectiveness* (resolution) was evaluated in terms of the within-subject Goodman-Kruskal gamma correlation between the assessed confidence and the correctness of each answer (Nelson, 1984). Gamma averaged .81, .83, and .92, for the older group, the Young-DA group, and the Young-FA group, respectively, $F(2, 57) = 3.20$, $MSE = 0.02$, $p < .05$, $\eta^2 = .10$. Thus, both the older adults and the Young-DA group exhibited poorer monitoring than the Young-FA group. However, the monitoring resolution of the older adults was comparable to that of the Young-DA group. This pattern of results indicates, in line with Rhodes and Kelley's (2005) results, that age-related differences in monitoring resolution are eliminated when the quality of encoding is equated. Hence, age-related monitoring differences may in fact stem from differences in the efficiency of encoding processes. The results also suggest, however, that part of the age related reduction in memory accuracy, observed in comparing the older and Young-DA groups, stems from sources other than differences in monitoring resolution and/or encoding quality.

As mentioned earlier, the use of the confidence rating scale, rather than probability assessments of correctness, precluded the calculation of calibration bias scores (but see comparable measure in the later path analysis). Nonetheless, comparison of the mean confidence rating of the older adults (3.9) to that of the Young-DA group (3.7) does not reveal a significant difference between the two groups, $F(1, 38) = 2.07$, $MSE = 0.30$, *ns*, $\eta^2 = .05$. Given the comparable forced-report quantity performance of the two groups (reported previously), there is no evidence of an age-related difference in over- or underconfidence (the interaction between age group and measure, forced-report quantity vs. confidence, was not significant, $F < 1$).

As noted earlier, effective monitoring should enhance memory accuracy only to the extent that the control decision (i.e., whether or not to volunteer each answer) is sensitive to the monitoring output. To assess *control sensitivity*, we calculated within-subject gamma correlations between subjective confidence and the decision to volunteer an answer. These correlations were found to differ significantly between the groups. $F(2, 57) = 4.20$, $MSE = 0.01$, $p < .05$, $\eta^2 = .13$. The relationship between confidence and volunteering was less strong for the older participants (mean gamma = .90) than for both the Young-FA participants (mean gamma = .99) and the Young-DA participants (mean gamma = .96).

In addition, the older participants chose to volunteer significantly more answers (mean = 19.7) than did the Young-DA participants (mean = 15.9), $F(1, 57) = 6.73$, $MSE = 22.02$, $p < .05$, $\eta^2 = .15$. Given that the two groups exhibited comparable memory quantity performance and provided equally high confidence ratings in the forced-report phase, this pattern indicates that the older adults employed a more liberal *control policy* than their younger counterparts. This difference was also implied in the different accuracy–quantity tradeoff patterns observed earlier in comparing the different accuracy gains and quantity costs of free versus forced reporting exhibited by the two groups.

We turn next to examination of the results of the neurocognitive measures collected for the older group. In order to assess the potential role of executive functioning in the age-related memory and metamemory deficits, we calculated the correlations across participants within the older age group, between the memory measures, metacognitive measures, the neurocognitive indices obtained from WCST and the verbal fluency test, and age (in months).

As shown in Table 1, age differences within the older age group were found to be negatively correlated with the positive indices of executive functioning (verbal fluency, categories achieved in WCST) and positively correlated with the negative indices (total errors and preservation errors in WCST). Thus, the older the participant, the worse his or her performance on executive tests. In order to avoid the confound of neuropsychological

TABLE 1
Correlations between memory/metamemory indices and measures of executive functioning of the older participants

	Age	*Memory retention*	*Memory accuracy*	*Monitoring resolution*	*Control sensitivity*
FAS	−.68*	.58*	.62*	.43	.59*
WCSTc	−.53*	.24	.57*	.39	.42
WCSTt	.54*	−.30	−.58*	−.38	−.53*
WCSTp	.53*	−.46*	−.70*	−.44*	−.74*
Age	—	−.57*	−.63*	−.45*	−.42

*$p < .05$. FAS = Word fluency; WCSTc = WCST categories achieved; WCSTt = WCST total errors; WCSTp = WCST perseverative errors.

functioning with age, we examined the relationships between the executive measures and the cognitive measures using second-order partial correlations to partial out the age factor. These data, presented in Table 2, show that the executive measure of perseverative errors on WCST is strongly and negatively correlated with both memory accuracy ($r = -.56$) and control sensitivity ($r = -.67$), and that control sensitivity is correlated with the FAS index as well ($r = .46$).

With the aim of gaining a clearer picture of the direct and indirect contributions of age and executive functioning to free-report memory accuracy, and how these are mediated by memory and metamemory components, a series of path analyses were conducted (see Figure 3).[3] Based on Koriat and Goldsmith's (1996b) framework, each path model assumed that free-report accuracy was affected directly by forced-report quantity correct (the amount of correct information that is accessible in memory), monitoring resolution (within-participant gamma correlation between confidence rating and actual correctness of the answer), mean confidence, answer withholding rate (percentage of answers withheld under free report), and control sensitivity (within-participant gamma correlation between confidence rating and the decision to volunteer/withhold the answer). In addition, monitoring resolution was assumed to depend in part on the amount and quality of accessible information in memory (see Kelley & Sahakyan, 2003; Koriat, 1993, 1995; Rhodes & Kelley, 2005). Hence, age or

[3] Because of the small sample sizes, these path analyses were conducted using least-squares multiple regression rather than structural equation modelling (Kline, 1998). Power analyses based on Green (1991), with power set at .80, indicated adequate sample size to detect partial correlations ≥.43 in Models A and B and ≥.57 in Model C. Thus, the nonsignificant path coefficients in these models should be interpreted with caution, as they may be concealing low-to-moderate sized effects. (Note that the path coefficients are standardised beta coefficients, which are generally lower than the corresponding partial correlations.)

TABLE 2
Partial correlations between memory/metamemory indices and measures of executive functioning of the older participants

	Memory retention	*Memory accuracy*	*Monitoring resolution*	*Control sensitivity*
FAS	.32	.34	.19	.46*
WCSTc	−.09	.37	.19	.25
WCSTt	.00	−.38	−.18	−.39
WCSTp	.23	−.56*	−.26	−.67*

*$p < .05$. FAS = Word fluency; WCSTc = WCST categories achieved; WCSTt = WCST total errors; WCSTp = WCST perseverative errors.

executive functioning might affect monitoring resolution directly or indirectly via an effect on forced-report quantity correct. Of course, mean confidence was assumed to be strongly determined by forced-report quantity correct. Hence, any additional effect of age or executive functioning on mean confidence would indicate an effect that could not be explained by differences in the actual correctness of the answers, and would therefore reflect either differences in the use of the confidence scale (i.e., in assigning numbers to subjective confidence levels) or differences in monitoring calibration bias (over- or underconfidence). Similarly, the answer withholding rate was assumed to be strongly determined by mean confidence. Hence, any additional effect of age or executive functioning on this measure would indicate a difference in the withholding rate that could not be explained by a difference in mean confidence alone, and would therefore reflect a more conservative (positive effect) or more liberal (negative effect) control policy.

The first two path models (Figure 3, Models A and B) allowed for the possibility that each of the included cognitive or metacognitive variables might mediate the effects of age group, in comparing the older participants to the Young-DA group (Model A), or in comparing the older participants to the Young-FA group (Model B). The third model (Model C), focusing on the older age group alone, examined whether some of the effects of age within the older age group might be mediated by differences in executive functioning, which in turn might be mediated by any or all of the cognitive or metacognitive factors. Possible direct effects of age group (Models A and B), chronological age (Model C), and executive functioning (Model C) on free-report accuracy were also examined.

Beginning with the analysis comparing the older age group to the Young-DA group (Figure 3, Model A), we see that the cognitive and metacognitive factors together accounted for 87% of the variance in free-report memory accuracy, with no remaining direct effect of age group. In fact, the overall effect of age group on free-report accuracy ($r = -.28$) was mediated entirely

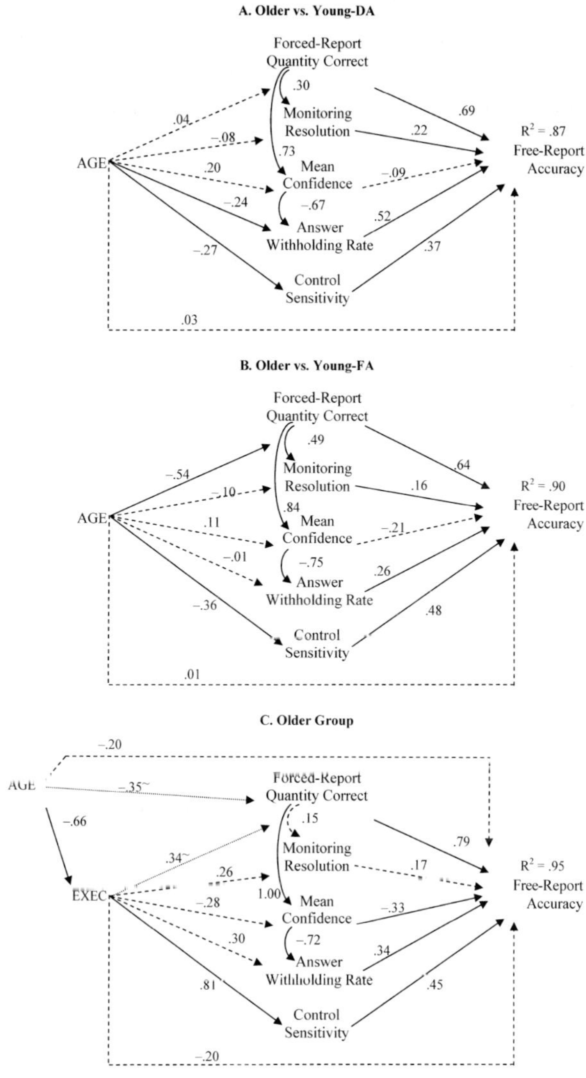

Figure 3. Path models examining the effects of age (Model A: Older vs. Young-DA participants; Model B: Older vs. Young-FA participants; Model C: chronological age within the older group) and executive functioning (EXEC; Model C only) on free-report accuracy performance, and the mediation of these effects by memory and metamemory components. Coefficients for each path represent standardised β weights. Statistically significant coefficients/paths are designated by solid arrows, and nonsignificant coefficients/paths are indicated by dashed arrows. The two coefficients/paths in Model C marked by a " ~" and dotted arrows are nonsignificant individually, but together comprise a significant regression model. Also in Model C, for the sake of clarity, nonsignificant paths between age and several of the cognitive and metacognitive variables have been omitted. See text for further details.

by the two metacognitive control variables: withholding rate and control sensitivity, with the indirect effects of age group via these two variables calculated as −.12 and −.10, respectively. Thus, the older participants tended to be more liberal in their reporting, and to base their reporting less strongly on their subjective confidence than did the Young-DA participants, with negative consequences for free-report accuracy stemming from both differences. Other variables affecting free-report accuracy that were not affected by age group in this analysis were forced-report quantity correct and monitoring resolution. The lack of age effect on forced-report quantity correct reflects the success of the divided-attention manipulation in equating forced-report performance (presumably by equating the quality of memory encoding) between the two age groups. Although not related to age group in this analysis, the unique contribution of monitoring resolution beyond that of forced-report quantity correct is worth noting, because it reinforces the general theoretical claim that effective memory monitoring is not just a matter of "good memory" (for a similar result, see Rhodes & Kelley, 2005).

Turning to the analysis comparing the older age group to the Young-FA group (Figure 3, Model B), the pattern of results is somewhat more complex. Once again, the cognitive and metacognitive factors together accounted for a very large proportion of the variance in free-report memory accuracy (90%), with no remaining direct effect of age group. Moreover, once again part of the overall effect of age group on free-report accuracy ($r = -.42$) was mediated by control sensitivity (indirect effect = −.17). In this comparison, however, there was no direct age effect on the answer withholding rate, and hence no indication of an age effect on the control policy. Instead, several indirect effects of age on free-report accuracy were mediated by forced-report quantity correct, with negative age effects stemming from the decreased accessibility of correct information per se (indirect effect = −.35) and from an ensuing decrease in monitoring effectiveness (indirect effect = −.04). Interestingly, these negative age effects were offset to a small degree by a positive indirect effect, in which lower accessibility of correct information leads to lower mean confidence, leading to more withholding of answers, leading to higher free-report accuracy (indirect effect = .09).

In the preceding two analyses, we examined the effects of age group on the various cognitive and metacognitive variables, and how these might mediate age-related effects on free-report accuracy. In this final analysis (Figure 3, Model C), we examined the extent to which age-related effects within the older group may be mediated by differences in executive functioning. To index executive functioning, we used a composite score based on the mean of the FAS score and WCST perseverance error score, after first standardising these scores and then reversing the sign of WCST perseverance error score (so that high values of the composite score would reflect good executive functioning). Unlike in the preceding analyses, chronological age (in months) was used to tap the potential age-related effects within the older group.

It can be seen that in this analysis, the entire path model accounted for fully 95% of the variance in free-report accuracy. Notably, although both executive functioning and age yielded large overall effects on free-report accuracy ($r = .73$ and $-.63$, respectively), once the cognitive and metacognitive factors were included in the model, the residual direct effect of executive functioning ($-.20$) was no longer significant, and once executive functioning was included in the model, the residual direct effect of age ($-.20$) was also no longer significant. In fact, the effects of executive functioning on memory accuracy in this analysis were mediated entirely by the included cognitive and metacognitive variables, whereas the effects of age were mediated mostly, if not entirely, by executive functioning. Examining first the effects of executive functioning, the most notable result is that control sensitivity was again found to mediate age-related differences in memory accuracy, now being shown to mediate the effects of executive functioning (indirect effect = .36). In contrast, after partialling out the relevant variables, the unique effects of executive functioning on forced-report quantity correct, monitoring resolution, mean confidence (calibration), and answer withholding rate (control policy), were not significant, though this may be due in part to the small sample size ($N = 20$). Presumably, despite the nonsignificant path coefficient (.34), some of the effect of executive functioning on memory accuracy is mediated by forced-report quantity correct. This is because the executive-functioning and age variables together accounted for a significant and moderately large proportion of the variance in forced-report quantity correct ($R^2 = .40$). Yet, with both variables included in the model, neither the executive functioning nor the age coefficient individually reached statistical significance.

Turning to the age variable, notwithstanding the problem just mentioned in interpreting the nonsignificant direct effect of age on forced-report quantity correct (versus the indirect effect of age on this variable via executive functioning), it is fair to say that much of the age effect on free-report memory accuracy observed in this analysis is mediated by the executive functioning composite score. This includes the indirect effect mediated by executive functioning and control sensitivity as well as the possible indirect effects mediated by executive functioning and forced-report quantity performance.

Taken together, the results of all three path analyses converge on the conclusion that diminished control sensitivity is an important mediator of the observed old-age decline in free-report memory accuracy, and this in turn stems from an old-age decline in executive functioning. This is in addition to inconsistent evidence of effects stemming from the use of a more liberal control policy (found in Model A but not in Models B and C) and to the effects due to an age-related decline in memory per se.

DISCUSSION

The present findings replicate those of numerous studies, demonstrating an age-related decline in the amount of retrieved information (for reviews, see Anderson & Craik, 2000; Balota, Dolan, & Duchek, 2000). More illuminating are the findings regarding memory accuracy, particularly when memory quantity was equated across the two age groups by dividing attention at study for the younger group. On the whole, these findings reveal a link between decreased memory accuracy, poorer executive functioning, and ageing within a general theoretical framework specifying the mediating role of metacognitive processes. Several differences were found between older and younger adults, both in memory accuracy and in its metacognitive determinants. First, the older participants exhibited lower free-report accuracy than did either group of younger participants. Second, the monitoring resolution of the older adults was lower than that of the Young-FA adults, but not lower than that of the Young-DA adults. This pattern suggests that the impaired monitoring (and ensuing consequences for memory accuracy) may be due to deficient memory encoding by older adults and Young-DA adults alike (see also Kelley & Sahakyan, 2003; Rhodes & Kelley, 2005).

Third, the higher volunteering rate of the older participants compared to the Young-DA participants, given the comparable level of retention and confidence of the two groups, suggests that they may have set a more lax criterion for volunteering information. This, together with the finding of a smaller reduction in memory quantity performance stemming from the exercise of free-report option by the older participants compared to the Young-DA participants, could be taken to reflect a general difference between older and younger adults in control policy. This possibility is consistent with previous findings demonstrating that older adults are less likely than younger adults to withhold answers when given the option of free report, even though this leads them to higher rates of false memory (see Jacoby et al., 2005; Kelley & Sahakyan, 2003). One reason why older adults might be reluctant to utilise the option of free report is the desire to "save face" by providing a reasonable amount of information despite their poor memory retention (cf. the "minimum informativeness" criterion recently proposed by Ackerman & Goldsmith, in press). This reluctance might be reinforced by metaknowledge that their memory quantity performance is generally poor (Hertzog & Hultsch, 2000) and by low self expectations with regard to their memory performance (Kausler, 1991). In other words, older adults may tend to adopt a liberal report criterion in an attempt to compensate for relatively low memory quantity, even though this comes at a cost in memory accuracy. In contrast, young adults would be more likely to attribute low memory quantity performance to external, situational factors. Indeed, the Young-DA participants in the present experiment could easily blame their relatively low memory quantity performance on the difficulty of attending to the presented information with an interfering tone-counting task.

Similar patterns of relatively low forced-report quantity performance accompanied by a relatively liberal control policy have been found in other special populations. For example, young children are particularly reluctant to withhold answers in response to memory questions and show a greater tendency than adults to provide wrong answers even when they are reminded that they have the option to say "don't know" (e.g., Cassel, Roebers, & Bjorklund, 1996). Thus, Koriat, Goldsmith, Schneider, and Nakash-Dura (2001) found a developmental trend, in which younger children exhibited both inferior memory quantity performance and a more liberal control policy than older children, leading to lower free-report accuracy as well.

The final age-related difference in metacognitive functioning observed in the current study is the finding of somewhat diminished control sensitivity in the older participants, indicating a reduced reliance on subjective confidence in deciding which answers to volunteer and which to withhold. As brought out in the path analyses, this difference in control sensitivity was responsible for some of the observed age-related accuracy reduction, and was quite robust, mediating age-related accuracy differences in all three analyses. This finding is particularly interesting in light of the strong correlation found between control sensitivity and measures of executive functioning within the older group. Taken together, the results suggest that the age-related reduction in memory accuracy results not only from poor memory retention and a consequential decline in memory monitoring, but also from a decline in metacognitive control (reduced sensitivity and perhaps a more lax control policy as well), which seems to be related to a decline in executive functioning, one of the important functions of the frontal lobe (Moscovitch & Winocur, 1995).

The concept of control sensitivity is an important feature of Koriat and Goldsmith's (1996b) theoretical framework, distinguishing it from similar frameworks such as signal-detection theory (see Goldsmith & Koriat, 2003, 2008). However, there are methodological (and hence interpretational) issues concerning the assessment of control sensitivity that must be considered. On the one hand, a procedure in which participants make their control decision immediately after providing a confidence judgement, on an item-by-item basis, might be suspected of demand characteristics, creating an artificially high correlation between the subjective measure and actual behaviour. On the other hand, eliciting the control decisions in a second phase, after the confidence ratings for all the items have been provided (and subsequently removed), as we did in the present study, also poses potential problems in interpreting the results.

One such problem (raised by an anonymous reviewer), is that despite the temporal separation, some participants may nonetheless remember the confidence ratings that they provided in the first phase when making their control decision in the second phase, which may in turn guide that decision. If so, age-related differences in control sensitivity might actually reflect poorer memory for the first-phase confidence judgements on the part of the older participants compared to the young participants. Another possibility is that participants' confidence in their answers might change somewhat from one phase to the next, and that the older participants' confidence may be less stable than that of the younger participants. Regarding the memory issue, we believe that given the nearly perfect correlations between confidence and volunteering for the young participant groups in this study (gamma averaging .97), as well as in other studies (e.g., Koriat & Goldsmith, 1996b), and the large number of confidence ratings that would need to be remembered (30 in this study, up to 90 in previous studies), it is doubtful that memory for one's previously provided confidence ratings could be contributing much variance. With regard to the stability issue, we note that the difference in control sensitivity was found between the older participants and the Young-DA participants (as well as the Young-FA participants), who were equated on memory retention. This reduces the possibility that confidence in one group would be less stable than in the other, but we acknowledge that this issue must remain open until it is examined more directly in future research.

To the extent that the observed age-difference in control sensitivity is real, it joins other recent evidence suggesting that control sensitivity is an important factor to consider in explaining memory performance in special populations. For example, in a series of studies, Koren and colleagues (Koren et al., 2004, 2005; Koren, Seidman, Goldsmith, & Harvey, 2006) adapted Koriat and Goldsmith's (1996b) framework and methodology to examine the performance of first-episode schizophrenic patients on a metacognitive free-report version of the WCST. In that adaptation, patients rated their confidence in each sort, and decided whether or not they wanted that sort to count towards their performance payoff. Several of the metacognitive measures from the adapted task were found to correlate more strongly with clinical measures relevant to real-world functioning ("insight into illness" and "competence to consent to treatment") than did traditional neuropsychological measures. Most prominent was control sensitivity, which was more highly correlated with the clinical measures of insight than any of the standard neuropsychological measures that were examined (Koren et al., 2004).

In a similar vein, Danion et al. (2001) used Koriat and Goldsmith's (1996b) metacognitive free-forced paradigm to compare schizophrenic patients with healthy controls on semantic (general-knowledge) memory tasks and found significantly lower control sensitivity for the schizophrenic patients (.83) compared to the healthy controls (.94). Interestingly, a similar reduction in control sensitivity was found with healthy participants who were under the influence of lorezapam (Massin-Krauss, Bacon, & Danion, 2002). Taken together, these lines of research point to an impaired relationship between subjective experience and behaviour associated with mental illness and the effects of psychoactive drugs that is similar to the one we found for normal older adults.

Diminished control sensitivity is reminiscent of what Stuss and Benson (1987) have called a dissociation between self-consciousness and self-knowledge, which is typical of patients with prefrontal damage (West, 1996). For example, this is the type of behaviour that frontal patients tend to exhibit when making perseverative errors on the WCST. The WCST requires the person to sort a series of cards based on a continually changing rule. When a category shift occurs, patients frequently continue to sort the cards to the now incorrect category, even as they express with each sort that this response is inappropriate (Duncan, 1995; Heaton, 1981). This suggests that the individual is aware that he or she is committing errors in behaviour, but is unable to modify that behaviour based on this knowledge. Thus, diminished control sensitivity could perhaps derive from a general age-related difficulty in inhibiting prepotent responses. This capacity has been attributed to the frontal lobe (see, e.g., Miyake et al., 2000; Rabbitt, Lowe, & Shilling, 2001), and has been suggested to be impaired among older adults (see, e.g., Zacks, Hasher, & Li, 2000), and perhaps among older adults with reduced executive functioning in particular (Davidson & Glisky, 2002).

Older adults' diminished control sensitivity may also stem in part from low memory self-efficacy (Hertzog & Hultsch, 2000), mentioned earlier in connection with the possibility of a general age-related relaxation of control policy. If older adults are distrustful of their memory monitoring as well as of their memory per se, this might make them less likely to rely on their monitoring output to guide their memory reporting.

Hence, an optimistic implication of our results is that part of the reduction in memory accuracy in old age may be avoidable: Training older adults to rely more on their monitoring output, and perhaps to be more conservative in their control policies, could help improve their free-report accuracy.

REFERENCES

Ackerman, R., & Goldsmith, M. (in press). Control over grain size in memory reporting—with and without satisficing knowledge. *Journal of Experimental Psychology: Learning, Memory and Cognition*.

Anderson, N. D., & Craik, F. I. M. (2000). Memory in the aging brain. In F. I. M. Craik & E. Tulving (Eds.), *The Oxford handbook of memory* (pp. 411–425). New York: Oxford University Press.

Balota, D. A., Dolan, P. O., & Duchek, J. M. (2000). Memory changes in healthy older adults. In F. I. M. Craik & E. Tulving (Eds.), *The Oxford handbook of memory* (pp. 395–409). New York: Oxford University Press.

Barnes, A. E., Nelson, T. O., Dunlosky, J., Mazzoni, G., & Narens, L. (1999). An integrative system of metamemory components involved in retrieval. In D. Gopher & A. Koriat (Eds.), *Attention and performance XVII: Cognitive regulation of performance: Interaction of theory and application* (pp. 287–313). Cambridge, MA: MIT Press.

Butler, K. M., McDaniel, M. A., Dornburg, C. C., Price, A. L., & Roediger, H. L. (2004). Age differences in veridical and false recall are not inevitable: The role of frontal lobe function. *Psychonomic Bulletin and Review, 11*, 921–925.

Cassel, W. S., Roebers, C. E. M., & Bjorklund, D. F. (1996). Developmental patterns of eyewitness responses to repeated and increasingly suggestive questions. *Journal of Experimental Child Psychology, 61*, 116–133.

Chan, J. C. K., & McDermott, K. B. (2007). The effects of frontal lobe functioning and age on veridical and false recall. *Psychonomic Bulletin and Review, 14*, 606–611.

Craik, F. I. M., & Anderson, N. D. (1999). Applying cognitive research to problems of aging. In D. Gopher & A. Koriat (Eds.), *Attention and performance XVII: Cognitive regulation of performance: Interaction of theory and application* (pp. 583–615). Cambridge, MA: MIT Press.

Danion, J. M., Gokalsing, E., Robert, P., Massin-Krauss, M., & Bacon, E. (2001). Defective relationship between subjective experience and behavior in schizophrenia. *American Journal of Psychiatry, 158*, 2064–2066.

Davidson, P. S. R., & Glisky, E. L. (2002). Neuropsychological correlates of recollection and familiarity in normal aging. *Cognitive, Affective and Behavioral Neuroscience, 2*, 174–186.

Duncan, J. (1995). Attention, intelligence, and the frontal lobes. In M. S. Gazzaniga (Ed.), *The cognitive neurosciences* (pp. 721–733). Cambridge, MA: MIT Press.

Fernandez-Duque, D., Baird, J. A., & Posner, M. I. (2000). Executive attention and metacognitive regulation. *Consciousness and Cognition, 9*, 288–307.

Glisky, E. L., Polster, M. R., & Routhieaux, B. C. (1995). Double dissociation between item and source memory. *Neuropsychology, 9*, 229–235.

Glisky, E. L., Rubin, S. R., & Davidson, P. S. R. (2001). Source memory in older adults: An encoding or retrieval problem? *Journal of Experimental Psychology: Learning, Memory, and Cognition, 27*, 1131–1146.

Goldsmith, M., & Koriat, A. (1999). The strategic regulation of memory reporting: Mechanisms and performance consequences. In D. Gopher & A. Koriat (Eds.), *Attention and performance XVII: Cognitive regulation of performance: Interaction of theory and application* (pp. 373–400). Cambridge, MA: MIT Press.

Goldsmith, M., & Koriat, A. (2003). Dolphins on the witness stand? The comparative psychology of strategic memory monitoring and control. *Behavioral and Brain Sciences, 26*, 345–346.

Goldsmith, M., & Koriat, A. (2008). The strategic regulation of memory accuracy and informativeness. In A. Benjamin & B. Ross (Eds.), *The psychology of learning and motivation* (Vol. 48, pp. 1–60). London: Academic Press.

Goldsmith, M., Koriat, A., & Pansky, A. (2005). Strategic regulation of grain size in memory reporting over time. *Journal of Memory and Language, 52*, 505–525.

Goldsmith, M., Koriat, A., & Weinberg-Eliezer, A. (2002). Strategic regulation of grain size memory reporting. *Journal of Experimental Psychology: General*, *131*, 73–95.

Green, S. B. (1991). How many subjects does it take to do a regression analysis? *Multivariate Behavioral Research*, *26*, 499–510.

Greenwood, P. M. (2000). The frontal aging hypothesis evaluated. *Journal of the International Neuropsychological Society*, *6*, 705–726.

Hart, R. P., Kwentus, J. A., Wade, J. B., & Taylor, J. R. (1988). Modified Wisconsin Sorting Test in elderly normal, depressed and demented patients. *The Clinical Neuropsychologist*, *2*, 49–56.

Heaton, W. C. (1981). *Wisconsin Card Sorting Test*. Odessa, TX: Psychological Assessment Resources.

Henkel, L. A., Johnson, M. K., & de Leonardis, D. M. (1998). Aging and source monitoring: Cognitive processes and neuropsychological correlates. *Journal of Experimental Psychology: General*, *127*, 251–268.

Hertzog, C., & Dunlosky, J. (2004). Aging, metacognition, and cognitive control. In B. H. Ross (Ed.), *The psychology of learning and motivation: Advances in research and theory* (pp. 215–247). San Diego, CA: Elsevier.

Hertzog, C., & Hultsch, D. F. (2000). Metacognition in adulthood and old age. In F. I. M. Craik (Ed.), *The handbook of aging and cognition* (2nd ed., pp. 417–466). Mahwah, NJ: Lawrence Erlbaum Associates, Inc.

Higham, P. A. (2002). Strong cues are not necessarily weak: Thomson and Tulving (1970) and the encoding specificity principle revisited. *Memory and Cognition*, *30*, 67–80.

Higham, P. A. (2007). No special K! A signal detection framework for the strategic regulation of memory accuracy. *Journal of Experimental Psychology: General*, *136*, 1–22.

Higham, P. A., & Tam, H. (2005). Generation failure: Estimating metacognition in cued recall. *Journal of Memory and Language*, *52*, 595–617.

Jacoby, L. L. (1999). Deceiving the elderly: Effects of accessibility bias in cued-recall performance. *Cognitive Neuropsychology*, *16*, 417–436.

Jacoby, L. L., Bishara, A. J., Hessels, S., & Toth, J. P. (2005). Aging, subjective experience, and cognitive control: Dramatic false remembering by older adults. *Journal of Experimental Psychology: General*, *134*, 131–148.

Jacoby, L. L., Debner, J. A., & Hay, J. F. (2001). Proactive interference, accessibility bias, and process dissociations: Valid subject reports of memory. *Journal of Experimental Psychology: Learning, Memory, and Cognition*, *27*, 686–700.

Jacoby, L. L., & Rhodes, M. G. (2006). False remembering in the aged. *Current Directions in Psychological Science*, *15*, 49–53.

Janowsky, J. S., Shimamura, A. P., & Squire, L. R. (1989). Source memory impairment in patients with frontal lobe lesions. *Neuropsychologia*, *27*, 1043–1056.

Jennings, J. M., & Jacoby, L. L. (1993). Automatic versus intentional uses of memory: Aging, attention, and control. *Psychology and Aging*, *8*, 283–293.

Kato, T. (1985). Semantic-memory sources of episodic retrieval failure. *Memory and Cognition*, *13*, 442–452.

Kausler, D. H. (1991). *Experimental psychology, cognition, and human aging* (2nd ed.). New York: Springer-Verlag.

Kelley, C. M., & Sahakyan, L. (2003). Memory, monitoring, and control in the attainment of memory accuracy. *Journal of Memory and Language*, *48*, 704–721.

Kline, R. B. (1998). *Principles and practice of structural equation modeling*. New York: Guilford Press.

Koren, D., Poyurovsky, M., Seidman, L. J., Goldsmith, M., Wenger, S., & Klein, E. M. (2005). The neuropsychological basis of competence to consent in first-episode schizophrenia: A pilot metacognitive study. *Biological Psychiatry*, *57*, 609–616.

Koren, D., Seidman, L. J., Goldsmith, M., & Harvey, P. D. (2006). Real-world cognitive—and metacognitive—dysfunction in schizophrenia: A new approach for measuring (and remediating) more "right stuff". *Schizophrenia Bulletin, 32*, 310–326.

Koren, D., Seidman, L. J., Poyurovsky, M., Goldsmith, M., Viksman, P., Zichel, S., & Klein, E. (2004). The neuropsychological basis of insight in first-episode schizophrenia: A pilot metacognitive study. *Schizophrenia Research, 70*, 195–202.

Koriat, A. (1993). How do we know that we know? The accessibility model of the feeling of knowing. *Psychological Review, 100*, 609–639.

Koriat, A. (1995). Dissociating knowing and the feeling of knowing: Further evidence for the accessibility model. *Journal of Experimental Psychology: General, 124*, 311–333.

Koriat, A., Ben-Zur, H., & Sheffer, D. (1988). Telling the same story twice: Output monitoring and age. *Journal of Memory and Language, 27*, 23–39.

Koriat, A., & Goldsmith, M. (1994). Memory in naturalistic and laboratory contexts: Distinguishing the accuracy-oriented and quantity-oriented approaches to memory assessment. *Journal of Experimental Psychology: General, 123*, 297–315.

Koriat, A., & Goldsmith, M. (1996a). Memory metaphors and the real-life/laboratory controversy: Correspondence versus storehouse conceptions of memory. *Behavioral and Brain Sciences, 19*, 167–228.

Koriat, A., & Goldsmith, M. (1996b). Monitoring and control processes in the strategic regulation of memory accuracy. *Psychological Review, 103*, 490–517.

Koriat, A., Goldsmith, M., & Halamish, V. (2008). Control processes in voluntary remembering. In I. H. L. Roediger (Ed.), *Cognitive psychology of memory* (Vol. 2, pp. 307–324). Oxford, UK: Elsevier.

Koriat, A., Goldsmith, M., & Pansky, A. (2000). Toward a psychology of memory accuracy. *Annual Review of Psychology, 51*, 481–537.

Koriat, A., Goldsmith, M., Schneider, W., & Nakash-Dura, M. (2001). The credibility of children's testimony: Can children control the accuracy of their memory reports? *Journal of Experimental Child Psychology, 79*, 405–437.

Koriat, A., Lichtenstein, S., & Fischhoff, B. (1980). Reasons for confidence. *Journal of Experimental Psychology: Human Learning and Memory, 6*, 107–118.

Koutstaal, W. (2006). Flexible remembering. *Psychonomic Bulletin and Review, 13*, 84–91.

Lichtenstein, S., Fischhoff, B., & Phillips, L. D. (1982). Calibration of probabilities: The state of the art to 1980. In D. Kahneman, P. Slovic, & A. Tversky (Eds.), *Judgment under uncertainty: Heuristics and biases* (pp. 306–334). New York: Cambridge University Press.

Massin-Krauss, M., Bacon, E., & Danion, J. M. (2002). Effects of benzodiazepine lorazepam on monitoring and control processes in semantic memory. *Consciousness and Cognition, 11*, 123–137.

McDaniel, M. A., Glisky, E. L., Rubin, S. R., Guynn, M. J., & Routhieaux, B. C. (1999). Prospective memory: A neuropsychological study. *Neuropsychology, 13*, 103–110.

Miyake, A., Friedman, N. P., Emerson, M. J., Witzki, A. H., Howerter, A., & Wager, T. D. (2000). The unity and diversity of executive functions and their contributions to complex "frontal lobe" tasks: A latent variable analysis. *Cognitive Psychology, 41*, 49–100.

Moscovitch, M., & Winocur, G. (1992). The neuropsychology of memory and aging. In F. I. M. Craik & T. A. Salthouse (Eds.), *The handbook of aging and cognition* (pp. 315–372). Hillsdale, NJ: Lawrence Erlbaum Associates, Inc.

Moscovitch, M., & Winocur, G. (1995). Frontal lobes, memory, and aging. In J. Grafman, K. J. Holyoak, & F. Boller (Eds.), *Structure and functions of the human prefrontal cortex* (pp. 119–150). New York: New York Academy of Sciences.

Moscovitch, M., & Winocur, G. (2002). The frontal cortex and working with memory. In D. T. Stuss & R. T. Knight (Eds.), *Principles of frontal lobe function* (pp. 188–209). New York: Oxford University Press.

Nelson, T. O. (1984). A comparison of current measures of the accuracy of feeling-of-knowing predictions. *Psychological Bulletin*, *95*, 109–133.

Nelson, T. O., & Narens, L. (1990). Metamemory: A theoretical framework and new findings. In G. H. Bower (Ed.), *The psychology of learning and motivation: Advances in research and theory* (Vol. 26, pp. 125–123). San Diego, CA: Academic Press.

Payne, B. K., Lambert, A. J., & Jacoby, L. L. (2002). Best laid plans: Effects of goals on accessibility bias and cognitive control in race-based misperceptions of weapons. *Journal of Experimental Social Psychology*, *38*, 384–396.

Perfect, T. (1997). Memory aging as frontal lobe dysfunction. In M. A. Conway (Ed.), *Cognitive models of memory: Studies in cognition* (pp. 315–339). Cambridge, MA: MIT Press.

Perfect, T. J., & Stollery, B. (1993). Memory and metamemory performance in older adults: One deficit or two? *Quarterly Journal of Experimental Psychology: Human Experimental Psychology*, *46A*, 119–135.

Rabbitt, P. M. A., Lowe, C., & Shilling, V. (2001). Frontal tests and models for cognitive ageing. *European Journal of Cognitive Psychology*, *13*, 5–28.

Raz, N. (2000). Aging of the brain and its impact on cognitive performance: Integration of structural and functional findings. In F. I. M. Craik & T. Salthouse (Eds.), *The handbook of aging and cognition* (2nd ed., pp. 1–90). Mahwah, NJ: Lawrence Erlbaum Associates, Inc.

Rhodes, M. G. (2004). Age-related differences in performance on the Wisconsin Card Sorting Test: A meta-analytic review. *Psychology and Aging*, *19*, 482–494.

Rhodes, M. G., & Kelley, C. M. (2005). Executive processes, memory accuracy, and memory monitoring: An aging and individual difference analysis. *Journal of Memory and Language*, *52*, 578–594.

Roediger, H. L., & Geraci, L. (2007). Aging and the misinformation effect: A neuropsychological analysis. *Journal of Experimental Psychology: Learning, Memory, and Cognition*, *33*, 321–334.

Salthouse, T. A., Atkinson, T. M., & Berish, D. E. (2003). Executive functioning as a potential mediator of age-related cognitive decline in normal adults. *Journal of Experimental Psychology: General*, *132*, 566–594.

Schwartz, B. L. (1994). Sources of information in metamemory: Judgments of learning and feelings of knowing. *Psychonomic Bulletin and Review*, *1*, 357–375.

Shimamura, A. P. (2000). Toward a cognitive neuroscience of metacognition. *Conciousness and Cognition*, *9*, 313–323.

Souchay, C., & Isingrini, M. (2004). Age related differences in metacognitive control: Role of executive functioning. *Brain and Cognition*, *56*, 89–99,

Souchay, C., Isingrini, M., & Espagnet, L. (2000). Aging, episodic memory feeling-of-knowing, and frontal functioning. *Neuropsychology*, *14*, 299–309.

Stuss, D. T., & Benson, D. F. (1987). The frontal lobes and control of cognition and memory. In E. Perecman (Ed.), *The frontal lobes revisited* (pp. 141–158). New York: IRBN Press.

Stuss, D. T., Craik, F. I. M., Sayer, L., Franchi, D., & Alexander, M. P. (1996). Comparison of older people and patients with frontal lesions: Evidence from word list learning. *Psychology and Aging*, *11*, 387–395.

Vilkki, J., Servo, A., & Surma-aho, O. (1998). Word list learning and prediction of recall after frontal lobe lesions. *Neuropsychology*, *12*, 268–277.

Waltz, J. A., Knowlton, B. J., Holyoak, K. J., Boone, K. B., Mishkin, F. S., de Menezes Santos, M., et al. (1999). A system for relational reasoning in human prefrontal cortex. *Psychological Science*, *10*, 119–125.

West, R. L. (1996). An application of prefrontal cortex function theory to cognitive aging. *Psychological Bulletin*, *120*, 272–292.

Zacks, R. T., Hasher, L., & Li, K. Z. H. (2000). Human memory. In F. I. M. Craik (Ed.), *The handbook of aging and cognition* (pp. 293–357). Mahwah, NJ: Lawrence Erlbaum Associates, Inc.

EUROPEAN JOURNAL OF COGNITIVE PSYCHOLOGY
2009, 21 (2/3), 330–346

Psychology Press
Taylor & Francis Group

The effect of attentional set-shifting, working memory, and processing speed on pragmatic language functioning in Parkinson's disease

A. McKinlay

Psychology Department, University of Canterbury, New Zealand

J. C. Dalrymple-Alford

Psychology Department, University of Canterbury, and Van der Veer Institute for Parkinson's disease and Brain Research, New Zealand

R. C. Grace and D. Roger

Psychology Department, University of Canterbury, New Zealand

Parkinson's disease (PD) is traditionally associated with motor symptoms. However, impairments in language functioning may also accompany this disorder. The present study investigated pragmatic language deficits in PD and their relationship to cognitive functioning. Forty patients with PD were compared to age- and IQ-matched controls on measures of pragmatic language functioning using the Test of Language Competence–Expanded (TLC-E), and measures of attentional set-shifting, working memory, and processing speed. Overall, PD patients were impaired on aspects of language, working memory, and processing speed. Measures of cognition were significantly correlated with pragmatic language functioning. Path analyses revealed that deficits in pragmatic language functioning were mediated by verbal working memory and processing speed, but not attentional set-shifting. Regression analyses found that processing speed was a stronger determiner of pragmatic language performance than verbal working memory. Results suggest that pragmatic language deficits may be explained in terms of deficits in processing speed associated with the disease.

Keywords: Parkinson's disease; Language; Working memory; Processing speed; Attention.

Correspondence should be addressed to Audrey McKinlay, University of Canterbury, Private Bag 4800, Christchurch, New Zealand. E-mail: audrey.mckinlay@student.canterbury.ac.nz

We are indebted to neurologists Tim Anderson and John Fink for the referral of patients, advice on the interpretation of the UPDRS, and helpful comments on a draft of this manuscript. The research was supported by a grant from the Canterbury Medical Research Foundation.

http://www.psypress.com/ecp DOI: 10.1080/09541440802281266

Parkinson's disease (PD) is one of the most common neurodegenerative disorders in people over 50 years of age. Depletion of dopamine containing cells in the basal ganglia is considered to be a characteristic feature of the disorder (see Frank, 2005; Middleton & Strick, 2000, for review). As the basal ganglia are key to the execution of movement and cognitive tasks (Frank, 2005; Middleton & Strick, 2000), it is not surprising therefore that cognitive impairments are frequently reported in patients with PD, even in the absence of dementia (Pillon, Boller, Levy, & Dubois, 2001). Communication problems may also accompany PD, and include impairments in speech production and a range of language abilities, including comprehension and effective verbal expression (Grossman, Carvell, Stern, Gollomp, & Hurtig, 1992; Owen, 2004). However, there is considerable controversy regarding the degree to which language deficits in PD may be mediated by other cognitive skills (Murdoch, 2001).

Subtle cognitive deficits in PD resulting from the dysfunction of the basal ganglia are apparent early in the disease process, similar to that seen in patients who have experienced prefrontal lesions (Cooper, Sagar, Jordan, Harvey, & Sullivan, 1991; Frank, 2005; Royall et al., 2002). Difficulties with attentional control, working memory, processing speed, planning, problem solving, and memory have been reported (Pillon et al., 2001). Language-related deficits that have been reported in PD include reduced verbal fluency, difficulties with processing of past tense verbs, and impairments in detecting and correcting syntax errors (McNamara & Durso, 2003; Monetta & Pell, 2007; Ullman, 2001). The comprehension of sentences with complex or irregular grammatical structures is one of the most frequently reported deficits (Bodis-Wollner & Jo, 2006; Grossman, 1999; Grossman et al., 1991, 1992, 2003; Lieberman, Friedman, & Feldman, 1990; McNamara, Krueger, O'Quin, Clark, & Durso, 1996).

However, the degree to which language deficits in PD are dependent on the integrity of other cognitive skills is still being investigated (Murdoch, 2001). To date, researchers have found evidence of an association between impaired sentence comprehension in PD and a number of other cognitive tasks including attentional set-switching, inhibition, working memory and attention, and processing speed (Angwin, Chenery, Copland, Murdoch, & Silburn, 2005; Grossman et al., 2002, 2003; Hochstadt, Nakano, Lieberman, & Friedman, 2006). Indeed, Grossman and colleagues (1992) reported that working memory and attention accounted for over 97% of the variance in complex sentence comprehension for PD patients.

It seems likely that more complex aspects of language, such as the understanding of pragmatics, would be more dependent on other aspects of cognition. Pragmatics involves the ability to use and interpret verbal and nonverbal language appropriately within the social situation in which the communicative exchange occurs, requiring a degree of inference and interpretation (Perkins, 2005). Different aspects of pragmatic language are considered to be highly resource demanding (Monetta, Ouellet-Plamondon,

& Joanette, 2006). For example, the ability to interpret nonliteral elements of language such as metaphor, considered to be a part of pragmatic language, requires the comprehension of a false statement using cues from the current context (Glucksberg, 2003; Monetta & Pell, 2007).

Impairments in pragmatic language commonly result when the prefrontal cortex is compromised (see Martin and McDonald, 2003, for a review). Given that basal ganglia dysfunction has been associated with "frontal type" deficits, it would seem likely that pragmatic language problems would also be evident for individuals with PD. Moreover, given the complexity of skills associated with the comprehension of pragmatic language, it would seem likely that other cognitive skills would be implicated in its effective use. However, there is relatively little information regarding the association between pragmatic deficits and other cognitive functions for patients with PD.

The studies that have examined pragmatic language in PD have reported deficits when compared with healthy controls. For example, Lewis, Lapointe, Murdoch, and Chenery (1998) compared the language abilities of 20 nondemented PD patients (all Hoehn & Yahr Stage 3; Hoehn & Yahr, 1967) to healthy controls using the Boston Naming Test (BNT), the WORD Test (TWT; Jorgensen, Barrett, Huistingh, and Zachman, 1981), and the Test of Language Competence–Expanded Edition (TCL-E; Wiig & Secord, 1989). Parkinson's disease patients were significantly poorer at interpreting ambiguity, figurative language, and sentence construction. Furthermore, patients with lower levels of general cognitive functioning were more impaired than other PD patients.

McNamara and Durso (2003) examined the association between pragmatic language functions and frontal dysfunction, comparing 22 nondemented PD patients with healthy controls. Pragmatic skills were assessed using a formal pragmatic skills protocol devised by Prutting and Kirchner (1987). Two tests of frontal ability were also administered; the interference condition of the Stroop colour–word test to assess susceptibility to interference, and the Tower of London task as a test of planning ability. Significant deficits were evident for the PD group when compared to healthy controls on the test of pragmatic language ability and the test of susceptibility to cognitive interference. Deficits in pragmatic language ability were correlated with poorer performance on tests of planning and susceptibility to cognitive interference. These authors concluded that impairments in pragmatic language ability may be related to frontal lobe dysfunction.

Monetta and Pell (2007) examined the effects of verbal working memory deficits on metaphor; comparing 17 individuals with PD with mild to moderate motor symptoms to healthy controls. This study used a verbal working memory span task to assess working memory capacity, and a metaphor comprehension task following the methods of Gernsbacher, Keysar, Robertson, and Werner (2001). Parkinson's disease patients were less efficient at processing metaphorical information (as measured by accuracy and speed). Further, there was a strong relationship between pragmatic language ability and working memory. However, when patients were divided into two groups according to their working memory performance (impaired and unimpaired), only those with impaired working memory performance were impaired in the processing of metaphorical language. These authors concluded that efficient metaphor interpretation was dependent on intact working memory systems that enabled the efficient storage and processing of metaphorical information. Further, that working memory relied on the integrity of the frontostriatal systems, which are compromised in patients with PD.

The current literature suggests that pragmatic language skills are impaired as part of the neurodegenerative process associated with PD. This present study was designed to examine the degree to which any deficits in pragmatic language are mediated by different cognitive skills including working memory, processing speed, and attentional set shifting. These aspects of cognition were selected as they have frequently been found to be impaired in patients with PD, even in the early stages of the disease process (Cooper et al., 1991; Gabrieli, Singh, Stebbins, & Goetz, 1996; Lewis, Dove, Robbins, Barker, & Owen, 2003; Muslimovic, Post, Speelman, & Schmand, 2005). We hypothesised that compared to health controls, PD patients would show deficit in pragmatic language tasks. We further hypothesised that these deficits would be mediated by deficits in other areas of cognitive functioning.

METHODS

This study received approval from the Upper South B Regional Ethics Committee. Parkinson's patients in the Canterbury region of New Zealand who could be identified at the time of this study and had not been diagnosed with dementia, were invited by letter to participate.

Participants

Parkinson's patients. Participants were required to meet the following inclusion criteria: (1) a diagnosis of idiopathic Parkinson's disease, confirmed by a specialist neurologist; (2) assessed at the Hoehn and Yahr Stages 1–4 (Hoehn & Yahr, 1967; numbers of patients at each stage were as follows: Stage 1, $n = 8$; Stage 1.5, $n = 6$; Stage 2, $n = 7$; Stage 2.5, $n = 10$; Stage 3, $n = 7$; Stage 4, $n = 2$.); (3) aged between 50 and 80 years; (4) adequate or corrected hearing and vision (self-report checked by examiner); (5) stable on PD medication; (6) English as the primary spoken language; (7) no suspicion of dementia (Mini-Mental Status Exam, MMSE $= 25$; Demential Rating Scale–II, DRS-II, Jurica, Leitten, & Mattis, 2001; DSM-IV criteria, American Psychiatric Association, 2000).

The following exclusion criteria were applied: (1) currently involved in a therapeutic trial; (2) a history of: (a) moderate or severe head injury, (b) stroke or other neurological impairment, (c) other major medical illness, (d) significant psychiatric illness requiring hospitalisation, (e) major depressive episode in the previous 6 months; (3) diagnosis of, or special education for, a learning disability; (4) premorbid IQ estimated at < 85 using National Adult Reading Test (NART); (5) currently taking medications known to have a significant effect on the central nervous system (other than medications prescribed for the control of PD symptoms); (6) Beck Depression Inventory–II (BDI-II; Beck, Steer, & Brown, 1996) score of > 16.

Of the 115 letters that were posted, 6 (5.2%) of individuals with PD could not participate due to illness, 6 (5.2%) were deceased, 8 (6.9%) declined, 34 (29.6%) did not respond, and 21 (18.3%) did not meet the inclusion/exclusion criteria. Forty participants with PD who met the exclusion/inclusion criteria were available to participate in the study. All patients were on anti-Parkinsonian medication and were tested while on optimal levels of medication (self-report and examiner observation).

Controls. Controls were recruited from a number of sources including a previously established database, advertisements at local clubs (bowling, hiking, and table tennis), and businesses. All controls were given a brief outline of the study on first phone contact. In addition to adequate or corrected hearing and vision (self-report and checked by the examiner) and being aged between 50 and 80 years of age, the same exclusion criteria listed participants with PD also applied to the control group.

Procedure

Assessments were carried out at the University of Canterbury. Written consent was obtained from all participants at the beginning of testing after the study had been explained. Additional information pertinent to the inclusion/exclusion criteria was obtained from all participants using a semistructured interview. All tests were conducted according to standardised procedures. Each PD patient was individually matched to a healthy control in terms of age, premorbid IQ, and current mental status.

Measures

Clinical and demographic information

The NART was used to estimate premorbid IQ. Words were scored 0 for incorrect and 1 for correct pronunciation (Lezak, 1995). The BDI-II was used to assess mood. This test consists of 21 items; each question was rated

0–3 with higher scores indicating greater intensity of symptoms (Beck et al., 1996). The BDI-II has been validated for use with PD patients, with a cutoff of 16/17 being recommended (Leentjens, 2004). The MMSE provided information regarding current cognitive status (Folstein, Folstein, & McHugh, 1975). Two additional measures were used for patients with PD to provide information regarding motor impairment: (1) Unified Parkinson's Disease Rating Scale (UPDRS) motor section (Fahn & Elton, 1987) and (2) the Hoehn and Yahr, which was used to rate the stage of the disease (Hoehn & Yahr, 1967).

Language and cognitive assessment

Pragmatic language. Pragmatic language was assessed using the Test of Language Competence–Expanded Edition Level 2 (TLC-E). Five scores were generated using scoring instructions provided in the test manual (Wiig & Secord, 1989): (1) a total score (maximum = 189) and a score for each of the following subtests; (2) ambiguous sentences, used to assess the participant's ability to recognise lexical and structural ambiguities of a sentence (possible scores ranged from 0 to 39); (3) listening comprehension (making inferences) assessed the participants' ability to identify inferences in a series of short paragraphs (possible scores ranged from 0 to 36); (4) oral expression (recreating sentences) evaluated the ability to formulate a grammatically complete sentence that was appropriate for a given situation (possible scores ranged from 0 to 78); (5) figurative language designed to assess the ability to interpret metaphoric expressions (possible scores range from 0 to 36). For each of the subtests, a discontinue rule of failure to respond to three consecutive items was used.

Attentional set-shifting. This skill was assessed using the Intradimensional/Extradimensional Shift (ID/ED) from the Cambridge Neuropsychological Test Automated Battery (CANTAB; Owen, Roberts, Polkey, Sahakian, & Robbins, 1991). This test uses computer-generated visual stimuli to assess the individuals' ability to maintain attention to different examples within a particular perceptual dimension (e.g., shapes) while ignoring irrelevant information (e.g., lines). Without prior warning, the participant must then shift attention away from this relevant dimension and attend to a previously redundant dimension. In this present study all sections of the test were administered, but analysis of the results was based on the ID + ED trails as outlined by Hutton et al. (1998).

Working memory. The Daneman and Carpenter Reading Span test (Daneman & Carpenter, 1980) was used to assess verbal working memory (Waters & Caplan, 1996). This test requires the participant to read sentences, judge their veracity, and then retain the final word in the sentence. The number of sentences presented prior to recall of words varied from two to six. The reading span was assessed as the maximum number of words remembered, with at least two out of three trials correctly recalled (possible scores ranged from 1 to 6). The test was discontinued if a participant was unable to remember the last word from any of the sentences in a trial set.

Processing speed. Word naming and colour naming from the Delis Kaplan Executive Function System (D-KEFS; Delis, Kaplan, & Kramer, 2001) were used to assess this skill. Age-adjusted scores were used with a mean of 10 and standard deviation of 3. Scores for colour naming and word reading were then averaged to provide a single score for speed of mental processing.

RESULTS

Differences in demographic and clinical characteristics were examined using *t*-tests and χ^2 as appropriate. Patients were well matched to healthy controls in terms of age and premorbid IQ (see Table 1), but differed in terms of symptoms consistent with low mood (as measured by the BDI-II) and current mental status (as measured by the MMSE), but no patient met the criteria for a depressive episode or dementia (DSM-IV criteria).

Table 2 shows the comparison between PD patients and matched controls on measures of language, working memory, processing speed, and attentional set-shifting using *t*-tests. PD patients performed more poorly in terms of their overall TLC-E score and for three out of the four subtests. Deficits

TABLE 1
Clinical and demographic characteristics, Parkinson's disease group versus controls

	Parkinson's disease (n = 40)		*Control group (n = 40)*			
	Mean	*SD*	*Mean*	*SD*	*t-value*	*p-level*
NART[1]	109.05	(10.13)	111.20	(10.30)	0.94	>.30
Education (years)[2]	13.94	(2.56)	13.76	(2.57)	−0.30	>.75
Age	66.15	(6.65)	66.58	(5.47)	0.31	>.75
MMSE[3]	28.65	(1.42)	29.58	(0.71)	3.67	<.001
BDI-II[4]	7.59	(4.34)	4.13	(3.39)	−3.96	<.001
PD onset[5]						
DRS-II[6]	10.06	(2.60)	11.14	(2.40)		
UPDRS[7]	28.46	(9.49)				

[1]National Adult Reading Test; [2]Total number of years formal education; [3]Mini-Mental Status Exam; [4]Beck Depression Inventory; [5]Years since diagnosis of Parkinson's disease; [6]Demential Rating Scale–II; [7]Unified Parkinson's Disease Rating Scale (motor score component).

TABLE 2
Comparisons between Parkinson's disease group and matched controls on measures of language functioning, information processing speed, working memory, and attention

	PD patients	*Controls*	*t*	*p*
TLC-E total[1]	155.95 (19.12)	167.28 (16.22)	2.86	<.01
Subtests				
Ambiguous sentence	31.18 (6.47)	32.35 (5.63)	0.87	>.35
Making inferences	25.73 (4.87)	29.73 (4.64)	3.76	<.001
Oral expression	68.70 (8.22)	72.78 (6.07)	2.52	<.02
Figurative language	30.25 (5.48)	33.10 (3.79)	2.71	<.01
Information processing speed[2]	9.66 (1.87)	11.34 (1.47)	4.46	<.0001
Reading span	1.66 (0.57)	2.46 (0.67)	5.73	<.0001
Attentional set-shifting	10.23 (2.13)	10.95 (2.25)	1.48	>.10

[1]Test of Language Competence–Expanded, total score; [2]age-adjusted scores (mean = 10, *SD* = 3).

were also evident for tests of processing speed and working memory. However, there was no significant difference between the groups on attentional set-shifting or for ability to interpret ambiguous sentences.

Table 3 shows the correlations (using Pearson correlations) for the combined sample (i.e., PD patients and controls) between pragmatic language functioning and processing speed, working memory, and attentional set-shifting. Significant positive correlations were found between each of the different aspects of cognition and pragmatic language. Significant negative correlations were also found between disease state (i.e., PD patients vs. controls) and measures of cognition and pragmatic language functioning, confirming the deficits shown by PD patients in Table 2.

Next, a series of path analyses were conducted to determine whether the pragmatic language deficits observed in the PD patients might be a secondary effect of deficits in cognitive functioning. Specifically, whether working memory, processing speed and attentional set-shifting might mediate the relationship between disease state and pragmatic language functioning evidenced in Table 3. TLC-E total score was used as the measure of pragmatic language functioning.

Four basic steps were followed in the models described here (Shrout & Bolger, 2002). First, the direct path in which the independent variable (in this case disease state) caused a change in another dependent variable (in this case pragmatic language) was calculated (represented by the solid arc in Figures 1 and 2). The relationship between disease state and a potential mediating variable (attentional set-shifting, processing speed and working memory) was then tested. Next, the relationship between the proposed

TABLE 3
Correlations between measures of language functioning, processing speed memory, and attentional set-shifting for the combined Parkinson's disease and control group ($n = 80$)

	TLC-E total	*Ambiguous sentences*	*Making inferences*	*Oral expression*	*Figurative language*	*Processing speed*	*Reading span task*	*Attentional set-shifting*
TLC-E total								
Ambiguous sentences	0.72***							
Making inferences	0.73***	0.39***						
Oral expression	0.78***	0.42***	0.42**					
Figurative language	0.82***	0.45***	0.60***	0.51***				
Processing speed	0.51***	0.27*	0.54***	0.48***	0.42***			
Reading span	0.36***	0.26*	0.35**	0.22	0.40***	0.39***		
Attentional set-shifting	0.44***	0.23*	0.37***	0.37***	0.35**	0.27*	0.15	
PD vs. control	−0.31**	−0.10	−0.40***	−0.28*	−0.29**	−0.45***	−0.54***	−0.09

*$p < .05$; **$p < .01$; ***$p < .001$.

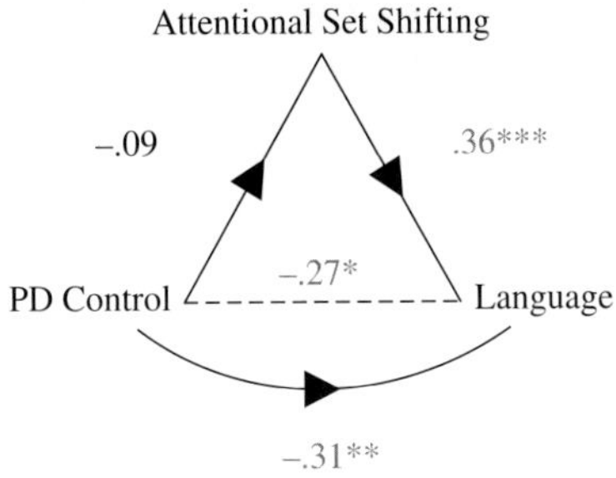

Figure 1. Path diagram where the intervening variable is attentional set-shifting.

mediating variable and pragmatic language was assessed. Finally, the change in the relationship between disease state and pragmatic language was calculated when the mediator was included. The resulting effect is the indirect path, signified by a dotted line in Figures 1 and 2. Sobel's z-test was used (Baron & Kenny, 1986) to test whether the difference in the relationship between disease state and pragmatic language when the mediator was included reflected a significant change.

As can be seen in Figure 1, there was no significant association between PD disease state and attentional set-shifting ability. Further, although performance on attentional set-shifting was significantly associated with language performance, there was no evidence of a significant mediating effect (Sobel's $z = 0.80$, $p > .40$) and the relationship between disease state and pragmatic language remained significant even after attentional set shifting ability was controlled for (see Table 4 for beta weights).

Figure 2 shows that there was a significant change in the relationship between disease state and pragmatic language functioning with the inclusion of either working memory or processing speed as a mediator (see Table 4 for full results). For both these models, the indirect pathway between disease

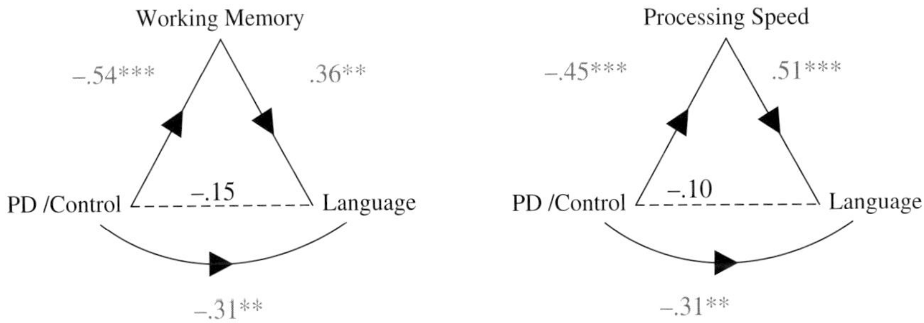

Figure 2. Path diagram where the intervening variable is working memory and separately processing speed.

TABLE 4
Regression coefficients for mediating variables

Variable	Step 1 (criterion: Lang) β	Step 1 (criterion: Lang) t	Step 2 (criterion: PS) β	Step 2 (criterion: PS) t	Step 3 (criterion: Lang) β	Step 3 (criterion: Lang) t
Group	−.31	−2.86**	−.45	−4.46***	−.10	−0.88 *ns*
Processing speed					.47**	4.32
			Step 2 (criterion: WM)		*Step 3 (criterion: Lang)*	
Group			−.54	−5.73***	−.16	−1.27 *ns*
Working memory					.27	2.16*
			Step 2 (criterion: ATT)		*Step 3 (criterion: Lang)*	
Group			−.09	−0.81 *ns*	−.27	−2.47**
Attentional set-shifting					.41	4.19***

Lang = language functioning; PS = processing speed; WM = working memory; ATT = attentional set-shifting.

state and pragmatic language functioning was no longer significant when the mediating variable was included, and the drop in association between the direct and indirect pathways was significant (Sobel's $z = 2.90$, $p < .01$ and $z = 3.4$, $p < .001$ for working memory and processing speed, respectively). Thus, results of the path analyses suggest that both working memory and processing speed, but not attentional set-shifting, can explain the deficits in pragmatic language functioning shown by the PD patients.

Because measures of working memory and processing speed were correlated, (see Table 3), multiple regression analysis was used to enable us to examine these two factors separately so that the effect of each could be estimated. We specifically wanted to test whether one of these variables might be primarily responsible for the pragmatic language deficits associated with PD. For these analyses, group (PD versus control) and verbal working memory (or processing speed) were entered at the first step, and processing speed (or verbal working memory) was entered at the second step. When group and verbal working memory were entered in the first step, processing speed was significantly related to the TLC-E ($\beta = .44$, R^2 change $= .15$, $p = .001$). However, when processing speed and group were entered on the first step, verbal working memory was not significantly related to the TLC-E ($\beta = .18$, R^2 change $= .02$, $p = .12$). These results suggest that processing speed is a stronger determiner of performance on the TLC-E than verbal working memory, and hence that the pragmatic language deficits associated with PD are best understood as being mediated by deficits in processing speed.

DISCUSSION

The goal of this study was to assess pragmatic language functioning in patients with PD compared to healthy older adults, and to examine the degree to which deficits that were observed could be explained by other cognitive processes. These processes included working memory, processing speed and attentional set-shifting. Patients with PD were found to perform significantly more poorly on pragmatic language tasks than healthy controls. Performances on pragmatic language tasks were significantly correlated with processing speed, verbal working memory, and attentional set-shifting. These three cognitive skills accounted for 13–26% of the variance on the TLC-E. Whereas path analyses indicated that both verbal working memory and processing speed mediated the relationship between disease status and higher order language functioning, multiple regressions confirmed that information processing speed was a stronger determiner of pragmatic language performance than verbal working memory. Overall, these results suggest that the pragmatic language deficits in PD are secondary to deficits in processing speed, more than likely reflecting the severe depletion of dopamine in the basal ganglia and subsequent deterioration of frontostriatal circuits that has been associated with deficits in executive functioning (Owen, 2004).

Our findings may indicate that processing speed declines more rapidly than working memory in individuals with PD compared to healthy older people, hence the stronger association between speed of processing and deficits in pragmatic language abilities. It is generally accepted that processing speed and working memory are interdependent, as processing speed plays a major role in working memory efficiency (Salthouse, 1994; Verhaeghen & Salthouse, 1997). For example, if processing speed is slowed, a higher demand is placed on the storage system of the working memory system. Therefore, impaired speed of processing ability could be viewed as underlying the cognitive deficits seen in PD.

However, as Verhaeghen and Salthouse (1997) point out, speed of processing and working memory share a high proportion of variance in different cognitive abilities, and neither appears to be a single determiner of age related declines. It therefore it seems likely that both processing speed and working memory contribute to complex cognitive activities such as the interpretation of pragmatic language in PD.

Another possible reason for our findings may be that the reading span task used was not a pure measure of working memory. Reading span tasks have been used as tests of working memory because they require active manipulation of information and concurrent item retention (Just & Carpenter, 1992). However, reading span tasks have been found to rely on many of the same processes as reading comprehension tasks (Engle,

Tuholski, Laughlin, & Conway, 1999), which makes it difficult to draw any strong conclusions in terms of the mediating value of working memory for pragmatic language skills. However, a working memory task that was not highly dependent on reading comprehension may have resulted in a different outcome to those reported in this study.

The comparisons between PD patients and matched controls in the present study are consistent with previous studies that have documented deficits in processing speed and working memory in PD patients (Berry, Nicolson, Foster, Behrmann, & Sagar, 1999; Lewis, Cools, et al., 2003; Lewis, Dove, et al., 2003; Lewis, Slabosz, Robbins, Barker, & Owen, 2005; Pillon et al., 1989). Further, PD patients have consistently been reported as experiencing difficulty in different components of language, particularly understanding complex sentences (Grossman et al., 2002; Hochstadt et al., 2006). Deficits in working memory and processing speed have previously been reported as affecting the accuracy of patients with PD with regard to understanding of complex sentences (Angwin et al., 2005; Grossman et al., 2002; Hochstadt et al., 2006). Given this evidence and the findings from our own investigations, it seems likely that both working memory and speed of processing contribute the effective understanding of pragmatic language.

Although relatively few studies have investigated outcomes for PD patients in terms of pragmatic language functioning, those that have reported deficits particularly for those experiencing cognitive problems (Lewis et al., 1998; McNamara et al., 1996; Monetta & Pell, 2007). Of particular interest is the study conducted by Lewis et al. (1998), which, contrary to this study, found evidence for deficits in the understanding of ambiguous sentences. However, patient characteristics may account for this apparent discrepancy. Lewis et al. did not explicitly exclude PD patients with dementia, and it is likely that interpretation of ambiguity is more impaired for these patients.

Pragmatic language functioning required in everyday communication is complex, with a considerable degree of novelty. It would be expected that these types of language interactions would rely more heavily on other cognitive skills such as of information processing working memory. The method of assessment used here enabled the examination of skills that closely resemble those used in everyday communication and their relationship with other cognitive skills. Nonetheless, it is pertinent to consider the limitations of this study. Although this study endeavoured to recruit a representative sample, patients were self-selected. Further, only nondemented patients with no illnesses apart from PD were included. It is likely that pragmatic language deficits would be more severe in patients with greater cognitive decline. Moreover, we individually matched participants in terms of age, education, and premorbid IQ, but we did not assess socioeconomic status, although it is highly correlated with cognitive ability.

Pragmatic language used in everyday communication requires the ability to understand meanings that extend beyond the actual words spoken. Understanding of ambiguity and inference of what is intended by the speaker is also required. Even subtle deficits in these areas of language may serve to increase isolation of PD patients from normal social interaction intensifying their reduced quality of life (Miller, Noble, Jones, & Burn, 2006). It is also likely that these types of difficulties may cause frustration for caregivers who may not understand the changes in comprehension and interpretation that are occurring for the patient. Understanding the exact nature of cognitive deficits, or intact skills, that could facilitate learning could potentially provide a means of intervention to ease any language problems. For example, education for professionals and caregivers regarding how to present information in an appropriate way to enhance communication could ease the frustration of caring for an individual who has difficulty communicating. Patients could be instructed in the use of strategies to clarify misunderstandings. Further, because effective communication appears to be linked with intact cognition, professionals could screen for cognitive decline as a marker for communication problems and take steps to intervene early in the disease process.

REFERENCES

American Psychiatric Association. (2000). *Diagnostic and Statistical Manual of Mental Disorders* (4th ed.). Washington, DC: American Psychiatric Association.

Angwin, A. J., Chenery, H. J., Copland, D. A., Murdoch, B. E., & Silburn, P. A. (2005). Summation of semantic priming and complex sentence comprehension in Parkinson's disease. *Cognitive Brain Research*, *25*, 78–89.

Baron, R. M., & Kenny, D. A. (1986). The moderator-mediator variable distinction in social psychological research: Conceptual, strategic, and statistical considerations. *Journal of Personality and Social Psychology*, *51*, 1173–1182.

Beck, A. T., Steer, R. A., & Brown, G. K. (1996). *Beck Depression Inventory* (2nd ed.). New York: Psychological Corporation.

Berry, E. L., Nicolson, R. I., Foster, J. K., Behrmann, M., & Sagar, H. J. (1999). Slowing of reaction time in Parkinson's disease: The involvement of the frontal lobes. *Neuropsychologia*, *37*(7), 787–795.

Bodis-Wollner, I., & Jo, M. Y. (2006). Getting around and communicating with the environment: Visual cognition and language in Parkinson's disease. *Journal of Neural Transmission Supplement*, *70*, 333–338.

Cooper, J. A., Sagar, H. J., Jordan, N., Harvey, N. S., & Sullivan, E. V. (1991). Cognitive impairment in early, untreated Parkinson's disease and its relationship to motor disability. *Brain*, *114*(5), 2095–2122.

Daneman, M., & Carpenter, P. (1980). Individual differences in working memory and reading. *Journal of Verbal Learning and Verbal Behavior*, *19*, 450–466.

Delis, D. C., Kaplan, E., & Kramer, J. H. (2001). *Delis Kaplan Executive Function System*. New York: Psychological Corporation.

Engle, R. W., Tuholski, S. W., Laughlin, J. E., & Conway, A. R. A. (1999). Working memory, short-term memory, and general fluid intelligence: A latent-variable approach. *Journal of Experimental Psychology: General*, *128*(3), 309–331.

Fahn, S., & Elton, R. L. (1987). *Unified Parkinson's Disease Rating Scale* (Vol. 2). Florham Park, NJ: Macmillan Health Care Information.

Folstein, M. F., Folstein, S. E., & McHugh, P. R. (1975). "Mini-mental state": A practical method for grading the cognitive state of patients for the clinician. *Journal of Psychiatric Research*, *12*(3), 189–198.

Frank, M. J. (2005). Dynamic dopamine modulation in the basal ganglia: A neurocomputational account of cognitive deficits in medicated and nonmedicated Parkinsonism. *Journal of Cognitive Neuroscience*, *17*(1), 51–72.

Gabrieli, J. D. E., Singh, J., Stebbins, G. T., & Goetz, C. G. (1996). Reduced working memory span in Parkinson's disease: Evidence for the role of a frontostriatal system in working and strategic memory. *Neuropsychology*, *10*(3), 322–332.

Gernsbacher, M. A., Keysar, B., Robertson, R. R. W., & Werner, N. K. (2001). The role of suppression and enhancement in understanding metaphors. *Journal of Memory and Language*, *45*, 433–450.

Glucksberg, S. (2003). The psycholinguistics of metaphor. *Trends in Cognitive Neuroscience*, *7*(2), 92–96.

Grossman, M. (1999). Sentence processing in Parkinson's disease. *Brain Cognition*, *40*(2), 387–413.

Grossman, M., Carvell, S., Gollomp, S., Stern, M. B., Vernon, G., & Hurtig, H. I. (1991). Sentence comprehension and praxis deficits in Parkinson's disease. *Neurology*, *41*(10), 1620–1626.

Grossman, M., Carvell, S., Stern, M. B., Gollomp, S., & Hurtig, H. I. (1992). Sentence comprehension in Parkinson's disease: The role of attention and memory. *Brain and Language*, *42*(4), 347–384.

Grossman, M., Cooke, A., DeVita, C., Lee, C., Alsop, D., Detre, J., et al. (2003). Grammatical and resource components of sentence processing in Parkinson's disease: An fMRI study. *Neurology*, *60*(5), 775–781.

Grossman, M., Zurif, E., Lee, C., Prather, P., Kalmanson, J., Stern, M. B., et al. (2002). Information processing speed and sentence comprehension in Parkinson's disease. *Neuropsychology*, *16*(2), 174–181.

Hochstadt, J., Nakano, H., Lieberman, A., & Friedman, H. (2006). The roles of sequencing and verbal working memory in sentence comprehension deficits in Parkinson's disease. *Brain and Language*, *97*, 243–257.

Hoehn, M. M., & Yahr, M. D. (1967). Parkinsonism: Onset, progression and mortality. *Neurology*, *17*(5), 427–442.

Hutton, S. B., Puri, B. K., Duncan, L. J., Robbins, T., Barnes, T. R. E., & Joyce, E. M. (1998). Executive function in first-episode schizophrenia. *Psychological Medicine*, *28*, 463–473.

Jorgensen, C., Barrett, M., Huistingh, R., & Zachman, L. (1981). *The WORD Test: A test of expressive vocabulary and semantics.* Moline, IL: LinguiSystems, Inc.

Jurica, P. J., Leitten, C. L., & Mattis, S. (2001). *DRS-2 Dementia Rating Scale-2: Professional manual.* Psychological Assessment Resources, Inc.

Just, M. A., & Carpenter, P. A. (1992). A capacity theory of comprehension: Individual differences in working memory. *Psychological Review*, *99*(1), 122–149.

Leentjens, A. F. (2004). Depression in Parkinson's disease: Conceptual issues and clinical challenges. *Journal of Geriatric Psychiatry and Neurology*, *17*(3), 120–126.

Lewis, S. J., Cools, R., Robbins, T. W., Dove, A., Barker, R. A., & Owen, A. M. (2003). Using executive heterogeneity to explore the nature of working memory deficits in Parkinson's disease. *Neuropsychologia*, *41*(6), 645–654.

Lewis, S. J., Dove, A., Robbins, T. W., Barker, R. A., & Owen, A. M. (2003). Cognitive impairments in early Parkinson's disease are accompanied by reductions in activity in frontostriatal neural circuitry. *Journal of Neuroscience, 23*(15), 6351–6356.

Lewis, S. J., Lapointe, L. L., Murdoch, B. E., & Chenery, H. J. (1998). Language impairment in Parkinson's disease. *Aphasiology, 12*(3), 193–206.

Lewis, S. J., Slabosz, A., Robbins, T. W., Barker, R. A., & Owen, A. M. (2005). Dopaminergic basis for deficits in working memory but not attentional set-shifting in Parkinson's disease. *Neuropsychologia, 43*(6), 823–832.

Lezak, M. D. (1995). *Neuropsychological assessment* (3rd ed.). Oxford, UK: Oxford University Press.

Lieberman, P., Friedman, J., & Feldman, L. S. (1990). Syntax comprehension deficits in Parkinson's disease. *Journal of Nervous and Mental Disease, 178*(6), 360–365.

Martin, I., & McDonald, S. (2003). Weak coherence, no theory of mind, or executive dysfunction? Solving the puzzle of pragmatic language disorders. *Brain and Language, 85*, 451–466.

McNamara, P., & Durso, R. (2003). Pragmatic communication skills in patients with Parkinson's disease. *Brain and Language, 84*, 414–423.

McNamara, P., Krueger, M., O'Quin, K., Clark, J., & Durso, R. (1996). Grammaticality judgments and sentence comprehension in Parkinson's disease: A comparison with Broca's aphasia. *International Journal of Neuroscience, 86*(1–2), 151–166.

Middleton, F. A., & Strick, P. L. (2000). Basal ganglia and cerebellar loops: Motor and cognitive circuits. *Brain Research and Brain Research Review, 31*(2–3), 236–250.

Miller, M., Noble, E., Jones, D., & Burn, D. (2006). Life with communication changes in Parkinson's disease. *Age and Ageing, 35*, 235–239.

Monetta, L., Ouellet-Plamondon, C., & Joanette, Y. (2006). Simulating the pattern of right-hemisphere-damaged patients for the processing of the alternative metaphorical meanings of words: Evidence in favour of a cognitive resources hypothesis. *Brain and Language, 96*, 171–177.

Monetta, L., & Pell, M. D. (2007). Effects of verbal working memory deficits on metaphor comprehension in patients with Parkinson's disease. *Brain and Language, 101*, 80–89.

Murdoch, B. E. (2001). Subcortical brain mechanisms in speech and language. *Folia Phoniatrica, 53*(5), 233–251.

Muslimovic, D., Post, B., Speelman, J. D., & Schmand, B. (2005). Cognitive profile of patients with newly diagnosed Parkinson disease. *Neurology, 65*(8), 1239–1245.

Owen, A. M. (2004). Cognitive dysfunction in Parkinson's disease: The role of frontostriatal circuitry. *Neuroscientist, 10*(6), 525–537.

Owen, A. M., Roberts, A. C., Polkey, C. E., Sahakian, B. J., & Robbins, T. W. (1991). Extra-dimensional versus intra-dimensional set shifting performance following frontal lobe excisions, temporal lobe excisions or amygdalo-hippocampectomy in man. *Neuropsychologia, 29*(10), 993–1006.

Perkins, M. R. (2005). Pragmatic ability and disability as emergent phenomena. *Cinical Linguistics and Phonetics, 19*(5), 367–377.

Pillon, B., Boller, F., Levy, R., & Dubois, B. (2001). Cognitive deficits and dementia in Parkinson's disease. In F. Boller & S. F. Cappa (Eds.), *Handbook of neuropsychology* (2nd ed., Vol. 6, pp. 311–371). New York: Elsevier Science BV.

Pillon, B., Dubois, B., Bonnet, A. M., Esteguy, M., Guimaraes, J., Lhermitte, F., et al. (1989). Cognitive slowing in Parkinson's disease fails to respond to levodopa treatment: The 15-objects test. *Neurology, 39*, 762–768.

Prutting, C. A., & Kirchner, D. M. (1987). A clinical appraisal of the pragmatic aspects of language. *Journal of Speech and Hearing Disorders, 52*(2), 105–109.

Royall, D. R., Lauterbach, E. C., Cummings, J. L., Reeve, A., Rummans, T. A., Kaufer, D. I., et al. (2002). Executive control function: A review of its promise and challenges for clinical research.

A report from the Committee on Research of the American Neuropsychiatric Association. *Journal of Neuropsychiatry and Clinical Neuroscience*, *14*(4), 377–405.

Salthouse, T. A. (1994). The aging of working memory. *Neuropsychology*, *8*(4), 535–543.

Shrout, P. E., & Bolger, N. (2002). Mediation in experimental and nonexperimental studies: New procedures and recommendations. *Psychological Methods*, *7*(4), 422–445.

Ullman, M. T. (2001). The declarative/procedural model of lexicon and grammar. *Journal of Psycholinguist Research*, *30*(1), 37–69.

Verhaeghen, P., & Salthouse, T. (1997). Meta-analyses of age-cognition relations in adulthood: Estimates of linear and nonlinear age effects and structural models. *Psychological Bulletin*, *3*, 231–249.

Waters, G. S., & Caplan, D. (1996). The capacity theory of sentence comprehension: Critique of Just and Carpenter (1992). *Psychological Review*, *103*(4), 761–772.

Wiig, E. H., & Secord, W. (1989). *Test of Language Competence–Expanded Edition*. New York: Psychological Corporation.

EUROPEAN JOURNAL OF COGNITIVE PSYCHOLOGY
2009, 21 (2/3), 347–365

Psychology Press
Taylor & Francis Group

Ageing and organisation strategies in free recall: The role of cognitive flexibility

Laurence Taconnat

Centre de Recherche sur la Cognition et l'Apprentissage and Imagerie Fonctionnelle, Université François-Rabelais de Tours, France

Naftali Raz

Institute of Gerontology and Department of Psychology, Wayne State University, Detroit, MI, USA

Capucine Toczé and Badiâa Bouazzaoui

Centre de Recherche sur la Cognition et l'Apprentissage and Imagerie Fonctionnelle, Université François-Rabelais de Tours, France

Hélène Sauzéon

Laboratoire de sciences cognitive, Université Victor Segalen, Bordeaux 2, France

Séverine Fay and Michel Isingrini

Centre de Recherche sur la Cognition et l'Apprentissage and Imagerie Fonctionnelle, Université François-Rabelais de Tours, France

The first goal of this experiment was to examine the effect of age on recall and clustering across three successive trials. Sixty-two young (age 20–40 years) and 62 elderly (age 60–80 years) adults learnt a categorised word list for subsequent recall. A clustering index was computed to assess organisational strategy. Results showed that elderly adults performed less well on the recall test and forgot more words across trials. They also indicated that their clustering index was lower than that of younger adults but increased more across trials. Clustering was only associated with the recall scores for the younger adults. Participants were also administered

Correspondence should be addressed to Laurence Taconnat, Département de Psychologie, UMR 6234, Université François-Rabelais, 3, rue des Tanneurs, 37000 Tours, France. E-mail: taconnat@univ-tours.fr

This study was supported by grants from the ANR–Agence Nationale pour la Recherche 2007: Cognitive ageing, strategic variations, and executive functions in arithmetic, memory, and skill acquisition. We thank Elizabeth Yates for reviewing the use of English language style in this paper.

http://www.psypress.com/ecp DOI: 10.1080/09541440802296413

cognitive tests (cognitive flexibility, cognitive speed, and categorical fluency) to explore the possible mediators of memory and organisational strategy performances. Younger adults performed better on all these tests. Statistical analyses revealed that the variable most closely associated with clustering was cognitive flexibility. This finding supports the view that the age-related decrement in strategic organisation is due to a decrease in cognitive flexibility.

Keywords: Ageing; Episodic memory; Processing speed; Executive functions; Cognitive flexibility; Mnemonic strategies.

Organising material by dividing it into smaller, more manageable units is one of the best ways to improve performance on free-recall tasks in which no external cue is provided to aid performance (Denney, 1974; Gershberg & Shimamura, 1995; Kausler, 1991). Use of such strategies in experimental settings can be quantified by clustering indexes showing semantic (categorical) or subjective organisation. The former reflects the degree to which participants recall semantically related words (examples of category, associates, synonyms), and the latter indicates the likelihood of participants recalling the same combination of words across multiple study trials.

Implementation of clustering as a mnemonic strategy may depend on the ability to organise information deliberately during recall and is frequently impaired following brain damage, especially when the lesion involves the prefrontal cortex and the adjacent white matter (e.g., Gershberg & Shimamura, 1995). Problems with applying optimal recall strategies have also been noted in schizophrenic patients (e.g., Brébion, David, Jones, & Pilowsky, 2004) and in elderly adults (e.g., West & Thorn, 2001). These instances of failure to deploy beneficial recall strategies are similar in one important respect: They all involve impairment of the frontal lobe structures (Holthausen et al., 2003; Raz, 2000). Prefrontal regions of the brain are believed to support goal-directed strategic cognitive operations, known collectively as executive functions (Moscovitch & Winocur, 2002; Parkin & Walter, 1992; Shimamura, 2002). Intact executive functions are vital for performing a large number of tasks that rely on control and coordination of multiple processes, notably free recall (Buckner, 2003; Parkin, Yeomans, & Bindschaedler, 1994; Velanova, Lustig, Jacoby, & Buckner, 2007).

Similarities between patterns of memory performance in patients with frontal lobe lesions and elderly adults have led to the frontal hypothesis of age-related memory decline (West, 1996). According to this hypothesis, age-related differences in memory arise from a decline in prefrontal cortex functioning, which may be particularly sensitive to the effects of ageing (Raz, 2000). The frontal/executive decline hypothesis of cognitive performance (West, 1996), and particularly memory, has received considerable empirical support (Moscovitch & Winocur, 1992; Parkin, 1997). One of the most prominent examples of the detrimental impact of prefrontal lesions on cognition is the deterioration of the ability to recall information without cognitive support (e.g., retrieval cues). Patients with frontal lobe lesions are particularly impaired when the tests depend on the use of memory strategies such as categorising word lists (e.g., Gershberg & Shimamura, 1995; Hirst & Volpe, 1988; Incisa della Rocchetta & Milner, 1993; Stuss et al., 1994). These disorders may reflect an impairment of executive control affecting selection and execution of organisational strategies (see Gershberg & Shimamura, 1995, and Stuss et al., 1994, for discussions about this point). Given the similarities between the patterns of memory impairment observed in patients with frontal lobe lesions and in elderly individuals, it is plausible that the deterioration of free recall might be due to a decrease in organisational strategies predicated by a specific impairment of executive functions.

The role of executive functions in the age-related decline of controlled processes of memory (Buckner, 2003; Bugaiska et al., 2007; Velanova et al., 2007), and particularly in mnemonic strategies (i.e., processes implemented to optimise memory performance), has been amply demonstrated (Bryan, Luszcz, & Pointer, 1999, Bunce, 2003; Taconnat et al., 2006, Taconnat, Clarys, Vanneste, Bouazzaoui, & Isingrini, 2007). However, the role of executive functions in organisational strategies has been explored mainly in patients with frontal lobe lesions but not in healthy elderly adults. Studies investigating age-related differences in clustering have yielded contradictory results. In some samples, clustering was not affected by age (e.g., Park, Smith, Dudley, & Lafronza, 1989; Rankin, Karol, & Tuten, 1984; Sauzéon, Claverie, & N'Kaoua, 2006), whereas other studies have shown decreased clustering with ageing (e.g., Denney, 1974; Howard, McAndrews, & Lagasa, 1981; West & Thorn, 2001; Zivian & Darjes, 1983). This discrepancy may stem from multiple causes, including differences in instructions given to the participants before performing the task, list length, typicality of the category examples, number of categories in the list, or the size of the samples studied (see Kausler, 1991, for a review of factors that may affect clustering scores).

The apparent lack of clear agreement among the studies may also reflect noncontrolled individual differences in implementing organisational strategy. For instance, when Sauzéon et al. (2006) found no age-related difference in a categorical clustering index computed to quantify the clustering strategy (Adjusted Ratio Clustering, ARC; Roenker, Thompson, & Brown, 1971), they observed exceptionally high variability among the older participants, for whom the coefficient of variation (standard deviation-to-mean ratio) exceeded 1.6, making detection of group differences highly unlikely. The source of this high variability in organisational strategy was not identified. In the light of the frontal/executive view of cognitive ageing outlined earlier, it is possible that at least some of that variability could be attributed to age-related decline in executive functions. Moreover, as executive functions represent a multidimensional construct, examination of their role in successful recall should involve multiple executive indices. The major constructs that fall under the rubric of "executive" functions are updating, inhibition, and shifting (Miyake et al., 2000). Cognitive flexibility is a common feature of these executive functions and refers to an ability to adapt cognitive behaviour to changing contexts in order to maximise success in a particular cognitive task (Ridderinkhof, Ullsperger, Crone, & Nieuwenhuis, 2004). Shifting (or switching) is believed to reflect cognitive flexibility, as both require a rapid transition between tasks and reconfiguration of task sets in response to environmental changes. Failure to shift a strategy (lack of cognitive flexibility) results in perseverative behaviour, and ability to transcend perseveration is thus important for effective strategic management of cognitive performance (Ridderinkhof, Span, & van der Molen, 2002; Ridderinkhof et al., 2004).

This paper focuses on the effect of ageing on an encoding strategy (clustering) known to enhance recall, and on the role of executive function therein. To this end, the present study was designed to explore the effect of age-related reduction in cognitive flexibility on the implementation of organisational strategy during free recall. It was expected that older adults would exhibit difficulties on tasks that depend on a strategy based on an age-sensitive function, such as cognitive flexibility (Ridderinkhof et al., 2002). However, ageing is also associated with significant declines in processing speed, irrespective of executive deficits (Salthouse, 1996), and advanced age is linked to significant declines in categorical fluency (Winocur, Moscovitch, & Stuss, 1996), which might be related to categorical clustering. We therefore tested the specificity of the cognitive flexibility hypothesis by comparing its effect with those of perceptual-motor speed and categorical fluency. Moreover, it was expected that if clustering is used as a strategy to improve recall, it should on the one hand be significantly and positively associated with recall, and on the other hand prevent the words in a recall trial being forgotten. However, because elderly adults experience difficulty carrying out most mnemonic strategies, we hypothesised that the link between clustering and recall would be stronger in young adults than in their older counterparts.

To test these assumptions, and to explore the evolution of recall and clustering in young and older adults, we related the indices of three age-sensitive cognitive measures (i.e., cognitive flexibility, speed of processing, and categorical fluency) to the amount of clustering and recall observed across three trials.

METHOD

Participants

The sample consisted of 124 healthy French adults living in a medium-sized metropolitan area. The participants were divided into two age groups: 62 younger (age 20–40 years, 26 women) and 62 older adults (age 60–81 years, 47 women). Four of the older participants were excluded from the sample due to their very low recall scores (less than five words recalled), and the statistical analyses were thus conducted on the scores of 62 young and 58 older adults, i.e., 120 participants. All the elderly participants lived at home and were recruited from leisure clubs and the Senior Citizens' University. The young participants were recruited from leisure clubs and through referrals by the elderly participants. In order to minimise a possible cohort effect and because none of the older adults had a high level of education, none of the young participants were recruited from higher education institutions. Participants were all volunteers, and were individually interviewed to exclude any with a history of alcoholism, undergoing treatment for psychiatric illness, or taking psychoactive medication. None of the elderly participants were institutionalised. The two groups were matched on their performances on the Mill Hill vocabulary test (Raven, Court, & Raven, 1986), number of years of formal education, self-reported health score (measured by using a 5-point scale from 0 ("bad health") to 5 ("very good health"), and depression scores on the HADS (Hospital Anxiety and Depression Scale; Zigmond & Snaith, 1983). These variables were controlled because verbal ability may affect verbal learning, level of formal education may affect learning strategies, and depression, generally found to be linked to self-evaluated health, is known to affect motivation to learn. The characteristics of each group are presented in Table 1. The older adults were also screened on the Mini-Mental State Examination (MMSE;

TABLE 1
Participants' characteristics in each group

	Age group		
	Young (n = 62) *M (SD)*	*Elderly (n = 58)* *M (SD)*	*t(118)*
Age (in years)	27.58 (5.60)	69.29 (5.16)	
Vocabulary	24.35 (3.56)	26.10 (4.57)	1.88*
Formal education (in years)	12.17 (2.11)	11.55 (2.74)	1.40
Self-reported health	3.64 (1.10)	3.65 (1.09)	0.007
Depression	7.61 (3.80)	7.19 (3.32)	0.64

*$p = .06$.

Folstein, Folstein, & McHugh, 1975), with the cutoff threshold set at 27 points to minimise the risk of including people with preclinical dementia. After the experiment, participants were informed about the general goal of the research.

As shown in Table 1, the age groups were matched on all measures, and a nonsignificant trend was only noted for the Mill Hill Vocabulary scores. As that small difference favoured the older participants, any age-related differences emerging in the dependent variables (i.e., clustering and recall) biased towards the younger adults would not be attributable to differences in verbal ability.

Materials and procedure

The experiment was conducted in two sessions, 3 to 5 days apart depending on the participants' availability, and no participants dropped out of the study. During the first session, participants were screened and interviewed. They performed the experimental episodic memory task and about half of the battery of paper-and-pencil cognitive tests. During the second session, they completed the cognitive test battery.

Experimental task: Episodic memory and clustering. Participants were shown once a categorised 20-word list (five categories of four words). The words were arranged and presented in pseudorandom order so that two words from the same category were never presented sequentially. Participants were not informed about the possible structuring of lists. The words for the five categories were selected from Marchal and Nicolas's (2003) table, constructed from category classes generated by young and elderly adults. The categories were matched with respect to word length, word frequency (Brulex database; Content, Mousty, & Radeau, 1990), and typicality of semantic category, similar for both young and elderly people. The words were 5–8 letters long, with 2–3 syllables, and were all concrete nouns. The mean frequency value of the words was 19.23 (the complete list of words is presented in the Appendix). The stimuli were presented on a computer screen, for 5 s each. After the list presentation, participants performed a letter comparison task (XO) for 45 s. This task served both as an interference task to prevent the recency effect and as a measure of processing speed. After the XO task, the participants were asked to say as many words as they could recall, and their replies were recorded by the experimenter. In this way, any difficulty in writing was avoided, particularly in older adults. The participants were asked to recall the list three times without relearning it, with 30 s between each repetition, with the aim of evaluating the evolution or stability of memory and clustering across time. At the end of learning and recall, participants relaxed for a few minutes before taking the remaining tests.

The *Adjusted Ratio Clustering* score (ARC) developed by Roenker et al. (1971) was used as a measure of categorical organisation at recall. It ranges from 0 to 1; a score of 0 indicates chance clustering and a score of 1 refers to perfect clustering. It is computed according to the following formula: $ARC = [R - E(R)]/[maxR - E(R)]$, where R is the total number of category repetitions, max R is the maximum possible number of category repetitions, and E(R) is the expected (chance) number of category repetitions" (Roenker et al., 1971, p. 46). It adjusts for the differences in total number of items recalled, which is important considering that young adults are likely to recall more words than older participants. Thus, ARC scores are relatively independent of the recall score, inasmuch as a low score at recall may lead to a high ARC score if the few words are recalled in an organised fashion.

Cognitive assessment. Three cognitive test scores were selected, designed specifically to evaluate different cognitive functions such as executive functions, speed, and categorical fluency (one score for each function). These cognitive abilities were selected because they are known to be related to age and to the dependent variables studied here. In order to identify which variables were most associated with clustering and recall, the association of each with performance on clustering and recall needed to be explored.

Cognitive flexibility. To assess cognitive flexibility we used the Wisconsin Card Sorting Test (WCST), which is sensitive to frontal lobe lesions and is thought to be a valid measure of executive functions (Lezak, 1995; Miyake et al., 2000; Spreen & Strauss, 1998). This test was administered and scored according to the standard procedure using two packs of 64 cards (Heaton, Chelune, Talley, Kay, & Curtiss, 1993; Lezak, 1995). The specific measure retained here was the number of perseverative errors, which are those most affected by age and the most representative of cognitive flexibility (Kaplan, Sengör, Gürvit, Genç, & Güzelis, 2006). Perseveration reflects difficulty in adaptively discontinuing a prepotent response or use of a previously reinforced strategy when its use is no longer beneficial. The number of perseverative errors thus seems to be an appropriate measure of the ability to use the best strategy to learn a categorised word list, where clustering is required to improve mnemonic performance. A high score on this test reflects low cognitive flexibility.

Processing speed. Processing speed was assessed using the letter-comparison test (Salthouse, 1990), in which participants were presented with a page containing pairs of letters (X-O). They were instructed to decide as fast as possible whether the two members of the pair were identical or not, and to tick the "identical" or "different" column accordingly. The dependent measure was the number of items answered correctly within 45 s. This test was also used as an interference task between learning and recall (see the earlier Procedure section).

Categorical fluency test. The categorical fluency test (from the Controlled Oral Word Association Test; Benton, Hamsher, & Sivan, 1983) was used to assess organisation in semantic memory. In this test, participants were required to say in 60 s as many different words as possible within a certain category (here: animals, fruits, and vegetables). This test has been found to be sensitive to level of frontal functional activity (Frith, Friston, Liddle, & Frackowiak, 1991; Gourovitch, Kirkby, & Goldberg, 2000). However, it has also been shown to be associated with temporal lobe activity (Pihlajamäki et al., 2000). For this reason, it was examined separately from the WCST, an executive task more specifically (although not exclusively) associated with the frontal brain regions. The categorical fluency test was intended to gauge the dependence of clustering strategy use on semantic and episodic organisation ability. It is sensitive to normal age-related cognitive decline (Winocur et al., 1996). The participants' score retained here was the total number of correct words generated across all three trials divided by three.

RESULTS

Effects of age and trials on clustering and recall

The descriptive statistics and age group comparisons of the cognitive variables are presented in Table 2.

Age-related differences in free recall. A 2 (age group) × 3 (trial) mixed analysis of variance was performed on the recall scores. The analysis revealed a main effect of age group, $F(1, 118) = 142.00$, $p < .0001$, $MSE = 0.047$, indicating that younger participants performed better than their older counterparts across the trials. A significant main effect of trial, $F(2, 236) = 13.16$, $p < .001$, $MSE = 0.006$, corresponded to the reduction in recall scores over trials. However, a significant Age group × Trial interaction, $F(2, 236) = 15.55$, $p < .01$, $MSE = 0.006$, indicated that performance decline was limited to the older participants, the younger participants maintaining a stable performance.

Age differences in use of clustering strategies. Inspection of the distribution of ARC scores across trials revealed clear departure from normality.

TABLE 2
Means (and standard deviation) of proportion of recall and clustering for each age group and trial

	Younger (n = 62)	*Older (n = 58)*	*t(118)*
Clustering (ARC)			
First trial	0.70 (0.28)	0.39 (0.25)	6.16*
Second trial	0.74 (0.24)	0.65 (0.32)	1.53
Third trial	0.84 (0.21)	0.79 (0.29)	1.06
Recall			
First trial	0.64 (0.10)	0.46 (0.15)	7.47*
Second trial	0.64 (0.11)	0.32 (0.15)	12.78*
Third trial	0.63 (0.11)	0.34 (0.16)	11.26*

$^*p < .001$.

Some participants attained very high scores indicating consistent use of clustering, whereas others showed limited use of that strategy. Thus, ARC scores were not amenable to parametric statistical analysis similar to the one performed on free-recall data. Comparison of the proportions of participants who used clustering at the 0.9–1.0 level (near or at the maximum possible) differed significantly between the age groups. In Trial 1, 34% of the young adults used clustering at the maximum level, whereas only 8.6% of the older adults did so, $\chi^2(1) = 11.26$, $p < .001$. However, on the later trials (2 and 3), the group difference disappeared. The proportion of consistent users of clustering among the older participants increased to 41%, whereas among the young group it remained stable at 36%, $\chi^2(1) = 0.50$, *ns*. On the third trial, 52% of the young and 56% of the old participants recorded ARC scores above 0.9, a nonsignificant difference, $\chi^2(1) = 0.56$, suggesting a more widespread use of clustering regardless of age. Thus, while the older adults gradually used the "right strategy", their performance diminished, whereas that of younger adults remained similar across the successive trials.

Age differences in the cognitive measures

The descriptive statistics for these measures are presented in Table 3. The comparisons show significant differences between the age groups on all cognitive variables, especially in the number of perseverative errors.

Association between recall and strategy use: Age group differences. To examine the possible links between use of clustering and success in free recall as well as possible age-related differences therein, we analysed free-recall scores as a function of age group and clustering use. Because of the irregular

TABLE 3
Means (and standard deviation) of cognitive function measures for the two age groups

	Younger (n = 62)	*Older (n = 58)*	*t(118)*
WCST-EP	10.87 (7.57)	25.41 (14.54)	6.93*
Speed	35.90 (7.12)	29.22 (9.29)	4.41*
Fluency	45.63 (10.46)	36.39 (12.51)	4.39*

*$p < .001$. WCST-EP: Number of perseverative errors in the Wisconsin Card Sorting Test, the measure of cognitive flexibility. Speed: Number of pairs completed in the letter comparison test. Fluency: Number of words generated in the Categorical Fluency Test.

pattern of the distribution described earlier, Clustering Use was categorised into a dichotomous "yes/no" variable with "yes" corresponding to ARC scores above 0.9. Each group was divided into two subgroups, accordingly. This procedure was applied at each trial. The age range of each group was large; thus, the mean age of both young adult groups and both older adult groups were examined. Mean age was similar for the two groups of younger adults for each trial (27.27 years vs. 28.14 years for those who clustered the best and least respectively, in Trial 1, 27.37 years vs. 27.97 years in Trial 2, and 26.76 years vs. 28.31 years in Trial 3). For the two groups of older adults, mean ages were 69.20 years for those who clustered the best and 68.71 years for those who clustered the least in Trial 1, 67.66 versus 69.53 in Trial 2, and 67.93 versus 69.84 in Trial 3. Thus, there is no reason to suspect that a difference in age is responsible for a possible difference in recall between participants who use the clustering strategy and those who do not.

In Trial 1, a significant age group difference in recall was observed, $F(1, 116) = 43.44$, $p < .001$, $MSE = 0.02$. The clustering use was marginally significant, $F(1, 116) = 3.17$, $p = .07$, $MSE = 0.05$, showing that participants who clustered the words recalled slightly more words than those who did not. The Age group × Clustering use interaction was significant, $F(1, 116) = 5.19$, $p < .05$, $MSE = 0.05$. Analyses of simple effects showed that only the young people who used clustering strategies most performed better than those who did not use the strategy (0.73 vs. 0.59, $p < .01$). No difference related to strategy use was observed in the older group (0.41 vs. 0.42, *ns*). In Trial 2, the age-related difference in recall scores was also significant, $F(1, 116) = 162.62$, $p < .0001$, $MSE = 0.018$. Neither a main effect of clustering use nor an interaction between age and clustering use were observed. In Trial 3, the effect of age remained strong and significant, $F(1, 116) = 126.80$, $p < .0001$, $MSE = 0.019$. There was no main effect of clustering use, $F(1, 116) = 0.63$, *ns*. However, the Age group × Clustering use interaction was significant, $F(1, 116) = 5.93$, $p < .05$, $MSE = 0.019$. Analysis of simple effects showed that, as in Trial 1, only the young people who used clustering strategies most performed better than their counterparts who did not use the strategy (0.67 vs. 0.59, $p < .01$). No difference related to strategy use was observed in the older group (0.32 vs. 0.37, *ns*). Thus, the use of clustering as a recall strategy was beneficial for the younger but not for the older participants.

Associations among all the variables were assessed using the nonparametric Spearman correlation coefficient ρ. The results are presented in Tables 4 and 5. The analyses were conducted separately for the young and older groups because the profiles of results differed in the two groups (i.e., there was a significant interaction between age group and clustering use on recall). As the age range within the groups was broad, we examined the potential links between the age of participants within each group and the cognitive variables. Based on studies showing that the use of encoding strategies relies on executive functions, we assumed that the organisation would be specifically correlated with the number of perseverative errors on the WCST. Better recall was expected to be associated with higher clustering scores, on the assumption that organisation is an encoding strategy that benefits recall. However, as shown by the previous analysis, recall and clustering were correlated only among the younger adults. On the other hand, free recall, which has been shown to depend on executive functions (e.g., Parkin et al., 1994), was expected to show positive links with the measure of cognitive flexibility.

The correlational analyses showed that age was not significantly correlated with the different variables. This indicates that cognitive performance did not vary as a function of age within each group. As expected, recall correlated significantly and positively with the clustering index in the younger adult group (for the first, second, and third trials, respectively: $\rho = .59$, $p < .001$, $\rho = .45$, $p < .01$, and $\rho = .27$, $p = .05$, see Table 4). These results indicate that the more the young participants used clustering, the more they recalled. These findings corroborate the results from the ANOVA (simple effects), which showed that use of clustering as a recall strategy was beneficial for the younger adults.

In the older adult group, recall on each trial and the corresponding ARC scores did not correlate significantly (see Table 5). However, surprisingly, the ARC score from the third trial was negatively correlated with the two previous recall scores. Thus, participants who clustered best in Trial 3 recalled fewer words in Trials 1 and 2. This could indicate that the older adults were able to cluster better when they applied the strategy to fewer have recalled words. In contrast to younger adults, speed of processing was related to the recall score in Trial 1 (and marginally correlated in Trial 2) in the older adults. This finding is in agreement with studies that show a central involvement of processing speed in memory (e.g., Perrotin, Isingrini, Souchay, Clarys, & Taconnat, 2006).

TABLE 4
Correlation matrix between cognitive variables and dependent variables: Young group ($N = 62$)

	Recall 1	*Recall 2*	*Recall 3*	*ARC 1*	*ARC 2*	*ARC 3*	*WCST-PE*	*Speed*	*Fluency*
Recall 2	70.***								
Recall 3	.51***	.69***							
ARC 1	.59**	.45**	.27*						
ARC 2	.48**	.46**	.23$^+$	.50**					
ARC 3	.49**	.41**	.39*	.62**	.69***				
WCST-PE	−.25$^+$	−.21	−.35**	−.27*	−.30*	−.32*			
Speed	.12	.22	.14	.12	.02	.21	−.09		
Fluency	−.12	.06	.22	.03	.18	.31*	−.36*	.19	
Age	.07	.17	.18	.05	.09	.06	−.12	.16	−.08

$^+p < .1$, $*p < .05$, $**p < .01$, $***p < .001$.

TABLE 5
Correlation matrix between cognitive variables and dependent variables: Older group ($N = 58$)

	Recall 1	*Recall 2*	*Recall 3*	*ARC 1*	*ARC 2*	*ARC 3*	*WCST-PE*	*Speed*	*Fluency*
Recall 2	.58***								
Recall 3	.57***	.87***							
ARC 1	−.16	−.15	−.20						
ARC 2	−.12	.06	.07	.10					
ARC 3	−.35*	−.27*	−.25$^+$	.23$^+$	.39**				
WCST-PE	−.12	−.17	−.26*	−.46***	−.44**	−.28*			
Speed	.42**	.22	.20	.15	.27*	.33*	−.22$^+$		
Fluency	.17	.04	.08	.07	.05	.13	.09	.31**	
Age	.20	.19	.12	.12	.19	.16	.05	−.21	−.17

$^+p < .1$, $*p < .05$, $**p < .01$, $***p < .001$.

The number of perseverative errors on the WCST was also correlated with the recall scores. In both groups the correlation was higher for the third trial than for Trials 1 and 2. One possible explanation of this finding is that the third trial took place a longer time after the learning stage than the previous trials and that executive processes required a longer time to gain influence on memory performance (see Leng & Parkin, 1989). The score on the categorical fluency test did not correlate with the recall scores. This lack of correlation may indicate that the retrieval of category classes from semantic memory and the recall of words in episodic memory are independent cognitive processes.

Clustering was significantly and negatively correlated with the number of perseverative errors on the WCST for each group and on each trial. Thus, as expected, use of clustering was associated with greater cognitive flexibility. For the older participants, at the second and third trials, clustering was marginally correlated with processing speed, a variable known as a marker of general age-related decline. In the younger group, clustering was correlated with the categorical fluency score on the third trial, suggesting that use of a clustering strategy for episodic recall might be related to the efficiency of word retrieval from categories stored in semantic memory, but only after the words were recalled twice.

GENERAL DISCUSSION AND CONCLUSION

This study investigated the influence of age, executive functions, categorical fluency, and processing speed on clustering strategy and free recall. While replicating the substantial age-related deficit in free recall, we also observed that older adults were less likely to use a clustering strategy than young participants. Moreover, the benefits of clustering were only apparent among the young participants. Although age-related deficits were observed in cognitive flexibility, processing speed, and categorical fluency, cognitive flexibility (less propensity for perseveration) was the variable the most reliably associated with better clustering for both age groups. Thus, it is possible that reduced executive control prevents the elderly from reaping the strategic support benefits that are apparent among younger adults.

The well-established effect of age on free-recall was replicated in the present study. The effect of age on clustering was also found, in agreement with some previous research on clustering strategy and ageing (e.g., Denney, 1974; Howard et al., 1981; West & Thorn, 2001; Zivian & Darjes, 1983). However, this result is inconsistent with reports that elderly adults can cluster as well as their younger counterparts (e.g., Park et al., 1989; Rankin et al., 1984; Sauzéon et al., 2006). This discrepancy might stem from differences in sample composition. The present study, which used a relatively large sample (62 younger and 58 older participants), had sufficient statistical power to reveal even relatively small effects (see Park et al., 2002). Samples that include participants from senior centres or in nursing care facilities, or people with low educational attainment, may lead to overestimation of the age effects (see Hedden & Gabrieli, 2004). In our sample, the older adults had a similar educational level as the younger group and had slightly higher vocabulary test scores.

Overall, these results show that both recall and the use of clustering strategies that support recall among the young diminish with age. An interesting finding concerns the trial-by-trial changes in the effects of age on clustering and on recall. First, the results reveal that the elderly adults forgot words across trials, whereas the younger adults did not; but, at the same time, they show that both elderly and young adults clustered more across successive trials. Taken alone, this result would suggest that although the elderly experienced difficulty in applying a clustering strategy at the first recall, they somehow caught up and used it as extensively as the younger adults. Thus, one would expect that with the aid of a strategy proven successful in the young, older adults would be able to improve their recall. Unfortunately, this expectation is not borne out by the data: the elderly improved their clustering while they lost words across trials. Moreover, when looking at quality of recall, it transpires that the words lost in Trial 2 (the elderly forgot words between Trials 1 and 2, whereas recall was the same in Trials 2 and 3) were those that were not included in clusters (i.e., they were isolated words). Thus, although clustering to some extent prevented forgetting, the words that were not recalled in an organised way in Trial 1 were not reorganised in the subsequent recalls. Hence, virtually no benefits of this seemingly useful strategy were experienced by the older participants. Once the words had been lost, no strategy could help recover them. These findings highlight the importance of introducing useful strategies as early as possible in the learning process, and herein lies an important point to anyone who plans to teach "old dogs new tricks".

Because of the computation method of the clustering index (ARC; Roenker et al., 1971), the absence of isolated words inflated the index value, raising a question about its differential validity for normal and memory-impaired individuals. Organisation only works when you have material to organise. The finding of the differential benefits of clustering is in accordance with our hypothesis and with earlier observations (Denney, 1974). The age-related decrease in using controlled mnemonic strategies has already been observed in several previous studies of strategic encoding (e.g., Bryan et al., 1999; Taconnat et al., 2006; Taconnat & Isingrini, 2004) and strategic retrieval (Bugaiska et al., 2007; Bunce, 2003; Dunlosky & Hertzog, 1998; Taconnat et al., 2007). However, our findings indicate that lack of strategy use by the elderly is neither total nor unconditional; it just comes too late.

The question arises about what accounts for the dramatic age-related differences in free recall that start at the first trial and become unrecoverable in spite of using an appropriate strategy. Exploration of recall mediators revealed that the number of perseverative errors on the WCST was the variable most closely associated with clustering performance. This measure looks at cognitive flexibility, a function largely involved in the use of adaptive strategies (e.g., Ridderinkhof et al., 2002). The role of cognitive flexibility in the recall of a categorised word list might be to prevent recalling the learned words in the order they were presented (or recalled at the previous trial), but to reorganise the words on the basis of their semantic category, so that words of the same category are recalled together (clustering). In this case, the category name would serve as a retrieval cue, explaining why clustering helps recall. This suggests that the age-related decline in cognitive flexibility could explain the impairment in using organisational strategies, especially at the initial trial.

The specific, reliable association between the recall score and the number of perseverative errors, considered as the most representative of the executive function factors (Miyake et al., 2000), is consistent with the theoretical viewpoint that the frontal structures which mainly underlie executive functioning are involved in episodic memory (see Moscovitch & Winocur, 1992, 1995, 2002; Wheeler, Stuss, & Tulving, 1995). The findings are also broadly consistent with studies of healthy adults, in which age-related differences in episodic memory have been explained by differences in prefrontal cortical volumes and mediated via their effects on other executive functions, such as working memory (Head, Rodrigue, Kennedy, & Raz, 2008).

Reduced executive control may affect memory in many ways, one of which, as shown by our results, is delayed application of organisation strategy. In light of the associations between ageing, prefrontal decline, and mediators of episodic recall, this finding is in accordance with observations of patients with frontal lobe lesions who cluster and recall less than healthy adults (e.g., Gershberg & Shimamura, 1995).

In sum, on the basis of the findings presented here, we conclude that although clustering is a beneficial strategy for boosting free recall of verbal material, its benefits are time sensitive and age dependent. Moreover, it can be concluded that clustering in young and older adults is not exactly comparable. The young participants seem to use that strategy to enhance recall and to prevent forgetting by reorganising materials across the successive trials. The older adults appear to apply the same approach when they recall fewer words and forget the nonclustered words across the successive recall trials. Thus, if it is not applied at the very beginning of recall trials, as done by the younger participants, clustering yields no benefits. This crucial delay in deploying a useful strategy may be related to reduced cognitive flexibility and the ensuing inability to respond to changes in cognitive demands. Cognitive flexibility, which emerges as one of the best associated variables for clustering, is important in both young and older adults. However, because it is reduced in the latter, it is more likely to result in memory impairment mediated by the lack of strategic support. Future studies of memory rehabilitation methods need to take into account this aspect of age difference in the timing of a strategy application and its executive determinants.

REFERENCES

Benton, A. L., Hamsher, K., & Sivan, A. B. (1983). *Multilingual aphasia examination* (3rd ed.). Iowa City, IA: AJA Associates.

Brébion, G., David, A. S., Jones, H., & Pilowsky, L. S. (2004). Semantic organization and verbal memory efficiency in patients with schizophrenia. *Neuropsychology, 18*, 378–383.

Bryan, J., Luszcz, M. A., & Pointer, S. (1999). Executive function and processing resources as predictors of adult age differences in the implementation of encoding strategies. *Aging, Neuropsychology, and Cognition*, *6*(4), 273–287.

Buckner, R. L. (2003). Functional-anatomic correlates of control processes. *Journal of Neuroscience*, *23*(10), 3999–4004.

Bugaiska, A., Clarys, D., Jarry, C., Taconnat, L., Tapia, G., Vanneste, S., & Isingrini, M. (2007). The effect of aging in recollective experience: The processing speed and executive functioning hypothesis. *Consciousness and Cognition*, *16*, 797–808.

Bunce, D. (2003). Cognitive support at encoding attenuates age differences in recollective experience among adults of lower frontal lobe function. *Neuropsychology, 17*(3), 353–361.

Content, A., Mousty, P., & Radeau, M. (1990). BRULEX. Une base de données lexicales informatisée pour le français écrit et parlé. *L'Année Psychologique*, *90*, 551–566.

Denney, N. W. (1974). Evidence for developmental changes in categorization criteria for children and adults. *Human Development*, *17*, 41–53.

Dunlosky, J., & Hertzog, C. (1998). Aging and deficits in associative memory: What is the role of strategy production? *Psychology and Aging*, *13*, 597–607.

Folstein, M. F., Folstein, S. E., & McHugh, P. R. (1975). Mini Cognitive State": A practical method for grading the cognitive state of patients for the clinician. *Journal of Psychiatric Research*, *12*, 189–198.

Frith, C. D., Friston, K. J., Liddle, P. F., & Frakowiak, R. S. J. (1991). Willed action and the prefrontal cortex in man: A study with PET. *Proceedings of the Royal Society of London*, *244*, 241–246.

Gershberg, F., & Shimamura, A. (1995). Impaired used organizational strategies in free recall following frontal damage. *Neuropsychologia*, *13*(10), 1305–1333.

Gourovitch, M. L., Kirkby, B. S., & Goldberg, T. E. (2000). A comparison of rCBF patterns during letter and semantic fluency. *Neuropsychology, 14*, 353–360.

Head, D., Rodrigue, K. M., Kennedy, K. M., & Raz, N. (2008). Neuroanatomical and cognitive mediators of age-related differences in episodic memory. *Neuropsychology, 22*, 491–507.

Heaton, R. K., Chelune, G. J., Talley, J. L., Kay, G. C., & Curtiss, G. (1993). *Wisconsin Card Sorting Test: Manual*. Odessa, FL: Psychological Assessment Resources.

Hedden, T., & Gabrieli, J. D. E. (2004). Insights into the ageing mind: A review from cognitive neuroscience. *Nature Reviews Neuroscience*, *5*, 87–96.

Hirst, W., & Volpe, B. T. (1988). Memory strategies with brain damage. *Brain and Cognition*, *8*, 379–408.

Holthausen, E. A. E., Wiersma, D., Dingemans, P. M., Schene, A. H., Sitskoorn, M. M., & van der Bosh, R. J. (2003). Long-term memory deficits in schizophrenia: Primary or secondary dysfunction? *Neuropsychology*, *17*, 539–547.

Howard, D. V., McAndrews, M. P., & Lagasa, M. L. (1981). Semantic priming of lexical decisions in young and older adults. *Journal of Gerontology*, *36*, 707–714.

Incisa Della Rocchetta, A., & Milner, B. (1993). Strategic search and retrieval inhibition: The role of the frontal lobes. *Neuropsychologia*, *31*, 503–524.

Kaplan, G. B., Sengör, N. S., Gürvit, H., Genç, I., & Güzelis, C. (2006). A composite neural network model for perseveration and distractibility in the Wisconsin card sorting test. *Neural Networks*, *19*, 375–387.

Kausler, D. H. (1991). Episodic memory: Effortful phenomena. In: D. H. Kausler (Ed.), *Experimental psychology, cognition, and human aging* (2nd ed., pp. 365–430). New York: Springer-Verlag.

Leng, N. R. C., & Parkin, A. J. (1989). Actiological variation in the amnesic syndrome: Comparisons using the Brown-Peterson task. *Cortex*, *25*, 251–259.

Lezak, M. D. (1995). *Neuropsychological assessment*. Oxford: Oxford University Press.

Marchal, A., & Nicolas, S. (2003). Normes de production catégorielle pour 38 catégories sémantiques [Category generation norms for 38 semantic categories in young and older subjects]. *L'Année Psychologique*, *103*, 313–366.

Miyake, A., Friedman, N., Emerson, M., Witzki, A., Howerter, A., & Wager, T. (2000). The unity and diversity of executive functions and their contributions to complex frontal lobe tasks: A latent variable analysis. *Cognitive Psychology*, *41*, 49–100.

Moscovitch, M., & Winocur, G. (1992). The neuropsychology of memory and aging. In F. I. M. Craik & T. A. Salthouse (Eds.), *The handbook of aging and cognition* (pp. 315–371). Hillsdale, NJ: Lawrence Erlbaum Associates, Inc.

Moscovitch, M., & Winocur, G. (1995). Frontal lobes, memory, and aging. In J. Grafman, K. J. Holyoak, et al. (Eds.), *Annals of the New York Academy of Sciences* (Vol. 769, pp. 119–150) New York: New York Academy of Sciences.

Moscovitch, M., & Winocur, G. (2002). The frontal cortex and working with memory. In D. T. Stuss & R. T. Knight (Eds.), *Principles of frontal lobe function* (pp. 188–209). New York: Oxford University Press.

Park, D., Lautenschlager, G., Hedden, T., Davidson, S., Smith, A. D., & Smith, P. K. (2002). Models of visuospatial and verbal memory across the adult life span. *Psychology and Aging*, *17*, 299–320.

Park, D. C., Smith, A. D., Dudley, W. N., & Lafronza, V. N. (1989). Effects of age and a divided attention task presented during encoding and retrieval on memory. *Journal of Experimental Psychology: Learning, Memory, and Cognition*, *15*, 1185–1191.

Parkin, A., & Walter, B. M. (1992). Recollective experience, normal aging and frontal dysfunction. *Psychology and Aging*, *2*, 290–298.

Parkin, A., Yeomans, J., & Bindschaedler, C. (1994). Further characterization of the executive memory impairment following frontal lobe lesions. *Brain and Cognition*, *26*, 23–42.

Parkin, A. J. (1997). Normal age-related memory loss and its relation to frontal lobe dysfunction. In P. Rabbitt (Ed.), *Methodology of frontal and executive function* (pp. 177–190). Hove, UK: Psychology Press.

Perrotin, A., Isingrini, M., Souchay, C., Clarys, D., & Taconnat, L. (2006). Episodic feeling-of-knowing accuracy and cued recall in the elderly: Evidence for double dissociation involving executive functioning and processing speed. *Acta Psychologica, 122*, 56–73.

Pihlajamäki, M., Tanila, H., Hänninen, T., Könönen, M., Laakso, M., Partanen, K., et al. (2000). Verbal fluency activates the left medial temporal lobe: A functional magnetic resonance imaging study. *Annals of Neurology, 47*, 470–476.

Rankin, J. L., Karol, R., & Tuten, C. (1984). Strategy use, recall, and recall organization in young, middle-aged, and elderly adults. *Experimental Aging Research, 10*, 193–196.

Raven, J. C., Court, J. H., & Raven, J. (1986). *Manual for Raven's progressive matrices and vocabulary scales.* Oxford, UK: Oxford Psychologists Press.

Raz, N. (2000). Aging of the brain and its impact on cognitive performance: Integration of structural and functional findings. In F. I. M. Craik & T. A. Salthouse (Eds.), *The book of aging and cognition* (pp. 1–90). Mahwah, NJ: Lawrence Erlbaum Associates, Inc.

Ridderinkhof, K. R., Span, M. M., & van der Molen, M. W. (2002). Perseverative behavior and adaptive control in older adults: Performance monitoring, rule induction, and set shifting. *Brain and Cognition, 49*, 382–401.

Ridderinkhof, K. R., Ullsperger, M., Crone, E. A., & Nieuwenhuis, S. (2004). The role of medial frontal cortex in cognitive control. *Science, 306*, 443–447.

Roenker, D. L., Thompson, C. P., & Brown, S. C. (1971). Comparison of measures for the estimation of clustering in free recall. *Psychological Bulletin, 76*, 45–48.

Salthouse, T. A. (1990). Working memory as a processing resource in cognitive aging. *Developmental Review, 10*, 101–124.

Salthouse, T. A. (1996). The processing-speed theory of adult age differences in recognition. *Psychological Review, 103*, 403–427.

Sauzéon, H., Claverie, B., & N'Kaoua, B. (2006). Age differences in the organization and acquisition-forgetting processes in a multi-free-recall task. *Current Psychology Letters, 18*, 1.

Shimamura, A. P. (2002). Relational binding theory and the role of consolidation in memory retrieval. Memory retrieval and executive control processes. In D. T. Stuss & R. T. Knight (Eds.), *Principles of frontal lobe function* (pp. 210–220). New York: Oxford University Press.

Spreen, O., & Strauss, E. (1998). *A compendium of neuropsychological tests: Administration, norms, and commentary* (2nd ed.) (p. 1998). New York: Oxford University Press.

Stuss, D. T., Alexander, M. P., Palumbo, C. L., Buckle, L., Sayer, L., & Poghe, J. (1994). Organizational strategies with unilateral or bilateral frontal lobe injury in word learning tasks. *Neuropsychology, 8*, 355–373.

Taconnat, L., Baudouin, A., Fay, S., Clarys, D., Vanneste, S., Tournelle, L., & Isingrini, M. (2006). Aging and implementation of encoding strategies in the generation of rhymes: The role of executive functions. *Neuropsychology, 6*, 658–665.

Taconnat, L., Clarys, D., Vanneste, S., Bouazzaoui, B., & Isingrini, M. (2007). Aging and strategic retrieval in memory: The role of executive functions. *Brain and Cognition, 64*, 1–6.

Taconnat, L., & Isingrini, M. (2004). Cognitive operations in the generation effect on a recall test: Role of aging and divided attention. *Journal of Experimental Psychology: Learning, Memory, and Cognition, 30*(4), 827–837.

Velanova, K., Lustig, C., Jacoby, L. L., & Buckner, R. L. (2007). Evidence for frontally mediated controlled processing differences in older adults. *Cerebral Cortex, 17*, 1033–1046.

West, R. J. (1996). An application of prefrontal function theory to cognitive aging. *Psychological Bulletin, 120*, 272–292.

West, R. L., & Thorn, R. M. (2001). Goal-setting, self-efficacy, and memory performance in older and younger adults. *Experimental Aging Research, 27*, 41–65.

Wheeler, M. A., Stuss, D. T., & Tulving, E. (1995). Frontal lobe damage produces episodic memory impairment. *Journal of the International Neuropsychological Society, 1*, 525–536.

Winocur, G., Moscovitch, M., & Stuss, D. T. (1996). Explicit and implicit memory in the elderly: Evidence for double dissociation involving medial temporal- and frontal-lobe functions. *Neuropsychology, 10*, 57–65.

Zigmond, A. S., & Snaith, R. P. (1983). The Hospital Anxiety and Depression Scale. *Acta Psychiatrica Scandinavica, 67*, 361–370.

Zivian, M., & Darjes, R. W. (1983). Free recall by in-school and out-of-school adults: Performance and metamemory. *Developmental Psychology, 19*, 513–520.

APPENDIX

Words presented (in French with their English translation). The names of the categories were not given, and the words were presented randomly.

French words	*English translation*
Animaux	*Animals*
Lapin	Rabbit
Canari	Canary
Tortue	Tortoise
Renard	Fox
Légumes	*Vegetables*
Carotte	Carrot
Poireau	Leek
Tomate	Tomato
Oignon	Onion
Parties du corps	*Parts of body*
Jambe	Leg
Oreille	Ear
Cheveu	Hair
Epaule	Shoulder
Vêtements	*Clothes*
Bonnet	Cap
Manteau	Coat
Pantalon	Trousers
Chemise	Shirt
Véhicules	*Vehicles*
Bateau	Boat
Voiture	Car
Avion	Plane
Train	Train

EUROPEAN JOURNAL OF COGNITIVE PSYCHOLOGY
2009, 21 (2/3), 366–387

Psychology Press
Taylor & Francis Group

Cross-modal repetition priming in young and old adults

Soledad Ballesteros, Montserrat González, Julia Mayas, Beatriz García-Rodríguez, and José Manuel Reales
Universidad Nacional de Educación a Distancia, Madrid, Spain

Previous research with young adults has shown cross-modal repetition priming for familiar objects between vision and touch. The present study further investigated whether cross-modal priming between these two perceptual modalities is preserved in older adults (Experiment 1). The study also investigated whether within-modal and cross-modal priming for ecological sounds and pictures is preserved with age by comparing performance of younger and older adults (Experiment 2). The results from both experiments showed that the repetition priming exhibited by young adults was similar to that shown by the older participants. These behavioural findings on cross-modal visual, auditory, and haptic priming as well as other recent results from neuroimaging studies reviewed in this paper suggest the implication of areas in the occipital cortex that were previously considered modality specific. Cross-modal facilitation might occur in posterior extrastriate occipital areas that are well preserved in normal ageing.

Keywords: Ageing; Cross-modal priming; Multisensory processing; Touch; Vision; Audition.

An important question in psychology and neuroscience is how object features extracted from different perceptual modalities are integrated to form coherent object representations that can be identified (e.g., Amedi, von Kriegstein, van Atteveldt, Beauchamp, & Naumer, 2005; Molhom, Ritter, Javitt, & Foxe, 2004; Taylor, Moss, Stamatakis, & Tyler, 2006) and retrieved

Correspondence should be addressed to Soledad Ballesteros, Facultad de Psicología, Universidad Nacional de Educación a Distancia, Juan del Rosal, 10, 28040 Madrid, Spain. E-mail: mballesteros@psi.uned.es

This study was supported by the Comunidad de Madrid and the DGICYT grants 06/HSE/2004 and SEJ2004-00752/PSIC to SB. MG and JM were supported by predoctoral grants from UNED and Ministerio de Educación (AP2003-0639), respectively. We thank Susana Paz for her help with data collection. We thank Morton Heller for his comments on a previous version of this paper. Finally, we are very grateful to Fergus Craik and two anonymous reviewers for their thoughtful comments. Parts of this research were presented at the Cognitive Ageing Symposium organised by S. Ballesteros and L.-G. Nilsson, at the ninth European Congress of Psychology, Granada, Spain, 3–8 July 2005.

http://www.psypress.com/ecp DOI: 10.1080/09541440802311956

under explicit and implicit conditions (e.g., Ballesteros, 2008; Ballesteros, Reales, Mayas, & Heller, 2008; Easton, Greene, & Srinivas, 1997; Easton, Srinivas, & Greene, 1997; James et al., 2002; Reales & Ballesteros, 1999).

We normally perceive objects and events occurring in our world by means of multiple modalities. Although in the sighted, vision is considered the primary sensory modality used to interact with objects in the world, other perceptual modalities, specially touch and audition, provide us with important information about an object's structure, shape and size. In previous studies, we (Ballesteros & Reales, 2004; Reales & Ballesteros, 1999) speculated that visual and haptic object representations might be shared between these two perceptual modalities. Reales and Ballesteros (1999) used a cross-modal priming paradigm with young adults and showed that exposure to real three-dimensional (3-D) familiar objects in one modality facilitated naming in a second encounter with the same 3-D object presented to the other modality. This facilitation is called repetition priming (Graf & Schacter, 1985; Schacter, 1987; Tulving & Schacter, 1990) and it is indicated when performance attributable to an experience with the stimuli previously encountered improves when the same stimuli are repeated. Here, we present the results from two experiments conducted to investigate whether the representations of familiar objects encoded visually, auditory, or haptically are modality specific and if this information is preserved with age. As far as we know, this is the first study that explored cross-modal repetition priming in three different modalities in young and older healthy individuals.

In recent years, there has been a trend in psychology (e.g., Ballesteros & Reales, 2004; Demattè, Sanabria, Sugerman, & Spence, 2006; Spence, Ranson, & Driver, 2000; Reales & Ballesteros, 1999) and neuroscience (e.g., Amedi et al., 2005; James et al., 2002; Molholm et al., 2004; Newman, Klatzky, Lederman, & Just, 2005; Pascual-Leone & Hamilton, 2001; Sathian & Prather, 2006; Taylor et al., 2006; Thesen, Vibell, Calvert, & Osterbauer, 2004) towards the view that perception is typically multimodal. In object recognition, multisensory (visual and auditory) inputs from the same object produce benefits because multimodal object recognition is faster than unimodal object recognition. This behavioural enhancement is signalled by the visually evoked potential N1 associated with the early feature processing in the ventral visual stream (Molholm et al., 2004).

AGE-RELATED CHANGES IN MEMORY PROCESSES

A wealth of research suggests age-related declines in a number of cognitive processes (e.g., Craik & Byrd, 1982; Hasher & Zacks, 1988; Park, 1999; Park et al., 2002; Prull, Gabrieli, & Bunge, 2000). Age-related memory changes have been observed not only in cross-sectional but also in longitudinal studies (Dixon et al., 2004; Nilsson, 2003). However, not all types of memories deteriorate equally with age. In contrast to the decline found on episodic memory in older adults, age invariance has usually been reported in within-modal implicit memory studies conducted with words and pictures of objects (Ballesteros, Reales, & Mayas, 2007; Mitchell, 1989; Mitchell & Schmitt, 2006; Prull et al., 2000; Schacter, Cooper, & Valdiserri, 1992), as well as with objects presented haptically (Ballesteros & Reales, 2004). Young and older healthy adults often show the same levels of repetition priming although the latter may sometimes have difficulty in intentionally remembering new facts and events (e.g., La Voie & Light, 1994; Light, 1991; Park, 1999; Park & Shaw, 1992).

This dissociation between episodic memory and repetition priming tasks is consistent with the idea that different memory systems mediated these two types of memory tasks. These haptic results support previous findings reported using words and novel patterns presented either to audition or vision (e.g., Keane, Gabrieli, Growdon, & Corkin, 1994; Park et al., 1998; Postle, Corkin, & Growdon, 1996; Verfaellie, Keane, & Johnson, 2000).

CROSS-MODAL PRIMING: FINDINGS IN YOUNG ADULTS

Only a few behavioural studies have investigated cross-modal repetition priming between vision and touch in young adults. Easton, Srinivas, and Greene (1997) used verbal stimuli and found that when the confounding of simultaneous and successive processing was controlled by presenting words to both modalities sequentially, cross-modal priming was similar to within-modal priming. In another study, Easton, Greene, and Srinivas (1997) presented novel raised-shapes and familiar objects. Results showed robust although diminished cross-modal facilitation.

Reales and Ballesteros (1999) conducted a series of cross-modal (vision to touch and touch to vision) experiments with young adults in which they examined whether priming is modality specific when familiar objects were presented to touch and vision at encoding and test. The results showed that repetition priming is not modality specific as complete cross-modal facilitation between both modalities (touch and vision) was reported. Implicit memory for familiar objects assessed by a *speeded object naming implicit task* showed similar perceptual facilitation for visually and for haptically previously encoded objects in both within-modal and cross-modal conditions (Exps 1 and 2). Furthermore, a levels-of-processing manipulation did not produce an effect on either within-modal or cross-modal priming. Results also showed that cross-modal and within-modal priming were present half an hour after encoding (Exp. 3). Based on these results, we proposed that vision and touch afford converging, common, long-lasting, abstract structural representations of 3-D objects. The findings suggest that cross-modal repetition priming is sensitive to high-level structural features of object shape. Once built these structural descriptions of objects can be accessed either by vision or by touch.

To our knowledge, just a single published behavioural study (Greene, Easton, & LaShell, 2001) has investigated cross-modal priming for visual and auditory events in undergraduate students. The study showed that while visual study produced auditory priming, auditory study produced auditory priming (within-modal priming) but not visual priming.

EXPERIMENTS

The multisensory nature of the mental representations of objects and events that occur within a certain spatiotemporal structure can lead to behavioural advantages in terms of response time and accuracy (e.g., Newell, 2004). Perceptual modalities do not work in isolation. They provide complementary and redundant information about objects in the environment, which facilitate recognition accuracy and identification speed (Amedi et al., 2005; Millar, 1994). Multisensory integration is a crucial characteristic of human perception (Fort, Delpuech, Pernier, & Guiard, 2002). Numerous recent studies in intersensory integration and cross-modal associations have shown cross-modal links in information processing between auditory and somatosensory modalities (e.g., Soto-Faraco, Spence, & Kingstone, 2004; Spence et al., 2000), and even between olfaction and touch (Demattè et al., 2006). This suggests that the information extracted by different sense modalities is combined in certain ways to facilitate perception and action (see Zampini, Torresan, Spence, & Murray, 2007).

Electrophysiological studies have further demonstrated the links between the neural processing of auditory and somatosensory information (e.g., Eimer, Val Valzen, & Driver, 2002; Murray et al., 2005) and that vision can modulate somatosensory cortical processing (Taylor-Clarke, Kennet, & Haggard, 2002). Moreover, single unit recording studies have shown that neurons in the monkey's anterior parietal cortex respond to auditory and visual stimuli, provided that these stimuli in other modalities are associated with tactile information needed for performance of the task. So, it has been inferred that these cells, in addition to facilitate or priming the task, form part of a network that maintains the tactile stimulus within the focus of attention during the delay (see Zhou & Fuster, 2000, 2004).

In the present study, we also investigated whether cross-modal repetition priming for objects and auditory events is preserved in old age. Preserved cross-modal repetition priming is expected in older adults, as well as in young adults for objects and auditory events presented to three perceptual modalities well adapted to deal with object geometrical and event temporal structures. These modalities are vision, audition, and touch.

Experiment 1 assessed the effect of modality change for objects presented cross-modally from study to test in young and older adults. As mention earlier, previous research from our laboratory with young and older adult participants has shown normal within-modal haptic (Ballesteros & Reales, 2004) and visual object priming (Ballesteros et al., 2007) in older adults. Therefore, in Experiment 1 we included just the two cross-modal conditions (vision-to-touch and touch-to-vision).

Experiment 2 in the present series was designed first to find out whether cross-modal (audition-to-vision and vision-to-audition) perceptual priming for ecological auditory events and their corresponding visual pictures produced similar cross-modal and inter-modal priming. Second, and more importantly, we were interested to find out whether repetition cross-modal priming between these two modalities was maintained in the old age and whether it was similar to intra-modal priming. We anticipated that if similar structural descriptions underlie object perception in these modalities, cross-modal priming will be similar to within-modal priming.

EXPERIMENT 1

Method

Participants. Forty-eight participants took part in this experiment, 24 young adults, 6 men and 18 women (mean = 34.79 years, $SD = 7.25$; years of education = 15, $SD = 3.42$), and 24 older adults, 6 men and 18 women (mean = 69.54 years, $SD = 6.15$; years of education = 14, $SD = 5.77$), who were randomly assigned to one of two modality groups.

All participants were assessed in a session that lasted approximately 45 minutes. The older adults were all community-residing volunteers. The young adults were first-year university students who participated for course credit. All had normal or corrected to normal vision and were naïve as to the purpose of the experiment. The Mini-Mental State Examination (MMSE; Folstein, Folstein, & McHugh, 1975) score of the older adults was normal (29.28, $SD = 0.96$). Twelve young and twelve older adults encoded the objects visually. After performing a 5 minute distractor task, they were tested tactually. The other two groups of young and older participants encoded the object by touch and were tested visually.

Materials and equipment. The stimuli consisted of 40 familiar target objects (see Figure 1). Ten additional objects were used for practice trials and were not included in the analysis. The objects were selected from several

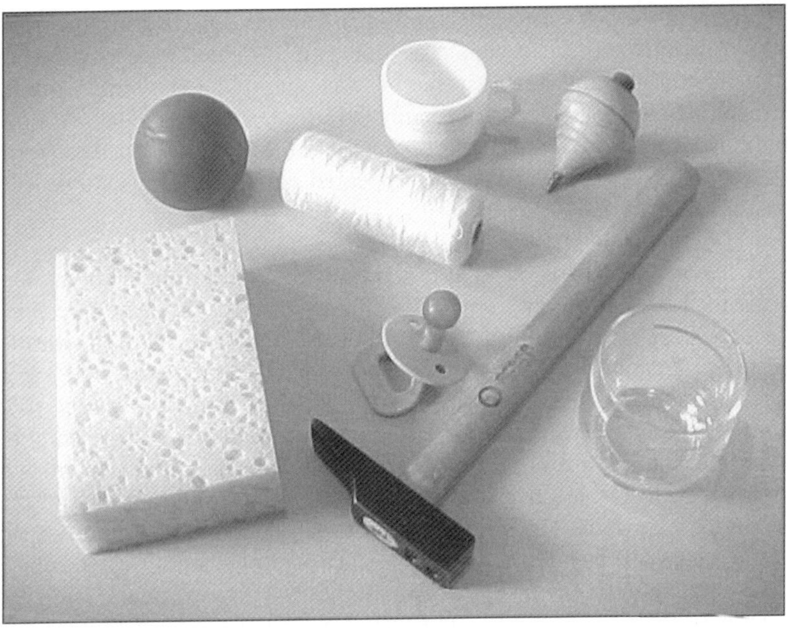

Figure 1. Some examples of the familiar objects used in Experiment 1.

basic-level categories (tools, personal care objects, household objects, and vegetables) and they neither produced special noises nor emitted special odours that would facilitate object identification. All the objects had a size that allows enclosing within the hands to facilitate haptic exploration and were easy to identify, although measures of familiarity, imagery, or degree of common features were not taken.

The objects were presented in a visual-haptic three-dimensional (3-D) object tachistoscope described in detail elsewhere (see Reales & Ballesteros, 1999). The apparatus was made in methacrylate with a liquid crystal window (size 13.7 × 13.7 cm) located centrally at the eye level of the seated participants. This window did not allow the participant to see the objects at any time during the haptic encoding condition. The presentation board was equipped with a piezosensor device located underneath at the centre of the presentation platform. The apparatus was interfaced with a PC computer for stimulus presentation and data collection. A voice key attached to the collar of the participant was also interfaced with the computer that recorded vocal reaction times. The key stopped the internal clock of the PC and measured reaction time.

Experimental design. The design consisted of a 2 (groups of participants: young adults and older adults) × 2 (cross-modal conditions: vision-to-touch and touch-to-vision) × 2 (study conditions: studied objects and nonstudied objects) mixed factorial design. The first two variables were manipulated between subjects and the last factor was manipulated within subjects. Participants were assigned randomly to the experimental cross-modal conditions. Furthermore, the 40 experimental objects were divided randomly in two sets of 20 objects each that appeared equally often as studied and nonstudied objects.

Procedure. Participants were tested individually in a quiet room. They were informed that they were participating in a study on object perception. The procedure was approved by the Ethical Committee of the Institution and all participants signed an informed consent form before the experimental session started. The session always started with a study phase followed by a distractor task that lasted 5 minutes. Then, the incidental test phase followed. According to the experimental condition, participants were presented with 20 objects, one by one, in a different random order, either visually or haptically. During the whole experimental session, participants had their eyes open as the tachistoscope did not allow them to see the objects in the haptic condition. In the haptic condition, participants explored each object with their hands for 10 s but they were instructed to name the object as soon as possible. The experimenter presented the objects, one by one at the centre of the presentation platform. A sound from the computer indicated to the participant to start the exploration of the object, introducing both hands through the aperture located at the bottom of the methacrylate panel. After 10 s, another sound from the computer indicated that he/she should give the answer. The task consisted of naming the object as soon as possible. Participants in the visual encoding condition looked at the object through the liquid crystal window of the tachistoscope for 10 s but they were instructed to name the object as soon as possible. When the study phase was over, participants performed the 5 min distractor task consisting of naming all friends and family members that came to mind.

During the testing phase, incidentally, participants performed a *speeded object naming task*. The session always started with 10 practice trials that did not enter into the statistical analysis. Participants whom at the study phase encoded the objects visually at test performed a haptic naming task, and those who studied the objects haptically performed a speeded visual naming task at test. Participants in the visual condition looked at the objects through the liquid crystal window of the apparatus whereas those in the haptic condition were asked to explore each object located in the presentation platform introducing their hands through the aperture. In this phase of the experiment 20 new objects were added to the objects that were already studied. The computer program produced a different random order for each participant.

In the haptic condition, the experimenter placed one object at a time at the centre of the presentation platform of the tachistoscope. A tone alerted the participant that the object was ready for haptic exploration. Latencies were automatically recorded from the time the hands started to explore the object to the naming response. In the visual condition, response times were recorded from the time the window allowed the participant to see the object located at the presentation platform until he or she produced the response. Each trial started with the participant's two forefingers placed on two placeholders. When the fingers were raised, the window allowed the participant to see the exposed object. A voice key located at the participant's collar stopped the internal clock of the computer and the program recorded the response time on a trial base.

Results and discussion

Response times corresponding to correct responses were the main dependent variable, but accuracy was recorded and errors were also analysed to check for speed-–accuracy tradeoffs. However, no such effect was found. Figure 2 displays the response times corresponding to the *speeded object naming test* as a function of the experimental condition (visual study-haptic test and haptic study-visual test), study condition (studied objects and nonstudied objects), and group (young adults and older adults). The results showed that studied objects (1609 ms) were named faster than nonstudied objects (1995 ms). Second, this pattern of results was similar in the two cross-modal conditions, haptic-to-visual (1301 and 1515 ms for studied and nonstudied stimuli presented visually at test, respectively) and visual-to-haptic (1917 ms

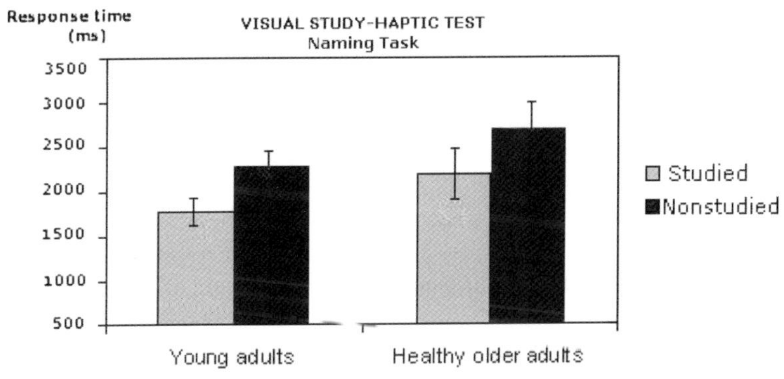

Figure 2. Response time (in seconds) in the cross-modal conditions: visual-study haptic-test condition (left) and in the haptic-study visual-test condition (right) for studied and nonstudied objects as a function of age (young adults and older adults). Error bars indicate the standard error of the mean.

and 2475 ms for studied and nonstudied stimuli presented haptically at test, respectively). Third, and more important, this pattern of results repeated across the two age groups, young adults (1287 and 1656 ms for studied and nonstudied, respectively) and older adults (1932 and 2334 ms for studied and nonstudied, respectively). On average the priming effect obtained for studied compared to nonstudied objects was 369 and 402 for young and older participants, respectively.

The three-factor mixed ANOVA conducted on correct latencies with group and condition as between-subjects variables and item type as the within-subject factor confirmed the previous description of the data. The main effect of item type was statistically significant, $F(1, 44) = 45.164$, $MSE = 79062.64$, $p < .01$. Studied objects were named reliably faster than nonstudied objects. The main effect of group was also statistically significant, $F(1, 44) = 10.54$, $MSE = 997436.98$, $p < .05$. Young adults named the objects significantly faster than the older adults. Importantly, the study condition by group interaction was not significant ($F < 1$), which means that young and older adults show similar levels of perceptual cross-modal priming. The main effect of condition was significant, $F(1, 44) = 14.943$, $MSE = 997436.98$, $p < .01$. Latencies were larger when the test modality was touch than when it was vision. The interaction between study condition and cross-modal condition was also significant, $F(1, 44) = 8.99$, $MSE = 79062.64$, $p < .05$. The interaction indicated that the facilitation was larger when the modality being tested was touch than when it was vision. No other interaction was significant. The absence of a three-way interaction suggests a complete transfer between vision and touch and that cross-modal priming is spared in older adults.

The mean percentage of errors for studied items was lower than for nonstudied items (1.50% and 3.22%, respectively). This pattern of results repeated in young (1.04% and 1.97%, respectively) and older adults (1.97% and 4.47%, respectively). Studied objects in both cross-modal conditions were identified more accurately than nonstudied ones.

The ANOVA conducted on errors confirmed the previous description showing the advantage of studied compared to nonstudied objects, $F(1, 44) = 12.11$, $MSE = 0.93$, $p < .01$. Participants were significantly more accurate for studied than for nonstudied objects. The main effect of group was also significant, $F(1, 44) = 5.9$, $MSE = 1.92$, $p < .01$. Older adults produced more errors than young adults. No other main effect or interaction was significant.

The significant cross-modal facilitation obtained in this experiment replicates previous findings with young adults (Reales & Ballesteros, 1999). Cross-modal priming was equivalent to within-modal priming, showing complete transfer between these two perceptual modalities well adapted to process object's shape and structure. The results suggest that similar structural descriptions mediated implicit memory for objects presented to vision and touch. Easton, Greene, and Srinivas (1997), using nonsense two-dimensional shapes and familiar objects, found significant cross-modal priming that was slightly quicker than within-modal priming.

Experiment 1 has shown that cross-modal (visual/haptic and haptic/visual) perceptual priming is age invariant. The facilitation observed in older adults and in young adults was similar. As far as we know, this is the first time that cross-modal priming between vision and touch has been reported in older adults. Previous results in the visual domain have shown age-invariance in object identification tasks (e.g., Ballesteros et al., 2007; Mitchell, 1989). The same finding was also reported in the haptic domain. Similar haptic priming was found in younger adults and older adults in a speeded object naming task (Ballesteros & Reales, 2004).

The results of Experiment 1 suggest that cross-modal repetition priming does not deteriorate with age as both groups showed the same level of transfer between these two perceptual modalities. Our previous findings suggested that the magnitude of haptic-to-visual priming was similar to that of visual-to-visual priming, and supported the hypothesis that vision and touch share common representations. Moreover, the finding that cross-modal (vision-to-touch and touch-to-vision) priming is preserved in ageing adults, suggests that the neural machinery involved in repetition object priming does not deteriorate with age.

EXPERIMENT 2

In Experiment 2, we assessed the effect of modality change in vision and audition, two modalities well adapted to deal with structure. The first goal of the experiment was to find out whether cross-modal perceptual priming between vision and audition differs from within-modal implicit priming. The second, but equally important goal was to investigate whether cross-modal priming between these two modalities is spared in normal ageing as we have just reported between vision and touch.

Method

Participants. One hundred and sixty healthy adults participated in a 40 to 45 minute experimental session. The participants were drawn from two age groups: 80 were young adults (32 men and 48 women) aged between 18 and 36 years (mean = 27.07, SD = 7, 25) and 80 were healthy older adults (35 men and 45 women) aged between 65 and 88 years (mean = 74.72, SD = 7.14). The young adults had a mean of 15.98 years of formal education (SD = 1.46) and the older adults had 13.90 years (SD = 1.48). Twenty participants from each age group were assigned randomly to one of the four experimental conditions. Young adults were first-year university students. Older adults were recruited from a private geriatric centre in Madrid. All participants had normal or corrected to normal vision and audition. They were naïve as to the purpose of the experiment and had not participated in any other perception or cognition experiment before. All participants were screened for previous history of neurological and psychiatric disorders and current medication used. All participants signed an informed consent form before the experiment started. Older adults were screened with the Mini-Mental State Exam (MMSE; Folstein et al., 1975) to ensure that they did not suffer from mild cognitive impairment or dementia. The scores obtained by the older adults in the MMSE were normal (mean 28.93, $SD = 1.07$).

Materials and equipment. Sixty ecologically familiar sound events and sixty corresponding pictures showing the actions that produced the sounds were used as stimuli. The sounds were selected from a larger set of 115 sounds obtained from several libraries (for more information, see Shafiro & Gygi, 2004). The results from a previous study conducted with 40 young adults and 40 older adults were used for the selection of the target stimuli (González & Ballesteros, 2006). All the stimuli were presented for 5 s. The sound format was PCM in stereo channel with a speed of 44 kHz and 16 bits of information. Auditory stimuli were presented binaurally through headphones connected to the headphone jack of the computer. Sound events correctly identified by more than 70% by the young and older adults in the previous study were selected as stimuli. A pilot study was also conducted to ensure that the pictures that corresponded to the sounds were identified equally well. The pictures with an accuracy superior to the 70% were selected as the visual stimuli. Examples are shown in Figure 3. The pictures were digitalised and saved in BMP format with a resolution of 640 × 480 pixels. The visual stimuli were presented on a 15-inch colour monitor of a PC compatible computer, which had a resolution of 640 × 480 pixels. The system was interfaced with a voice key to record the response time. The experiment was programmed using E-prime.

Experimental design. The experimental design consisted of a factorial design with study condition (studied and nonstudied stimuli) as the within-subject factor and three between-subjects factors: group (young adults and older adults), modality at study (audition and vision), and modality at test (audition and vision). Twenty participants were randomly assigned to each of the eight experimental conditions. In addition, for each participant the computer randomly selected 30 stimuli from a set of 60 stimuli which were presented during the study phase (studied stimuli). Fifteen of these were presented at the testing phase. For the nonstudied stimuli, the computer randomly selected 15 from the 30 remaining stimuli.

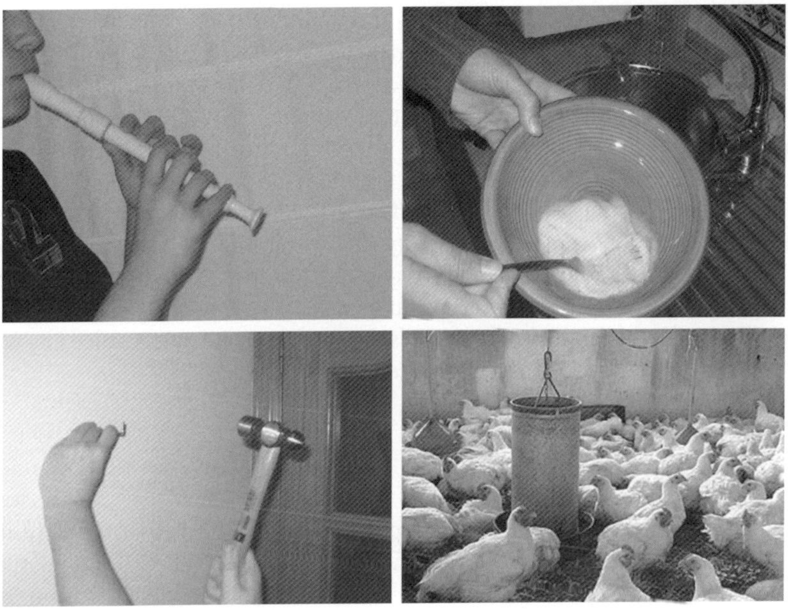

Figure 3. Examples of pictures used in Experiment 2. Upper left, flute playing; upper right, eggs beating; bottom left, hammer pounding; bottom right, hens cackling.

Procedure. Participants were tested individually in a quiet room and were informed that they were participating in a perceptual study. At the study phase, participants were presented with a series of 30 stimuli visually or auditory (according to the experimental condition). Participants in the auditory condition were allowed 5 s to listen to each sound but they were required to respond as quickly and accurately as possible. The computer generated a different random order for each participant. The session always started with 10 practice trials that did not entered into the analysis. During these trials, participants adjusted the volume of the loudspeakers until they felt comfortable. Observers who encoded the stimuli auditorily were asked to listen carefully and try to identify each sound as soon as possible. Observers in the visual condition were asked to look at the computer screen and name the visual event as fast and accurately as possible. As in the auditory condition, each picture was presented for 5 s. Each trial started with the presentation of a black fixation cross at the centre of a white screen that lasted for 500 ms followed by a sound or a picture (according to the experimental condition).

Between the study phase and the test phase, participants performed a 5 min distractor task, which consisted of naming as many names of cities as possible. After completing the distractor task, participants performed the test phase, which consisted of naming the sound or the picture as quickly as possible. In this part of the experiment, 15 studied (old) stimuli and 15 nonstudied (new) stimuli were presented in a different random order for each participant. Half of the young and half of the older participants who studied the stimuli through audition were tested auditorily (the within-modal groups); the other half were tested visually (the between-modal groups). Similarly, half of the younger and half of the older participants who studied the stimuli visually were tested visually (the within-modal groups); the other half were tested auditorily (the cross-modal groups). Response times were automatically recorded from the stimulus onset to the naming response. The experimenter registered the naming response after each trial. A voice key was used to stop the clock of the computer.

Results and discussion

As in Experiment 1, latencies corresponding to correct responses were the main dependent variable. Accuracy was also analysed to check for a possible speed–accuracy tradeoff. Figure 4 displays the mean latencies from the implicit memory test as a function of group (young adults and older adults), study condition (studied or nonstudied), and modality (intra-modal or cross-modal). Three main findings from latencies are important to note. First, there is a large priming effect for studied stimuli (1860 ms) compared to nonstudied stimuli (2339 ms). Second, although this pattern of results repeated in both age groups, latencies were affected by age as older adults were slower than young adults, both for studied (1942 ms and 1534 ms, respectively) and for nonstudied stimuli (2738 ms and 2187 ms, respectively). Note that young and older adults exhibited an advantage for studied compared to nonstudied stimuli. Third, within-modal (573 ms) and cross-modal repetition (486ms) priming effects were comparable in magnitude.

A four-factor mixed ANOVA was conducted with group, study modality, and test modality as between-subjects variables, and study condition as the within-subjects factor. Response times corresponding to correct responses were included in the ANOVA that confirmed the previous description of the data. Studied stimuli were named significantly faster (at both the auditory and the visual tests) than nonstudied stimuli. The main effect of study condition was also statistically significant, $F(1, 152) = 61.905$, $MSE = 296964.380$, $p < .001$. Studied stimuli were named reliably faster than new stimuli. The main effect of group was also significant, $F(1, 152) = 53.392$, $MSE = 786805.66$, $p < .001$. This effect indicates that young adults named the stimuli significantly faster than the older adults. The interaction between group and study condition was not significant ($F < 1$). This lack of interaction indicates that young and older adults named the studied stimuli

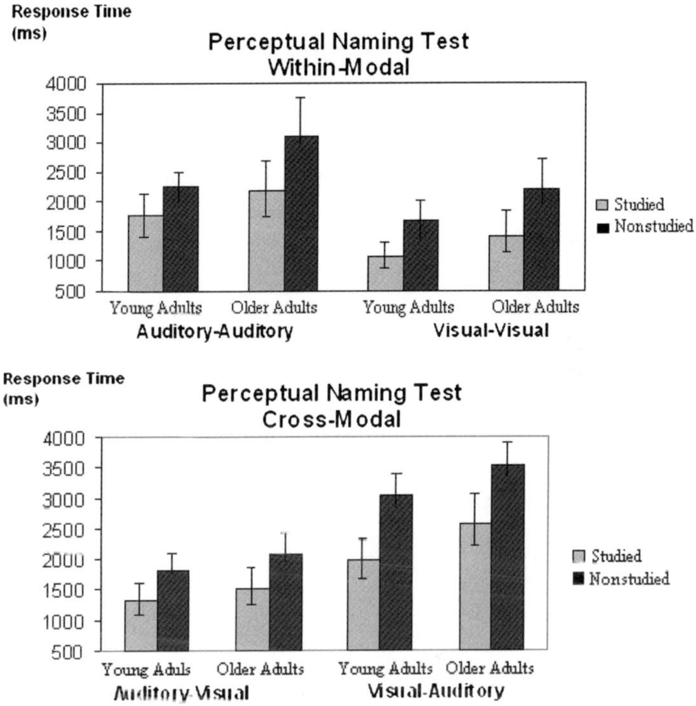

Figure 4. Response time (in ms) in the within-modal (top) and cross-modal conditions (bottom) in the perceptual naming test as a function of study condition (studied and nonstudied stimuli), study and test modality, and group (young and older adults). Error bars indicate the standard error of the mean.

faster than the nonstudied stimuli. The interaction between study condition and modality at test was significant, $F(1, 152) = 5.721$, $MSE = 296964.380$, $p < .05$. The interaction indicates that the facilitation was larger when the modality at test was audition than when it was vision. No other interaction was significant.

An additional ANOVA conducted on errors showed that the main effect of study condition, $F(1, 152) = 72.418$, $MSE = 0.626$, $p < .001$, was significant. The percentage of errors for studied stimuli was lower (2.51%) than for nonstudied stimuli (3.26%). Group was significant, $F(1, 152) = 66.342$, $MSE - 3.011$, $p < .001$. Young adults (2.09%) were more accurate than older adults (3.68%). The interaction between study condition and group was not significant. Fewer errors occurred for studied than for nonstudied stimuli in both groups. The main effect of the modality at test was significant, $F(1, 152) = 59.250$, $MSE = 3.011$, $p < .001$. There were more errors when the modality at test was audition (3.66%) than when it was vision (2.13%). Modality at study was also significant, $F(1, 152) = 9.403$, $MSE = 3.011$, $p < .003$. Fewer errors occurred in the visual presentation (2.08%) than in the auditory presentation (3.14%).

The results showed that there was no speed–accuracy tradeoff effect between latency and accuracy. Studied stimuli were identified both faster and more accurately than nonstudied stimuli. More importantly, repetition priming was preserved in ageing as young adults and older adults showed reliable and similar facilitation for studied compared to nonstudied stimuli, both in response times and in accuracy. However, older adults made more errors and required more time than young adults to identify the stimuli in all experimental conditions (within-modal as well as in cross-modal conditions). Importantly, these results showed that cross-modal perceptual priming (vision-to-audition and audition-to-vision) was similar to within-modal (vision-to-vision and audition-to-audition) priming not only in young adults but also in older adults. Auditory identifications required more time than visual identifications. Also, accuracy was lower in the auditory condition than in the visual condition.

GENERAL DISCUSSION

Two experiments explored whether the representations that mediate cross-modal priming are shared between modalities well adapted to deal with objects and auditory events produced by these objects and whether the facilitation was preserved in healthy ageing. The results from both experiments suggest that: (1) cross-modal repetition priming for familiar objects presented to touch and vision showed similar facilitation in older adults as in younger adults (Exp. 1); (2) ecological sound object-related repetition priming was equivalent in magnitude for auditorily and visually studied stimuli in both, within-modal as well as in cross-modal conditions; this facilitation occurred in younger as well as in older adults (Exp. 2); and (3) the perceptual facilitation occurred in response time as well as in accuracy, showing that there were no speed–accuracy tradeoff (Exps 1 and 2).

These findings extend previous results with young adults (Reales & Ballesteros, 1999) showing that cross-modal priming was similar to within-modal priming when familiar objects were presented visually or haptically to the auditory events produced by objects and their corresponding pictures. The cross-modal facilitation observed here suggests that the representations supporting repetition priming are not modality specific and might depend on high-level structural features that define an object's shape and its spatiotemporal structure.

The results suggest that repetition priming for objects presented to vision or touch, and the sounds produced by them, is not modality specific. Stimuli presented to a modality at study were identified faster and more accurately when the same stimuli were presented later at test to the other modality compared to new stimuli. This shows that the magnitude of priming between these modalities is similar to the magnitude of within-modal priming (when the stimuli were presented to the same modality). The present results support the idea that vision, touch, and audition share common object representations. Moreover, young adults and older adults showed similar magnitudes of cross-modal priming, suggesting that not only within-modal priming, but also cross-modal priming is preserved in normal ageing.

The present findings support the multiple memory systems proposal (Tulving & Schacter, 1990) and have implications for theories of adult memory and cognitive ageing. While the structural perceptual object system is spared with age, the episodic memory system that relies on the medial-temporal lobe is impaired. In contrast to the age-related decline on a number of cognitive functions, within-modal and cross-modal repetition priming (as a measure of implicit memory) is spared in older adults. This finding could be valuable in applied settings for developing training and rehabilitation programs for the old.

To our knowledge, this is the first study that reports complete and symmetrical cross-modal priming for ecological sounds and their corresponding visual pictures in younger and older adults. The complete cross-modal facilitation reported in this study between vision and audition contrasts with the results from a study conducted with young adults by Greene et al. (2001). These researchers have reported that visual study facilitated perceptual identification on both visual and auditory tests. However, auditory study facilitated perceptual identification in auditory tests but not in visual tests. The different results may be accounted for a number of experimental differences, including the smaller number of trials in Greene et al.'s study, the type of stimuli (filmed events vs. pictures), the experimental design (within-subjects vs. between-subject), and the selection of the dependent variable (accuracy vs. response time). The coordination between two or more sensory systems in object recognition (e.g., vision, touch, and audition) is the most common way to process information about objects in the world, rather than an exception.

In the burgeoning literature on brain imaging, stimulus repetition is associated with decreases in cortical activation in brain areas related to object processing (for reviews, see Henson, 2003; Schacter, Wig, & Stevens, 2007). The candidates are extrastriate regions in the occipital cortex and fusiform regions bilaterally (Eger, Henson, Driver, & Dolan, 2003). This area has been identified as the lateral occipital complex (LOC) that plays an important role in visual object recognition (Grill-Spector, Kourtzi, & Kanwisher, 2001). Recent functional imaging studies with objects explored haptically suggest further that these brain areas that were once thought to deal specifically with vision are in fact considered as polimodal sensory areas (Amedi, Jacobson, Hendler, Malach, & Zohary, 2002; Amedi, Malach, Hendler, Peled, & Zohary, 2001; Amedi et al., 2005; Pascual-Leone & Hamilton, 2001; Pascual-Leone et al., 2006; Reed, Shohalm, & Helgren, 2004). Furthermore, Newman et al. (2005) have shown further that LOC is involved in processing shape, regardless of whether the question posed by the experimenter related to a material (rough, hardness) or a geometric (shape, volume) characteristic.

In a fMRI study with young adults, James et al. (2002) showed that the haptic exploration of 3-D nonsense objects produced activation when the same objects were later presented visually not only in the somatosensory cortex but also in LOC and in the medial occipital (MOC) areas of the visual cortex. Importantly, these two areas were equally activated in the cross-modal (haptic-visual) priming condition and in the within-modal (vision-vision) priming condition. These results supported the idea that these two modalities share common representations. Moreover, structural imaging studies using longitudinal measures of 5-year change in regional brain volumes in healthy ageing adults have shown that the prefrontal cortex, the hippocampus, and the association cortices shrunk substantially with age, whereas the primary visual cortex did not show any change with age (Raz, 2000; Raz et al., 2005).

The posterior lateral temporal cortex is considered a multisensory region that is activated under multisensory processing (Beauchamp, Lee, Argall, & Martin, 2004; Wallace, Ramachandran, & Stein, 2004). Regions in the ventral occipitotemporal cortex (VOT) located ventral to LOC process abstract stimulus properties such as the object category that is accessible via touch and vision (3-D object structure). The claustrum may also play an important role in cross-modal matching as the modality-specific areas can interact via the claustrum (Hadjikhani & Roland, 1998). Furthermore, higher order temporal and occipital areas respond to coincident sounds and pictures regardless of their semantic relationship, whereas the right claustrum/insula region is differentially activated in association with multi-sensory integration of conceptually related common objects (Naghavi, Eriksson, Larsson, & Nyberg, 2007).

The complete cross-modal repetition priming (visual/auditory, auditory/visual, visual/haptic, and haptic/visual) found in younger and older adults is congruent with the idea that common representations are processed in multimodal areas of the occipital cortex and the lateral temporal cortex. Thus on the basis of the previous findings by Reales and Ballesteros (1999) and those of Richardson-Klavehn and Gardiner (1996), we conclude that cross-modal object priming is based on the structural features of object's shape that can be accessed either by vision or by touch. We proposed that similar structural descriptions may mediate object priming in vision and touch. These characteristics of objects might be shape and structure. The regions involved in auditory/visual recognition of familiar objects are the lateral temporal cortex (especially the superior temporal sulcus) that is a multisensory region (Beauchamp et al., 2004; Wallace et al., 2004), and the ventral temporal cortex.

The present cross-modal findings for familiar objects presented to vision and touch replicated previous results with young adults (Reales & Ballesteros, 1999) and extended previous unimodal visual (Ballesteros et al., 2007) and haptic implicit memory findings (Ballesteros & Reales, 2004) with ageing participants to cross-modal priming. They also extend cross-modal priming to the auditory modality, the third modality involved in object recognition. Further research is needed to clarify whether the observed cross-modal priming is preserved in the very old.

It could be argued that the effects might be due to lexical, semantic, or strategic processes as participants named the stimuli. However, it is worthy to note that Reales and Ballesteros (1999), Exp. 1) manipulated level of encoding at study and did not found any effect of this variable in within-modal or in cross-modal priming. The lexical/semantic explanation conflicts also with results in the verbal domain showing that cross-modal priming in normal adults presents no advantage of deep over shallow processing when the shallow encoding task requires lexical access (Richardson- Klavehn & Gardiner, 1996). Moreover, another experiment (Reales & Ballesteros, 1999, see Footnote 2) did not support the hypothesis. In that study, participants named familiar objects presented haptically followed by incidental speeded word-fragment completion. Even though participants at study directed their attention to the stimuli as lexical units, priming was not found when they were presented with the corresponding fragmented words. To completely rule out the lexical effect, additional studies are worth pursuing in which words would be included to see if presenting words produces the same cross-modal results.

In conclusion, the results from the two experiments reported here suggest that cross-modal repetition priming is not modality specific and support the structural description hypothesis not only in younger adults but also in older, healthy adults. Older adults, although slower and more error prone than younger adults, did not differ in the magnitude of cross-modal priming for objects presented to three different perceptual modalities: vision, touch, and audition. These modalities are well adapted to deal with object identification and as reviewed by Amedi et al. (2005), visual, tactile, and auditory object information activate cortical association areas that were previously believed to be modality specific. Today, there is an increased emphasis on the relationship between the senses, and a very interesting blurring of the lines between psychology and neuroscience (Heller & Ballesteros, 2006).

REFERENCES

Amedi, A., Jacobson, G., Hendler, T., Malach, R., & Zohary, E. (2002). Convergence of visual and tactile shape processing in the human lateral occipital complex. *Cerebral Cortex*, *12*, 1202–1212.

Amedi, A., Malach, R., Hendler, T., Peled, S., & Zohary, E. (2001). Visuo-haptic object-related activation in the ventral visual pathway. *Nature Neuroscience*, *4*, 324–330.

Amedi, A., von Kriegstein, K., van Atteveldt, N. M., Beauchamp, M. S., & Naumer, M. J. (2005). Functional imaging of human cross-modal identification and object recognition. *Experimental Brain Research*, *166*, 559–571.

Ballesteros, S. (2008). Implicit and explicit memory effects in haptic perception. In M. Grunwald (Ed.), *Human haptic perception: Basics and applications* (pp. 183–198). Boston: Birkhäser Verlag.

Ballesteros, S., & Reales, J. M. (2004). Intact haptic priming in normal aging and Alzheimer's disease: Evidence for dissociable memory systems. *Neuropsychologia*, *44*, 1063–1070.

Ballesteros, S., Reales, J. M., & Mayas, J. (2007). Picture priming in aging and dementia. *Psicothema*, *2*, 239–244.

Ballesteros, S., Reales, J. M., Mayas, J., & Heller, M. A. (2008). Selective attention modulates visual and haptic repetition priming: Effects of aging and Alzheimer's disease. *Experimental Brain Research*, *189*, 473–483.

Beauchamp, M. S., Lee, K. E., Argall, B. D., & Martin, A. (2004). Integration of auditory and visual information about objects in superior temporal sulcus. *Neuron*, *41*, 809–823.

Craik, F. M. I., & Byrd, M. (1982). Aging and cognitive deficits: The role of attentional resources. In F. I. M. Craik & S. Trehub (Eds.), *Aging and cognitive processes* (pp. 191–211). New York: Plenum.

Demattè, M. L., Sanabria, D., Sugerman, R., & Spence, C. (2006). Cross-modal interactions between olfaction and touch. *Chemical Senses*, *31*, 291–300.

Dixon, R. A., Wahlin, A., Maitland, S. B., Hultsch, D. F., Hertzog, C., & Bäckman, L. (2004). Episodic memory change in late adulthood: Generalizability across samples and performance indices. *Memory and Cognition*, *32*, 768–778.

Easton, R. D., Greene, A. J., & Srinivas, K. (1997). Transfer between vision and haptics: Memory for 2-D patterns and 3-D objects. *Psychonomic Bulletin and Review*, *4*, 403–410.

Easton, R. D., Srinivas, K., & Greene, A. J. (1997). Do vision and haptics share common representations? Implicit and explicit memory within and between modalities. *Journal of Experimental Psychology: Learning, Memory, and Cognition*, *23*, 153–163.

Eger, E., Henson, R. N. A., Driver, J., & Dolan, R. J. (2004). BOLD repetition decreases in object-responsive ventral visual areas depend on spatial attention. *Journal of Neurophysiology*, *92*, 1241–1247.

Eimer, M., Val Velzen, J., & Driver, J. (2002). Cross-modal interactions between audition, touch and vision in endogenous spatial attention: ERP evidence on preparatory states and sensory modulations. *Journal of Cognitive Neuroscience*, *14*, 254–271.

Folstein, M. F., Folstein, S. E., & McHugh, P. R. (1975). Mini-Mental State: A practical method for grading the cognitive of patients for the clinician. *Journal of Psychiatric Research, 12*, 189–198.

Fort, A., Delpuech, C., Pernier, J., & Guiard, M.-H. (2002). Early auditory interactions in human cortex during nonredundant target identification. *Cognitive Brain Research, 14*, 20–30.

González, M., & Ballesteros, S. (2006, July). *Normas de identificación para 115 estímulos auditivos ambientales: Un estudio con jóvenes y mayores* [Identification norms for 115 auditory ecological stimuli: A study with young and older adults]. Poster presented at the VI Congreso de la Sociedad Española de Psicología Experimental, Santiago de Compostela, La Coruña, Spain.

Graf, P., & Schacter, D. L. (1985). Implicit and explicit memory for new associations in normal and amnesic subjects. *Journal of Experimental Psychology: Learning, Memory, and Cognition, 11*, 501–518.

Greene, A. J., Easton, R. D., & LaShell, L. S. R. (2001). Visual-auditory events: Cross-modal perceptual priming and recognition memory. *Consciousness and Cognition, 10*, 425–435.

Grill-Spector, K., Kourtzi, Z., & Kanwisher, N. (2001). The lateral occipital complex and its role in object recognition. *Visual Research, 41*, 1409–1422.

Hadjikhani, N., & Roland, P. E. (1998). Cross-modal transfer of information between the tactile and the visual representations in the human brain: A positron emission tomographic study. *Journal of Neuroscience, 18*, 1072–1084.

Hasher, L., & Zacks, R. T. (1988). Working memory, comprehension and memory: A review and a new view. In G. Bower (Ed.), *The psychology of learning and motivation* (Vol. 22, pp. 193–225). New York: Academic Press.

Heller, M. A., & Ballesteros, S. (2006). Introduction: Approaches to touch and blindness. In M. A. Heller & S. Ballesteros (Eds.), *Touch and blindness: Psychology and neuroscience* (pp. 1–24). Hillsdale, NJ. Lawrence Erlbaum Associates, Inc.

Henson, R. N. A. (2003). Neuroimaging studies of priming. *Progress in Neurobiology, 70*, 53–81.

James, T. W., Humphrey, G. K., Gati, J. S., Servos, P., Menon, R. S., & Goodale, M. A. (2002). Haptic study of three-dimensional objects activates extrastriate visual areas. *Neuropsychologia, 40*, 1706–1714.

Keane, M. M., Gabrieli, J. D. E., Growdon, J. H., & Corkin, S. (1994). Priming in perceptual identification of pseudowords is normal in Alzheimer's disease. *Neuropsychologia, 32*, 343–356.

La Voie, D., & Light, L. L. (1994). Adult age differences in repetition priming: A meta-analysis. *Psychology and Aging, 4*, 538–553.

Light, L. L. (1991). Memory and aging: Four hypotheses in search for data. *Annual Review of Psychology, 42*, 333–376.

Millar, S. (1994). *Understanding and representing space: Theory and evidence from studies with blind and sighted children*. Oxford, UK: Oxford University Press.

Mitchell, D. B. (1989). How many memory systems? Evidence from aging. *Journal of Experimental Psychology: Learning, Memory, and Cognition, 15*, 31–49.

Mitchell, D. E., & Schmitt, F. A. (2006). Long- and short-term implicit memory in aging and Alzheimer's disease. *Aging, Neurospsychology, and Cognition, 13*, 611–635.

Molhom, S., Ritter, W., Javitt, D. C., & Foxe, J. J. (2004). Multisensory visual-auditory object recognition in humans: A high density electrical mapping study. *Cerebral Cortex, 14*, 452–465.

Murray, M. M., Mohholm, S., Michel, C. M., Heslenfeld, J. D., Ritter, W., Javitt, D. C., et al. (2005). Grabbing your ear: Auditory–somatosensory interactions in early sensory cortices are not constrained by stimulus alignment. *Cerebral Cortex, 15*, 963–974.

Naghavi, H. R., Eriksson, J., Larsson, A., & Nyberg, L. (2007). The claustrum/insula region integrates conceptually related sounds and pictures. *Neuroscience Letters, 422*, 77–80.

Newell, F. N. (2004). Cross-modal object recognition. In G. Calvert, C. Spence, & B. E. Stein (Eds.), *The handbook of multisensory processes* (pp. 123–139). Cambridge, MA: MIT Press.

Newman, S. D., Klatzky, R. L., Lederman, S. J., & Just, M. A. (2005). An fMRI comparison of haptic and visual imagery processes. *Cognitive Brain Research*, *23*, 235–246.

Nilsson, L.-G. (2003). Memory function in normal aging. *Acta Neurologica Scandinavica*, *107*(Suppl. 179), 7–13.

Park, D. C. (1999). The basic mechanisms accounting for age-related decline in cognitive functioning. In D. C. Park & N. Schwarz (Eds.), *Cognitive aging: A primer* (pp. 3–21). Philadelphia: Taylor & Francis.

Park, D. C., Davidson, L., Lautenschlager, G., Smith, A. D., Smith, P., & Hedden, T. (2002). Models of visuospatial and verbal memory across the adult life span. *Psychology and Aging*, *17*, 299–320.

Park, D. C., & Shaw, R. J. (1992). Effect of environmental support on implicit and explicit memory in younger and older adults. *Psychology and Aging*, *7*, 632–642.

Park, S. M., Gabrieli, J. D. E., Reminger, S. L., Monti, L. A., Fleischman, D. A., & Wilson, R. S., et al. (1998). Preserved priming across study–test picture transformations in patients with Alzheimer's disease. *Neuropsychology*, *12*, 340–352.

Pascual-Leone A., & Hamilton, R. H. (2001). The metamodal organization of the brain. *Progress in Brain Research*, *134*, 427–445.

Pascual-Leone, A., Theoret, H., Merabet, L., Kauffman, T., & Schlaug, G. (2006). The role of visual cortex in tactile processing: A metamodal brain. In M. A. Heller & S. Ballesteros (Eds.), *Touch and blindness: Psychology and neuroscience* (pp. 171–196). Hillsdale, NJ: Lawrence Erlbaum Associates, Inc.

Postle, B. R., Corkin, S., & Growdon, J. H. (1996). Intact implicit memory for novel patterns in Alzheimer's disease. *Learning and Memory*, *3*, 305–312.

Prull, M. W., Gabrieli, J. D. E., & Bunge, S. A. (2000). Age-related changes in memory: A cognitive neuroscience perspective. In F. I. M. Craik & T. A. Salthouse (Eds.), *The handbook of aging and cognition* (2nd ed., pp. 91–153). Mahwah, NJ: Lawrence Erlbaum Associates, Inc.

Raz, N. (2000). Aging of the brain and its impact on cognitive performance: Integration of structural and functional findings. In F. I. M. Craik & T. A. Salthouse (Eds.), *Handbook of aging and cognition* (2nd ed., pp. 1–90). Mahwah: NJ: Lawrence Erlbaum Associates, Inc.

Raz, N., Lindenberger, U., Rodrigue, K. M., Kennedy, K. M., Head, D., Williamson, A., et al. (2005). Regional brain changes in aging healthy adults: General trends, individual differences and modifiers. *Cerebral Cortex*, *15*, 1676–1689.

Reales, J. M., & Ballesteros, S. (1999). Implicit and explicit representations of visual and haptic objects: A cross-modal study. *Journal of Experimental Psychology: Learning, Memory, and Cognition*, *20*, 1–25.

Reed, C. L., Shohalm, S., & Helgren, E. (2004). Neural substrates of tactile object recognition: An fRMI study. *Human Brain Mapping*, *21*, 236–246.

Richardson-Klavehn, & Gardiner, J. M. (1996). Cross-modality priming in stem completion reflects conscious memory but not voluntary memory. *Psychonomic Bulletin and Review*, *3*, 238–244.

Sathian, K., & Prather, S. C. (2006). Cerebral cortical processing of tactile form: Evidence from functional neuroimaging. In M. A. Heller & S. Ballesteros (Eds.), *Touch and blindness: Psychology and neuroscience* (pp. 157–170). Hillsdale, NJ: Lawrence Erlbaum Associates, Inc.

Schacter, D. L. (1987). Implicit memory: History and current status. *Journal of Experimental Psychology: Learning, Memory, and Cognition*, *13*, 501–518.

Schacter, D. L., Cooper, L. A., & Valdiserri, M. (1992). Implicit and explicit memory for novel visual objects in older and younger adults. *Psychology and Aging*, *2*, 299–308.

Schacter, D. L., Wig, G. S., & Stevens, D. (2007). Reductions in cortical activity during priming. *Current Opinion in Neurobiology*, *17*, 171–176.

Shafiro, V., & Gyri, B. (2004). How to select stimuli for environmental sound research and where to find them. *Behavioral Research, Methods, Instruments, and Computers*, *36*, 580–598.

Soto-Faraco, S., Spence, C., & Kingstone, A. (2004). Congruency effects between auditory and tactile motion: Extending the phenomenon of cross-modal dynamic capture. *Cognitive, Affective and Behavioral Neuroscience*, *4*, 208–217.

Spence, C., Ranson, J., & Driver, J (2000). Cross-modal selective attention: On the difficulty of ignoring sounds at the locus of visual attention. *Perception and Psychophysics*, *62*, 410–424.

Taylor, K. I., Moss, H. E., Stamatakis, E. A., & Tyler, L. K. (2006). Binding cross-modal object features in perirhinal cortex. *Proceedings of the National Academy of Sciences*, *103*, 8239–8244.

Taylor-Clarke, M., Kennet, S., & Haggard, P. (2002). Vision modulates somatosensory cortical processing. *Current Biology*, *12*, 233–236.

Thesen, T., Vibell, J., Calvert, G. A., & Osterbauer, R. (2004). Neuroimaging of multisensory processing in vision, audition, touch and olfaction. *Cognitive Processing*, *5*, 84–93.

Tulving, E., & Schacter, D. L. (1990). Priming and human memory systems. *Science*, *247*, 301–306.

Verfaellie, M., Keane, M. M., & Johnson, G. (2000). Preserved priming in auditory perceptual identification in Alzheimer's disease. *Neuropsychologia*, *38*, 1581–1592.

Wallace, M. T., Ramachandran, R., & Stein, B. E. (2004). A revised view of sensory cortex parcellation. *Proceedings of the National Academy of Sciences*, *101*, 2167–2172.

Zampini, M., Torresan, D., Spence, C., & Murray, M. M. (2007). Auditory–somatosensory interactions in front and rear space. *Neuropsychologia*, *45*, 1869–1877.

Zhou, Y.-D., & Fuster, J. M. (2000). Visuo-tactile cross-modal associations in cortical somatosensory cells. *Proceedings of the National Academy of Sciences*, *97*, 9777–9782.

Zhou, Y.-D., & Fuster, J. M. (2004). Somatosensory cell response to an auditory cue in a haptic memory task. *Behavioral Brain Research*, *153*, 573–578.

EUROPEAN JOURNAL OF COGNITIVE PSYCHOLOGY
2009, 21 (2/3), 388–405

Psychology Press
Taylor & Francis Group

Diabetes and elevated glycosylated haemoglobin: Episodic memory and utilisation of cognitive support

Erik Nilsson

Department of Clinical Neuroscience, Karolinska Institute, Stockholm, Sweden

Åke Wahlin

Department of Psychology, Stockholm University, Stockholm, Sweden

Associations between diabetes and episodic memory performance were examined under varying levels of cognitive support at encoding and retrieval in a population-based sample of persons 35–85 years old. Participants were divided into diagnostic groups: (1) persons with diabetes ($n = 125$), (2) persons without diabetes diagnosis but with elevated levels of glycosylated haemoglobin (HbA_{1c}; $n = 151$), and (3) persons without diabetes or elevated HbA_{1c} ($n = 2489$). Among participants 65 years of age and younger, Group 1 performed at significantly lower levels than Groups 2 and 3. Among participants 70 years of age or older, Group 2 performed at the lowest level. The results are discussed in relation to varying underdiagnosis of diabetes across age.

Keywords: Diabetes; Glycosylated haemoglobin; Episodic memory.

By definition, diabetes is an etiologically opaque group of diseases, where Type 2-diabetes is not caused by any known specific pathogenetic process (The Expert Committee on the Diagnosis and Classification of Diabetes Mellitus, 2003). Risk-factors for developing diabetes are: increasing age,

Correspondence should be addressed to Erik Nilsson, Department of Clinical Neuroscience, Karolinska University Hospital Huddinge, M56, S-141 86 Stockholm, Sweden. E-mail: erik.nilsson@sll.se

The Betula prospective cohort study is an ongoing study funded by the Bank of Sweden Tercentenary Foundation Grants 1988-0082:17 and J2001-0682; Swedish Council for Planning and Coordination of Research Grants D1988-0092, D1989-0115, D1990-0074, D1991-0258, D1992-0143, D1997-0756, D1997-1841, D1999-0739, and B1999-474; Swedish Council for Research in the Humanities and Social Sciences Grant F377/1988-2000; Swedish Council for Social Research Grants 1988-1990:88-0082 and 311/1991-2000; and Swedish Research Council Grants 2001-6654, 2002-3794, and 2003-3883. This study was also financed in part by a Swedish Research Council Grant 2002-2575, and a stipend from the Solstickan Foundation.

http://www.psypress.com/ecp DOI: 10.1080/09541440802333133

obesity, and lack of physical activity. Since age is a risk factor, it is reasonable to assume that Type 2-diabetes is more common in older populations than in younger. Type 1-diabetes is, due to a historical selective survival, actually more common in younger cohorts, but prevalence rates are very low (0.45–0.6% in Swedish estimations). Dunstan et al. (2002) examined diabetic status among 11,247 Australian residents aged 25 and older, and showed that prevalence figures are 0.3% in the 25–34 age range, and gradually increase with increasing age, up to 13.1% in the 55–64 age range, and 23% in the 75 and older age group. The Australian study also indicated an alarming underdiagnosis of diabetes. Among those diagnosed with diabetes in the study, about one third of the youngest age group, and more than half in the oldest age group were unaware of their diabetic status. A 50% underdiagnosis was also found in a Swedish study focusing on women 64 years of age (Brohall, Behre, Hulthe, Wikstrand, & Fagerberg, 2006). In the present study, we include an objective measure of long-term blood glucose level (HbA_{1c}). Although an elevated level of HbA_{1c} is not diagnostic for diabetes, it may indicate either that a subject has an increased risk of developing diabetes or that the subject is already in fulfilment of diagnostic criteria for diabetes, but has not been tested for the disease. It is reasonable to assume that the biological processes leading to diabetes-related cognitive impairment do not start at a discrete time-point, but rather are aggregated in response to the diabetic disease progression. Thus, whether the subjects with elevated levels of HbA_{1c} are actually undiagnosed diabetics or simply at increased risk of developing diabetes, analysing the performance of persons with elevated HbA_{1c} in the absence of formal diabetes diagnosis is informative.

The development of memory deficits in normal adulthood and ageing has been extensively studied. Tasks drawing on different memory systems seem to be differentially affected by ageing (Bäckman, Small, & Wahlin, 2001; Nilsson, 2003; Rönnlund, Bäckman, Lövdén, Nilsson, & Nyberg, 2000). There is a spectrum of differentially affected memory systems, with profound age differences in tests of episodic memory and working memory, smaller differences in semantic memory, and very small age differences in primary memory (Bäckman, Small, Wahlin, & Larsson, 2000). A variety of tasks assessing implicit memory, both using visual stimuli (e.g., Ballesteros, Reales, & Mayas, 2007; LaVoie & Light, 1994), and objects presented to the touch (Ballesteros & Reales, 2004), have been shown to be less affected by ageing than tasks assessing explicit memory. Even though ageing affects absolute performance differentially across memory systems, the general structure of memory systems seems to be age invariant (Nyberg et al., 2003). Some of the observed age differences may be accounted for by underlying abilities that are also changing with time. For example, there is compelling evidence that memory performance may be effected by ability to integrate contextual information. Related to this, it has been shown that age-related differences in memory performance may be reduced by adding organisational structure, richness of stimulus, or retrieval cues to the tests administered (Bäckman, Mäntylä, & Herlitz, 1990). Since it is likely impossible to control for all instances of present, incipient, or future disease, effects of the combined disease burden in the studied population may be difficult to separate from effects of normal ageing.

Effects of diabetes on cognition have been studied since the 1920s (Miles & Root, 1922), and structured cognitive assessments have been performed in this context since the 1970s (Bale, 1973). A recent systematic review of the literature (Areosa & Grimley, 2002) showed that both cross-sectional and longitudinal studies tend to demonstrate effects of diabetic status on cognitive functioning, with some discrepancies due to variable methodology and heterogeneity of studied populations. Given that only roughly half the patients who fulfil the diagnostic criteria for Type 2-diabetes are aware of their disease, the process by which diabetes diagnoses are set in studies may also introduce divergent results with regard to cognition. Many domains of cognitive function have been studied, but it seems that the most robust effects are found in tests of learning and verbal memory. The quality of cognitive assessment, as well as the cognitive domains studied, vary greatly. However, there is now sufficient evidence (Areosa & Grimley, 2002) to claim that diabetes causes an up to twofold increase in risk of cognitive impairment or dementia.

Diabetes is frequently associated with other vascular risk factors and diseases such as hypertension, dyslipidemia, cerebro- and cardiovascular disease (e.g., Elliott & Viberti, 1993; Kannel & McGee, 1979). Since these risk factors can also contribute to cognitive impairment (e.g., Kilander, Nyman, Boberg, Hansson, & Lithell, 1998), it is imperative to control for such conditions when studying the effects of diabetes on cognition (Strachan, Deary, Ewing, & Frier, 1997). Diabetes is also related to an increased risk of developing Alzheimer's disease (AD), and other dementias (see, e.g., Ott et al., 1996; Stewart & Liolitsa, 1999; Xu, Qiu, Wahlin, Winblad, & Fratiglioni, 2004). Since it has been shown in numerous studies that preclinical dementia is associated with cognitive impairment up to 10 years before dementia diagnosis (e.g., Lövden, Bergman, Adolfsson, Lindenberger, & Nilsson, 2005), it is important to account for the effect of incipient or preclinical dementia when studying cognitive repercussions of diabetes.

Almost all speculations on biological causes of cognitive impairment in diabetic patients focus on insulin (Wickelgren, 1998) or blood glucose variability (Convit, Wolf, Tarshish, & de Leon, 2003). Insulin action is possible through several mechanisms. Insulin receptors are present in the brain, with markedly elevated density in the hippocampus, olfactory bulb, cerebral cortex, cerebellum, and hypothalamus (Park, 2001; Unger, Livingston, & Moss, 1991), structures known to play important roles for memory proficiency (Squire, 1992). The acute effect of increased brain insulin levels on cognition seems to be beneficial under euglycaemic conditions (Kern et al., 2001) but nonbeneficial under hyperglycaemic conditions (Watson & Craft, 2006). This is another reason (besides the underdiagnosis previously described) for indicators of blood glucose regulation, such as HbA_{1c}, to be included in studies attempting to examine the impact of diabetes on cognitive functioning.

In two prior population-based studies of community-dwelling diabetic persons, we have documented diabetes-related cognitive deficits beyond the effects resulting from related vascular disorders. In the first study (Nilsson, Fastbom, & Wahlin, 2002), diabetes was found to affect performance on Mini-Mental State Examination (MMSE; Folstein, Folstein, & McHugh, 1975). In the second study, based on the same population and utilising an extensive cognitive test battery, diabetes related cognitive deficits in both episodic memory and verbal fluency were documented (Wahlin, Nilsson, & Fastbom, 2002). These effects were however found to vary as a function of semantic structure inherent in the test materials. Presence of semantic structure in the test materials may be viewed as an aspect of cognitive support that positively affects level of performance (Bäckman et al., 1990). Consequently, diabetes-related cognitive deficits were detected only when the episodic and verbal fluency tasks included low levels of support. In the present study, we further examine the effect of cognitive support. The tests used in the present study (see Methods and Appendix) were chosen to allow for two clarifications of the previous results. First, in the present study the material to be remembered is highly similar in the high and low support settings, allowing for more specific interpretation of the effect of cognitive support. Second, level of cognitive support is in the present study varied at both encoding and retrieval, allowing for both a dose–response analysis (high support/high support, high/low, low/high, and low/low), and for examining any effects specific to encoding support or retrieval support.

The effect of the level of education of the subject on performance in cognitive testing is well documented (see Bäckman, Small, Wahlin, & Larsson, 2000). When studying diseases with varying prevalences across levels of education, or indeed diseases where education-related prevalence is unknown, it is informative to consider level of education.

In the present study, we examine: (1) whether diabetes affects cognitive functioning differentially depending on age, (2b) whether elevated HbA_{1c}-levels are associated with impaired cognitive functioning in the absence of diabetes diagnosis, and (3) whether cognitive support at encoding or retrieval attenuates differences between diagnostic groups.

METHODS

Data collected in the Betula Prospective Cohort Study (Nilsson et al., 1997, 2004) were used. The Betula Project involves 2961 participants living in the city of Umeå in northern Sweden. The first sample (S1) comprises 1000 participants who were aged 35, 40, 45, 50, 55, 60, 65, 70, 75, and 80 years when first tested in 1988–1990 (the first Betula test occasion; T1). Participants belonging to sample 2 (S2; $n = 996$) were first tested in 1993–1995 (the second Betula test occasion; T2), and were in the same age at testing as the participants in S1. The sample 3 (S3; $n = 965$) participants were also tested for the first time in 1993–1995 (T2), but belonged to the age cohorts 40, 45, 50, 55, 60, 65, 70, 75, 80, and 85 years of age. In each of the three samples, there were about 100 participants in each age group. All participants ($N = 2961$) were diagnosed as nondemented at the time of first testing (American Psychiatric Association, 1987). Subjects have been retested at 5-year intervals, according to a special scheme to maximise the statistical utility of the collected data. In the present study, all data except dementia diagnoses are from the subjects' first test occasion. The project has been approved according to the ethical guidelines of the Swedish Council for Research in the Humanities and Social Sciences (§7/870303, 97–173). All participants have given informed consent.

Participants were randomly selected from the population (about 100,000). Thus, in the older cohorts, there is close to total participation in the study. Most subjects were tested on-site at the Betula offices in central Umeå, but in order to minimise drop-out and nonattendance some elderly participants were tested at home. The participants of Betula have been compared with the population of Sweden with regard to demographic factors, and the study population reflects the general levels of Sweden (Nilsson et al., 1997).

Participants who would become demented within 10 years after collection were excluded ($n = 183$). Of these, 12 persons were diabetics, 16 were nondiabetics with elevated levels of HbA_{1c}, and 155 were nondiabetic controls with normal levels of HbA_{1c}.

Importantly, prevalence of diabetes in the present study ($n = 125$, i.e., 4.5%) is comparable to the prevalence rates of Sweden.

Medical and laboratory examination

Participants took part in an extensive health examination, including detailed anamnesis about conditions (e.g., diabetes) requiring healthcare contacts, and a comprehensive laboratory assessment. A total of 55 ml of blood was used for blood chemistry testing (including HbA_{1c}).

Cognitive examination

Psychological assessment included tests of short-term and long-term memory processing (semantic memory, episodic memory, priming) and attention. The results analysed in this study were episodic memory assessments with varying degree of support at encoding (subject performed tasks and verbal tasks) and retrieval (cued recall and free recall). The information to be encoded was presented in a similar way in the subject performed tasks and the verbal tasks. In the subject performed task setting, the subject was instructed to perform the actions described in several imperative sentences, one at a time, when the sentences were presented on index cards. When an imperative sentence was presented (e.g., "roll the ball"), the subject was given the object mentioned in the sentence (e.g., a ball). Immediately after the subject's performance of the last action, the subject was asked to recall as many of the presented sentences as possible. In the verbal task setting, subjects were presented with similar imperative sentences, but instead of performing the actions described were instructed to read the sentences aloud to the experimenter. Immediately after the reading of the last sentence the subject was asked to recall as many sentences as possible. Following both the free recall of subject performed tasks and free recall of verbal tasks, subjects were presented with a cued recall task. In the cued recall task, the subjects were presented with category cues relating to the nouns of the presented imperative sentences. The sentences were counterbalanced across tests, such that the chance of the sentence "roll the ball" being presented as stimulus in the verbal task was equal to it being presented as stimulus in the subject performed task. Test order was varied, such that verbal tasks and subject performed tasks were equally likely to be tested first. Testing of cued recall always followed testing of free recall.

The cognitive assessment lasted between 1.5 and 2 hours. Each participant was tested individually.

A detailed description of the cognitive tests can be found in the Appendix. For an overview of the complete test battery, the reader may consult L.-G. Nilsson et al. (1997, 2004).

Diagnosis of dementia

In order to exclude persons who would later develop dementia, data from T3 (1998–2000) and T4 (2003–2005) were used. At those test occasions, persons fulfilling one or more of the following criteria were referred to a specialist in neuropsychiatry: (1) suspected dementia signs observed by experimenter or nurse, (2) MMSE score (Folstein et al., 1975) below 24, or (3) a decline of three or more MMSE points over the 5-year follow-up intervals. Based on thorough examination, and in accordance with the *Diagnostic and Statistical Manual of Mental Disorders* (American Psychiatric Association, 2000), a neuropsychiatrist made the clinical diagnosis of dementia—if warranted.

Diagnosis of diabetes and impaired glucose metabolism

Participants who reported having received medical care for diabetes were assigned to the group "Diabetics" ($n = 125$). All participants assigned to the group "Diabetics" had B-HbA$_{1c}$ levels above cutoffs for elevated HbA$_{1c}$. Participants with a B-HbA$_{1C}$ level greater than 6.6% in sample one, or greater than 5.3% for samples two or three, but no diagnosis of diabetes, were assigned to the group "Nondiabetics with elevated levels of HbA$_{1C}$" ($n = 151$). Participants with neither elevated HbA$_{1C}$ nor diagnosis of diabetes were assigned to the group "Nondiabetics" ($n = 2489$). The different levels of HbA$_{1C}$ required for inclusion in the "elevated" group reflect different laboratory procedures for HbA$_{1C}$ in the samples. Although individual HbA$_{1C}$ values are not perfectly correlated across the two methods, application of clinical cutoffs (Sacks et al., 2002) as a basis for dichotomisation largely reduces this potential problem. The clinical cutoffs are the values at which the result is considered pathological, and irrespective of methodological differences, the Sacks et al. study has shown that this value conveys much the same information. So whereas a difference of, e.g., two units may not be comparable between methods, dichotomising at the level considered pathological gives similar results under different laboratory methods. Information regarding diabetic status was missing in 13 cases. These were excluded.

Statistical analysis

Possibly interesting comorbid conditions (myocardial infarction, stroke, hypertension, unconsciousness, and eye disease) were subjected to a principal components factor analysis. The analyses resulted in a single factor (Eigenvalue: 1.397, percentage of variance: 27.9). The resulting factor scores were used as a control variable in the main analyses. Table 1 displays demographic, HbA$_{1C}$, and comorbid conditions data across groups.

Cognitive data were analysed by means of a 3 (diagnostic group) $\times$ 2 (age; ≤ 65 years, > 65 years) $\times$ 2 (education; ≤ 6 years, > 6 years) $\times$ 2 (encoding; verbal, cued) $\times$ 2 (retrieval; free, cued) repeated measures analysis of covariance (ANCOVA) model with the comorbidity factor scores serving as covariate. This model reflects the main and putative interaction effects among diagnostic group, age, education, and performance in cognitive tests with varying levels of encoding and retrieval support.

TABLE 1
Demographics, glycosylated haemoglobin (HbA_{1C}), and comorbidity across groups

		Nondiabetics	
Variable	*Diabetics* (*n* = 125)	*Elevated HbA1C* (*n* = 151)	*Normal HbA1C* (*n* = 2489)
Mean age (*SD*)*	66.92 (12.21)	66.89 (13.25)	56.94 (13.97)
Gender (% female)	58.4	58.9	53.8
Education*	8.03 (3.14)	8.38 (3.58)	10.37 (4.01)
HbA_{1C}*	7.73 (2.76)	6.58 (1.46)	5.00 (0.73)
Diseases (%)			
Circulatory*	48.8	39.1	27.5
Stroke*	10.4	7.3	3.0
Hypertension*	51.2	32.5	19.5
Unconsciousness	14.4	12.6	10.8
Eye disease*	29.6	20.5	14.8
Disease factor score*	0.81 (1.22)	0.34 (1.15)	−0.06 (0.95)

*Group differences significant at $p < .001$.

RESULTS

All between-subjects main effects were significant: diagnostic group, $F(2, 2752) = 4.06$, $p = .017$, partial eta$^2 = .003$; age group, $F(1, 2752) = 94.47$, $p < .001$, partial eta$^2 = .033$; education, $F(1, 2752) = 39.11$, $p < .001$, partial eta$^2 = .014$; as were the main effects of the CVD factor covariate, $F(1, 2752) = 57.09$, $p < .001$, partial eta$^2 = .014$. The diagnostic group effect was due to that nondiabetic controls performed at the highest level across all cognitive measures followed by the diabetics and the group with elevated HbA_{1c} levels (that did not differ from each other), the effect of age group was due to that the younger participants performed at a higher level, higher levels of education resulted in better performance, and the effect of CVD factor scores, finally, resulted from a negative association with overall memory performance such that a higher factor score resulted in worse memory performance.

Both within-subjects main effects were significant: encoding support, $F(1, 2752) = 1018.67$, $p < .001$, partial eta$^2 = .270$, and retrieval support, $F(1, 2752) = 400.41$, $p < .001$, partial eta$^2 = .127$. These effects were due to that both higher levels of encoding support and higher levels of retrieval support resulted in better memory performance.

An interaction effect of encoding by retrieval support, $F(1, 2752) = 8.82$, $p = .003$, was demonstrated. Figure 1 shows the differential effects of encoding and retrieval support, averaged over both tests with low and high encoding and retrieval support respectively. The interaction is explained

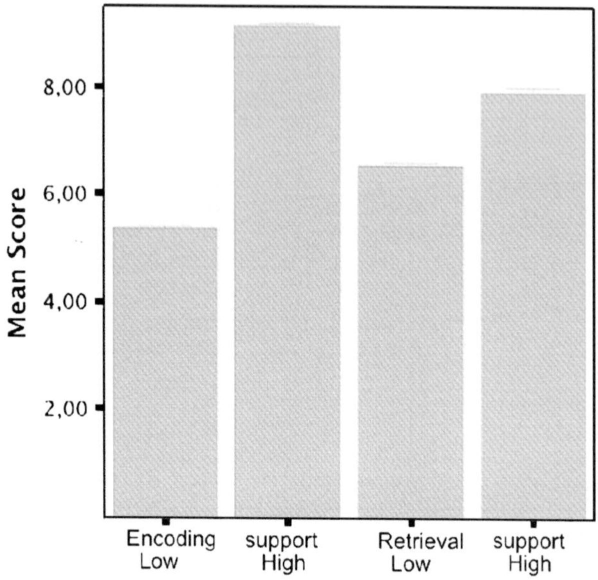

Figure 1. Performance across levels of support for all subjects (n =2948). Error bars represent standard error.

by a differential effect of support, such that retrieval support is more effective when encoding support is also high (see Table 2).

A significant three-way interaction was obtained for retrieval support by diagnostic group by age group, $F(2, 2752) = 4.02$, $p = .018$. Figure 2 illustrates the interaction showing, for the young age group, that nondiabetic controls performed at a slightly higher level than non diabetics with elevated levels of HbA_{1c} (mean difference [least significant different] = 0.49, $p = .047$), who in turn performed at a similar level as diabetics (mean difference = 0.25, $p = .499$). The performance difference between nondiabetic controls and diabetics was 0.74 ($p = .008$). In the old age group, however, we found that participants with elevated levels of HbA_{1c} but no diabetes diagnosis were performing at a slightly lower level than diabetics (mean difference = 0.50, $p = .135$), but at a significantly lower level than nondiabetic controls (mean

TABLE 2
Encoding by retrieval support means (*SE*)

	Encoding support	
Retrieval support	*Low*	*High*
Low	3.80 (0.11)	7.19 (0.12)
High	5.09 (0.14)	8.90 (0.11)

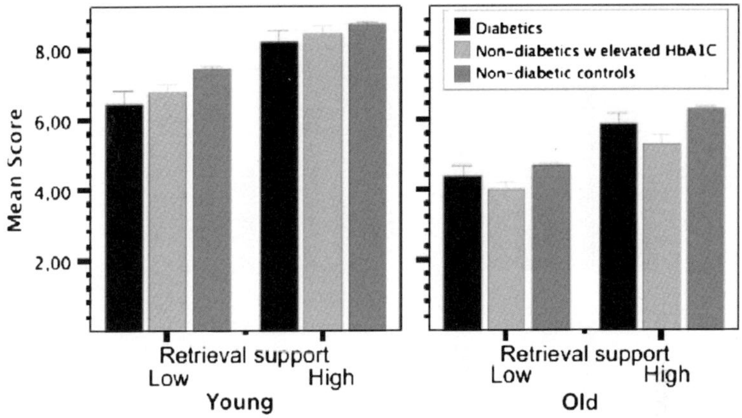

Figure 2. Performance across levels of retrieval support, age group, and diagnostic group. Young ($\leq$65 years) diabetics (n = 60), nondiabetics with elevated HbA_{1c} (n = 74), and controls (n = 1855) are represented in the left panel. Old ($\geq$70 years) diabetics (n = 77), nondiabetics with elevated HbA_{1c} (n = 93), and controls (n = 789) are represented in the right panel. Error bars represent standard error.

difference = 0.82, $p = .001$). The performance difference between nondiabetic controls and diabetics in the old age group was 0.32 ($p = .212$). Furthermore, collapsed across age groups, a larger performance difference as a function of low and high retrieval support was present in diabetics (mean difference = 1.58, $p < .001$) than in nondiabetics (mean difference = 1.36, $p < .001$). Participants with elevated levels of HbA_{1c} showed an intermediary difference (mean difference = 1.47, $p < .001$).

One four-way interaction was detected, namely encoding support by diagnostic group by age group by level of education, $F(2, 2752) = 3.19$, $p = .041$. Figure 3 illustrates this interaction, showing that the difference between diabetics and nondiabetics with elevated levels of HbA_{1c} was smaller among those with high education (mean difference = 0.35, $p = .295$) as compared to those with low education (diabetics vs. nondiabetics with elevated levels of HbA_{1c}, mean difference = 0.70, $p = .057$), whereas those with high education showed greater differences between other diagnostic groups (diabetics vs. nondiabetic controls, mean difference = 1.21, $p < .001$; nondiabetics with elevated levels of HbA_{1c} vs. nondiabetic controls, mean difference = 0.87, $p < .001$) than those with low education (diabetics vs. nondiabetic controls, mean difference = 0.19, $p = .500$; nondiabetics with elevated levels of HbA_{1c} vs. nondiabetic controls, mean difference = 0.89, $p = .001$). It is also clear that the Age × Diagnostic group interaction that was explored in Figure 2 was more pronounced among those with low education than among those with higher levels of education. Also, the effect of encoding support was—in absolute numbers—greatest among young

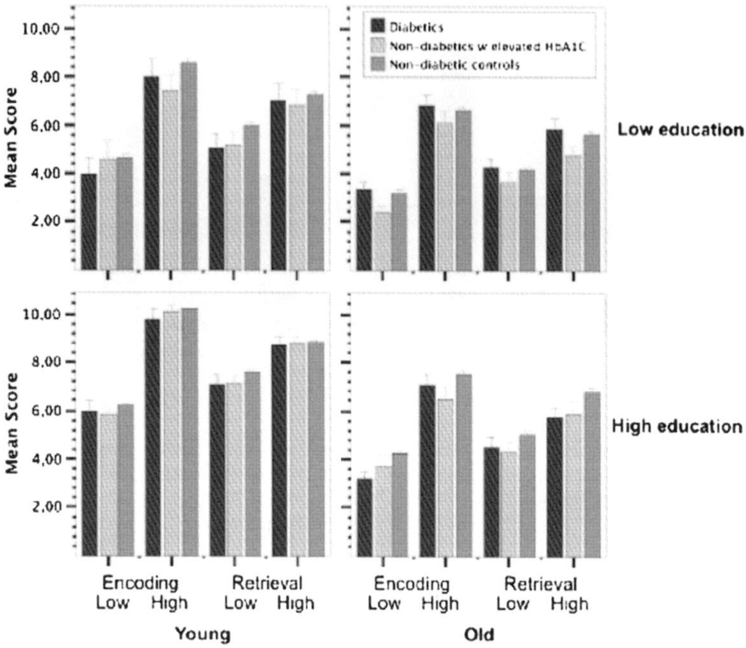

Figure 3. Performance across level of support, age diagnostic group, and education. Young persons ($\leq$65 years) with low education ($\leq$6 years) who are diabetic ($n = 20$), nondiabetic with elevated HbA_{1c} ($n = 17$), and controls ($n = 204$) are contrasted with young persons with high education ($>$6 years) who are diabetic ($n = 40$), nondiabetic with elevated HbA_{1c} ($n = 57$), and controls ($n = 1651$). Old persons ($\geq$70 years) with low education who are diabetic ($n = 42$), nondiabetic with elevated HbA_{1c} ($n = 55$), and controls ($n = 394$) are contrasted with old persons with high education who are diabetic ($n = 35$), nondiabetic with elevated HbA_{1c} ($n = 38$), and controls ($n = 395$). Error bars represent standard error.

persons with high level of education (mean difference = 3.96, $p < .001$), whereas retrieval support had the greatest impact among old persons with low education (mean difference = 1.44, $p < .001$). Finally, in order to examine the effects of elevated HbA_{1c} more closely, we repeated the main repeated measures ANCOVA with two modifications. In the first modified analysis, we included participants with elevated levels of HbA_{1c} in the group of nondiabetic controls, in such a way that the group comparison was between those with diagnosed diabetes and all others. The results showed no significant difference between the groups, $F(1, 2756) = 0.57$, $p = .452$. When we regrouped the participants such that persons with elevated levels of HbA_{1c} were included in the group of diabetics, the difference between groups was significant, $F(1, 2756) = 7.11$, $p = .008$, and actually larger than the corresponding effect in our original model.

DISCUSSION

We examined effects on episodic memory of diabetes at varying levels of encoding and retrieval support. Also, we took into account the under diagnosis of Type 2-diabetes in the population by assessing levels of HbA_{1c}. An important contribution of this study is that it assesses the cognitive impairment of diabetics in the general population. Whereas clinical populations from, for example, outpatient diabetes units at hospitals may provide diabetics that are more gravely ill, and as a consequence perform at a lower level in cognitive tests; diabetics sampled from the general population are arguably more representative of the diabetic population at large. Since the Betula samples are similar to the Swedish population on almost all demographic variables (Nilsson et al., 1997), it is reasonable to expect that the diabetics that were tested in this study are indeed representative of diabetics in Sweden.

The effects of age, education, and cardiovascular disease on cognitive performance were expected, given results from previous research (e.g., Bäckman et al., 2000, 2001; Nilsson, 2003). Importantly, the effects of cognitive support provided at retrieval seems to attenuate the difference between diabetics, nondiabetics with elevated levels of HbA_{1c}, and non-diabetic controls. Similar effects have been found in other diseases, as well as in normal ageing (Hassing, Wahlin, Winblad, & Bäckman, 1999; Wahlin, Bäckman, & Winblad, 1995). This indicates that participants can compensate for cognitive limitations imposed by disease and ageing by utilisation of cognitive support at retrieval. More specifically, the present findings add to the findings in our previous study (Wahlin et al., 2002) in showing that not just test materials but support provided at retrieval may attenuate cognitive performance deficits due to diabetes mellitus. The fact that retrieval support was more effective when encoding support was also provided was not unexpected. In general, more support generally results in better performance (e.g., Bäckman, Mäntylä, & Herlitz, 1990). Also, support provided at encoding allowing use of several sensory modalities will result in better encoding, which in turn will be maximally utilised in terms of memory performance in the case where these modalities are also tapped by support at retrieval. However, the findings of this study adds to this general picture by showing that utilisation of cognitive support in old age is moderated by diabetic status. Also, it expands the findings of Wahlin et al. (2002) where (utilising a much smaller sample) diabetes-related cognitive deficits among elderly persons were found to vary as a function of support inherent in the test materials.

The inclusion of a group of participants that have not received a proper diabetes diagnosis, but who demonstrate elevated levels of HbA_{1c}, was informative. It is well known that diabetes is underdiagnosed, especially in the elderly population (e.g., Dunstan et al., 2002). Thus, the group of nondiabetics with elevated levels of HbA_{1c} could very well comprise both persons who have not yet developed diabetes and persons who have indeed developed a condition that would fulfil the criteria of diabetes diagnosis if they were tested. Given the lower chance among older cohorts to be diagnosed with diabetes, even though they have a larger risk of actually being diabetic (e.g., Dunstan et al., 2002; Eliasson, Lindahl, Lundberg, & Stegamayr, 2002), it is reasonable to assume that the proportion of undiagnosed diabetics would be larger among the old. Indeed, in our data we find that the proportion of persons with elevated HbA_{1c} levels, but without diabetes diagnosis, is about threefold in the older age group. Persons with undiagnosed diabetes are not likely to receive optimum diabetes treatment, and are thus more likely to develop diabetes-related cognitive impairments. In light of this, the differential results regarding utilisation of retrieval support as a function of diabetes, nondiabetes with elevated HbA_{1c}, and nondiabetes among the young and the old are explainable. The $\leq$65-year-olds show the expected dose–response effect of glycaemic control—in the sense that the nondiabetic controls perform at the best level and show the least improvement in high retrieval support settings, followed by the performance of nondiabetics with elevated HbA_{1c}, and diagnosed diabetics—who show greater performance increases in the high retrieval support settings. The $\geq$70-year-olds demonstrate lowest performance among persons without diabetes diagnosis but with elevated HbA_{1c} levels, followed by those who have a diagnosis of diabetes, and show best performance among nondiabetic controls—without any apparent differences in utilisation of retrieval support. Cued recall is by necessity always tested after free recall, but it is unlikely that this influences the association between disease state, age, and utilisation of retrieval support. No differences have been noted as an effect of test order in previous examinations of the Betula test battery (see Nilsson et al., 1997, 2004). If the assumption that treatment of diabetes reduces risk of cognitive impairment (for discussion, see Areosa & Grimley, 2002) as well as the risk of other diabetes complications, it is reasonable to expect that those with diagnosed diabetes should—in cohorts where under diagnosis is a real problem—perform better since they receive treatment (see also Dunstan et al., 2002).

An important aspect of studying the effects of undiagnosed disease states, incipient diseases, or increased risk of developing disease, is that it adds to our understanding of ostensibly normal ageing. Whereas diabetes may be one of the most common underdiagnosed conditions, it is reasonable to assume that several other medical conditions that may affect cognition would also not be known by the subjects—or indeed asked about by study designers. Sisyphean attempts to fully diagnose and account for all medical conditions potentially related to cognition are obviously not advisable in ageing studies, but the general understanding that most diseases are continua is important for the interpretation of results in all studies of cognition. Some of the deleterious effect of most any disease could very well be expected to be present even in persons that do not themselves know that they are sick.

The analyses where we included participants with elevated levels of HbA_{1c} either in the group of nondiabetic controls or in the group of diabetics gave results that could be interpreted to mean that persons with elevated HbA_{1c} are more cognitively similar to diabetics than to nondiabetics. In light of this result, some of the divergent results reported in previous literature regarding cognitive repercussions of diabetes may be explained. In studies where diabetes diagnoses have been set utilising laboratory analyses, persons who fulfil diagnostic criteria for diabetes would be included in the diabetes group, and results can be expected to reveal lower performance in the diabetes group. Conversely, in studies that rely on self-reported diabetic status, persons who may in fact have diabetes may be included in the control group, thus diluting the results.

It should be noted that for inclusion into the group "diabetics" this study relies on self-reports of receiving medical care for diabetes. It could be argued that the inclusion of a group of participants with elevated HbA_{1c}, but no self-reported diabetes, reduces the impact of this potential limitation. This argument is also strengthened by the fact that including the persons with elevated HbA_{1C} in the group of diabetics only strengthened the association of cognitive performance and diabetic status. However, in view of the limitation of self-reports of receiving care for diabetes, the interpretations of the results for the group of participants with elevated levels of HbA_{1c} could be effected. The presented results could be consistent with a differentially self-reported illness, such that older participants who have impaired cognitive abilities would be less likely to correctly report their diabetic status—thus artificially worsening the apparent relative performance of the group with elevated HbA_{1C}. Given that persons who would later develop dementia are excluded, such an explanation is not likely. Note that the group of diabetics demonstrated the most elevated levels of HbA_{1C} (see Table 1), which may contradict assumptions of differentially self-reported disease leading to artificial results. Importantly, the proportion of persons reporting to have received care for diabetes is at the same level as in the general population (e.g., Henriksson et al., 2000). Note also that the proportion of persons with elevated levels of HbA_{1c} without diabetes diagnosis is similar to levels of underdiagnosis found in the studies in which diabetes was clinically diagnosed (Brohall et al., 2006; Dunstan et al., 2002). Furthermore, this study is limited by the fact that we lack data on diabetes duration, treatment, and severity. Although HbA_{1c} values of diagnosed diabetics could serve as a proxy of disease severity, it was judged to be of limited value for this study due to the fact that we had limited information regarding individual treatment strategies. Such information would of course add significantly to the interpretability of results. As a final caveat, we were not able to discriminate between subtypes of diabetes. However, on the basis of Swedish prevalence figures, a reasonable assumption is that the diabetics in the studied samples comprise almost exclusively Type 2-diabetics.

In sum, we have demonstrated that diabetics perform worse on cognitive testing than do nondiabetics. Persons who did not report diabetes but had elevated levels of HbA_{1c}, and could thus be viewed as persons who either are about to develop diabetes or already fulfil the diagnostic criteria for diabetes, performed at different levels under varying levels of retrieval support in relation to diabetics and nondiabetic controls depending on their age. Among persons 65 years of age or younger, diabetics performed at a lower level than nondiabetics with elevated levels of HbA_{1c} and nondiabetic controls—indicating a dose response effect of degree or duration of lacking metabolic control. However, among persons 70 years of age or older, the nondiabetics with elevated levels of HbA_{1c} performed at a lower level than both diabetics and nondiabetic controls. On a more general level—given under diagnosis in the old age groups—this indicates that undiagnosed, and thus untreated, diabetics are worse off than those who receive diagnosis and treatment. The differential results across age indicate that future studies of ageing and retrieval support, where control for diabetes related variation is desired, need to be performed with some care. If one were simply to—across age groups—statistically control for diabetic status, artificial results would be a distinct possibility. Excluding persons who are aware of their diabetic status does not seem like a good option, given underdiagnosis.

In view of the present results—which could be interpreted such that treatment of diabetes may, at least among the old, attenuate cognitive repercussions of diabetes—an important future field of medical study is intervention studies aiming at examining cognitive effects of improving glycaemic control among diabetes patients. This type of study should ideally be performed in a group of elderly diabetics, since undertreatment is more common among older than among younger diabetics. The details of how diabetic status differentially affects young and old also needs to be explored further, not only to expand the understanding of diabetes-related cognitive impairment, but also to facilitate interpretation of studies of ostensibly normal ageing.

REFERENCES

American Psychiatric Association. (1987). *Diagnostic and statistical manual of mental disorders* (3rd Rev. ed.). Washington, DC: Author.

American Psychiatric Association. (2000). *Diagnostic and statistical manual of mental disorders* (4th ed., text revision). Washington, DC: Author.

Areosa, S. A., & Grimley, E. V. (2002). Effect of the treatment of Type II diabetes mellitus on the development of cognitive impairment and dementia. *Cochrane Database of Systematic Reviews 2002*. Issue 4. Art. No.: CD003804. DOI: 10.1002/14651858.CD003804.

Bale, R. N. (1973). Brain damage in diabetes mellitus. *British Journal of Psychiatry, 122*(568), 337–341.

Ballesteros, S., & Reales, J. M. (2004). Intact haptic priming in normal aging and Alzheimer's disease: Evidence for dissociable memory systems. *Neuropsychologia, 42*(8), 1063–1070.

Ballesteros, S., Reales, J. M., & Mayas, J. (2007). Picture priming in normal aging and Alzheimer's disease. *Psicothema, 19*(2), 239–244.

Brohall, G., Behre, C. J., Hulthe, J., Wikstrand, J., & Fagerberg, B. (2006). Prevalence of diabetes and impaired glucose tolerance in 64-year-old Swedish women: Experiences of using repeated oral glucose tolerance tests. *Diabetes Care, 29*(2), 363–367.

Bäckman, L., Mäntylä, T., & Herlitz, A. (1990). The optimization of episodic remembering in old age. In P. B. Baltes & M. M. Baltes (Eds.), *Successful aging: Perspectives from the behavioral sciences* (pp. 118–163). New York: Cambridge University Press.

Bäckman, L., Small, B. J., & Wahlin, Å. (2001). Aging and memory: Cognitive and biological perspectives. In J. E. Birren (Ed.), *Handbook of the psychology of aging* (5th ed., pp. 349–377). San Diego, CA: Academic Press.

Bäckman, L., Small, B. J., Wahlin, Å., & Larsson, M. (2000). Cognitive functioning in very old age. In F. I. M. Craik & T. A. Salthouse (Eds.), *The handbook of aging and cognition* (2nd ed., pp. 499–558). Mahwah, NJ: Lawrence Erlbaum Associates, Inc.

Convit, A., Wolf, O. T., Tarshish, C., & de Leon, M. J. (2003). Reduced glucose tolerance is associated with poor memory performance and hippocampal atrophy among normal elderly. *Proceedings of the National Academy of Sciences of the USA, 100*(4), 2019–2022.

Dunstan, D. W., Zimmet, P. Z., Welborn, T. A., de Courten, M. P., Cameron, A. J., Sicree, R. A., et al. (2002). The rising prevalence of diabetes and impaired glucose tolerance: The Australian Diabetes, Obesity and Lifestyle Study. *Diabetes Care, 25*(5), 829–834.

Eliasson, M., Lindahl, B., Lundberg, V., & Stegamayr, B. (2002). No increase in the prevalence of known diabetes between 1986 and 1999 in subjects 25–64 years of age in northern Sweden. *Diabetic Medicine, 19*(10), 874–888.

Elliott, T. G., & Viberti, G. (1993). Relationship between insulin resistance and coronary heart disease in diabetes mellitus and the general population: A critical appraisal. *Baillieres Clinical Endocrinology and Metabolism, 7*(4), 1079–1103.

The Expert Committee on the Diagnosis and Classification of Diabetes Mellitus. (2003). Report of the Expert Committee on the Diagnosis and Classification of Diabetes Mellitus. *Diabetes Care, 26*(Suppl. 1), S5–S20.

Folstein, M. F., Folstein, S. E., & McHugh, P. R. (1975). "Mini-Mental State": A practical method for grading the cognitive state of patients for the clinician. *Journal of Psychiatric Research, 12*(3), 189–198.

Hassing, L., Wahlin, Å., Winblad, B., & Bäckman, L. (1999). Further evidence for the effects of vitamin B_{12} and folate status on episodic memory functioning: A population-based study of very old adults. *Biological Psychiatry, 45*, 1472–1480.

Henriksson, F., Agardh, C. D., Berne, C., Bolinder, J., Lonnqvist, F., Stenstrom, P., et al. (2000). Direct medical costs for patients with type 2 diabetes in Sweden. *Journal of Internal Medicine, 248*(5), 387–396.

Kannel, W. B., & McGee, D. L. (1979). Diabetes and glucose tolerance as risk factors for cardiovascular disease: The Framingham study. *Diabetes Care*, *2*(2), 120–126.

Kern, W., Peters, A., Fruehwald-Schultes, B., Deininger, E., Born, J., & Fehm, H.L. (2001). Improving influence of insulin on cognitive functions in humans. *Neuroendocrinology*, *74*(4), 270–280.

Kilander, L., Nyman, H., Boberg, M., Hansson, L., & Lithell, H. (1998). Hypertension is related to cognitive impairment: A 20-year follow-up of 999 men. *Hypertension*, *31*(3), 780–786.

LaVoie, D., & Light, L. L. (1994). Adult age differences in repetition priming: A meta-analysis. *Psychology and Aging*, *9*(4), 539–553.

Lövden, M., Bergman, L., Adolfsson, R., Lindenberger, U., & Nilsson, L.-G. (2005). Studying individual aging in an interindividual context: Typical paths of age-related, dementia-related, and mortality-related cognitive development in old age. *Psychology and Aging*, *20*(2), 303–316.

Miles, W., & Root, H. (1922). Psychologic tests applied to diabetic patients. *Archives of Internal Medicine*, *30*, 767–777.

Nilsson, E., Fastbom, J., & Wahlin, A. (2002). Cognitive functioning in a population-based sample of very old non-demented and non-depressed persons: The impact of diabetes. *Archives of Gerontology and Geriatrics*, *35*(2), 95–105.

Nilsson, L.-G. (2003). Memory function in normal aging. *Acta Neurologica Scandinavica*, *107*(Suppl. 179), 7–13.

Nilsson, L.-G., Adolfsson, R., Bäckman, L., de Frias, C. M., Molander, B., & Nyberg, L. (2004). Betula: A prospective cohort study on memory, health and aging. *Aging, Neuropsychology, and Cognition*, *11*(2–3), 134–148.

Nilsson, L.-G., Bäckman, L., Erngrund, K., Nyberg, L., Adolfsson, R., Bucht, G., et al. (1997). The Betula prospective cohort study: Memory, health, and aging. *Aging, Neuropsychology, and Cognition*, *4*(1), 1–32.

Nyberg, L., Maitland, S. B., Rönnlund, M., Bäckman, L., Dixon, R., Wahlin, Å., & Nilsson, L.-G. (2003). Selective adult age differences in an age-invariant multifactor model of declarative memory. *Psychology and Aging*, *18*, 149–160.

Ott, A., Stolk, R. P., Hofman, A., vanHarskamp, F., Grobbee, D. E., & Breteler, M. M. B. (1996). Association of diabetes mellitus and dementia: The Rotterdam study. *Diabetologia*, *39*(11), 1392–1397.

Park, C. R. (2001). Cognitive effects of insulin in the central nervous system. *Neuroscience and Biobehavioral Reviews*, *25*(4), 311–323.

Rönnlund, M., Bäckman, L., Lövdén, M., Nilsson, L.-G., & Nyberg, L. (2000). Five-year changes in recall across levels of support: Parallel age-related deficits. *International Journal of Psychology*, *35*(3–4), 366.

Sacks, D. B., Bruns, D. E., Goldstein, D. E., Maclaren, N. K., McDonald, J. M., & Parrott, M. (2002). Guidelines and recommendations for laboratory analysis in the diagnosis and management of diabetes mellitus. *Clinical Chemistry*, *48*, 436–472.

Squire, L. R. (1992). Memory and the hippocampus: A synthesis from findings with rats, monkeys, and humans. *Psychological Review*, *99*(2), 195–231.

Stewart, R., & Liolitsa, D. (1999). Type 2 diabetes mellitus, cognitive impairment and dementia. *Diabetic Medicine*, *16*(2), 93–112.

Strachan, M. W. J., Deary, I. J., Ewing, F. M. E., & Frier, B. M. (1997). Is type II diabetes associated with an increased risk of cognitive dysfunction? A critical review of published studies. *Diabetes Care*, *20*(3), 438–445.

Unger, J. W., Livingston, J. N., & Moss, A. M. (1991). Insulin receptors in the central nervous system: Localization, signalling mechanisms and functional aspects. *Progress in Neurobiology*, *36*(5), 343–362.

Wahlin, Å., Bäckman, L., & Winblad, B. (1995). Free recall and recognition of slowly and rapidly presented words in very old age: A community-based study. *Experimental Aging Research, 21*, 251–271.

Wahlin, Å., Nilsson, E., & Fastbom, J. (2002). Cognitive performance in very old diabetic persons: The impact of semantic structure, preclinical dementia, and impending death. *Neuropsychology, 16*(2), 208–216.

Watson, G. S, & Craft, S. (2006). Insulin resistance, inflammation, and cognition in Alzheimer's disease: Lessons for multiple sclerosis. *Journal of the Neurological Sciences, 245*(1–2), 21–33.

Wickelgren, I. (1998). Tracking insulin to the mind. *Science, 280*(5363), 517–519.

Xu, W. L., Qiu, C. X., Wahlin, Å., Winblad, B., & Fratiglioni, L. (2004). Diabetes mellitus and risk of dementia in the Kungsholmen project: A 6-year follow-up study. *Neurology, 63*(7), 1181–1186.

APPENDIX

Cognitive examination

The cognitive tests most relevant to the purposes of this study are the tests of episodic memory with varying levels of cognitive support at encoding and retrieval, respectively. The order of testing was reversed between Tests 1 and 2 for half of the participants in each age cohort.

1. Short sentences in imperative form (e.g., "roll the ball") were presented on index cards for 8 s each. Subjects were instructed to read the sentence back to the experimenter. Immediately after the presentation of the sentences, subjects were presented with a free recall test where they were asked to recall, during 2 minutes, as many of the sentences as possible.
2. Short sentences in imperative form were presented on index cards for 8 s. Subjects were instructed to perform the action described on each of the index cards. Immediately after the presentation of the sentences, subjects were presented with a free recall test where they were asked to recall, during 2 minutes, as many of the sentences as possible.
3. Immediately after each of the free recall tasks, cued recall tests were presented, in which the subjects were presented with category cues pertaining to the nouns of the sentences presented in Tests 1 and 2, respectively. Three minutes were allotted for these tasks.

Hence, there were four possible combinations of support (support at encoding, yes/no; support at retrieval, yes/no). All combinations of support were tested in each subject. In all four tests, possible performance scores varied between 0 and 16.

EUROPEAN JOURNAL OF COGNITIVE PSYCHOLOGY
2009, 21 (2/3), 406–427

Psychology Press
Taylor & Francis Group

A new look at aging and performance in the antisaccade task: The impact of response selection

Bettina Olk
School of Humanities and Social Sciences, Jacobs University Bremen, Bremen, Germany

Alan Kingstone
Department of Psychology, University of British Columbia, Vancouver, Canada

Aged adults respond more slowly and less accurately in the antisaccade task, in which a saccade away from a visual stimulus is required. This decreased performance has been attributed to a decline in the ability to inhibit prepotent responses with age. Considering that antisaccades also involve response selection, the present experiment investigated the contribution of inhibition and response selection. Young and aged adults were compared between conditions that required varying percentages of prosaccades, antisaccades, and no-go trials. The comparison between no-go (inhibition of a prosaccade) and antisaccade trials (inhibition of a prosaccade *and* selection of an antisaccade) showed significantly worse performance in the antisaccade task, especially for the older group, suggesting that they failed to select the antisaccade in a situation in which a competing, prepotent response is available. The impact of this response selection failure was underlined by an equivalent ability of both groups to impose inhibition.

Keywords: Oculomotor control; Aging; Saccades; Antisaccades; Inhibition; Competition; Response selection.

As the general population grows older, it is becoming increasingly important to understand how cognition is affected by the process of aging. One of the key cognitive functions that has been identified to decline as we age is the

---

Correspondence should be addressed to Bettina Olk, School of Humanities and Social Sciences, Jacobs University Bremen, P.O. Box 750 561, 28725 Bremen, Germany. E-mail: b.olk@jacobs-university.de

This work was supported by a fellowship of the Michael Smith Foundation for Health Research and a grant from the German Academic Exchange Service to Bettina Olk and by Canadian grants to Alan Kingstone from the Natural Sciences and Engineering Research Council, and the Social Science and Humanities Research Council.

http://www.psypress.com/ecp DOI: 10.1080/09541440802333190

ability to inhibit prepotent responses that may be incorrect in a particular situation (Butler & Zacks, 2006; Hasher, Zacks, & May, 1999; Sweeny, Rosano, Berman, & Luna, 2001). Well-documented failures in the elderly to inhibit eye movement responses are often put forward as evidence for this decline (Faust & Balota, 1997; Kramer, Hahn, Irwin & Theeuwes, 2000). Specifically, it has been demonstrated that when the task is to look away from a visual stimulus that is suddenly presented in peripheral vision, a response commonly referred to as "antisaccade", aged adults show a higher rate of erroneous saccades to the stimulus (the prepotent response which is called a "prosaccade") than younger participants (Abel & Douglas, 2007; Bojko, Kramer, & Peterson, 2004; Butler, Zack, & Henderson, 1999; Eenshuistra, Ridderinkhof, & van der Molen, 2004; Klein, Fischer, Hartnegg, Heiss, & Roth, 2000; Nieuwenhuis, Ridderinkhof, de Jong, Kok, & van der Molen, 2000; Olincy, Ross, Young, & Freedman, 1997; Sweeny et al., 2001) and also show prolonged saccadic reaction times, in particular for antisaccades (Abel & Douglas, 2007; Bojko et al., 2004; Eenshuistra et al., 2004; Klein et al., 2000; Nieuwenhuis et al., 2000; Olincy et al., 1997; Sweeny et al., 2001). This poorer performance in tasks requiring oculomotor control has commonly been attributed to the failure to inhibit the prepotent response to the visual stimulus, either directly due to a decline in the effectiveness of inhibitory processes with age (Butler & Zacks, 2006; Hasher et al., 1999; Sweeny et al., 2001) or, indirectly, due to either changes in working memory capacity or increasing "goal neglect" which then decrease the efficiency of inhibitory control (Colcombe et al., 2003; de Jong, 2001; Eenshuistra et al., 2004; Roberts, Hager, & Heron, 1994; Ryan, Shen, & Reingold, 2006).

In order to carry out correct antisaccades, it is without doubt essential to suppress the tendency to look at the visual stimulus before a correct eye movement can be made away from its location. Studies from different areas of research demonstrate that cognitively controlled inhibition is crucial to successful performance in the antisaccade task (Godijn & Kramer, 2006; Olk & Kingstone, 2003). For instance, studies using Transcranial Magnetic Stimulation (TMS) have shown that the modulation of activity in the frontal eye field (FEF) and the dorsolateral prefrontal cortex (dlPFC) is critical to inhibition and correct antisaccade performance (e.g., Olk, Chang, Kingstone, & Ro, 2006; Pierrot-Deseilligny, Rivaud, Gaymard, & Agid, 1991). Convergent with this evidence, patients with frontal lobe lesions demonstrate a marked inability to suppress unwanted prosaccades towards a visual stimulus (e.g., Everling & Fischer, 1998). However, there is at least one other control process involved in the antisaccade task besides inhibition, namely the selection of the correct saccadic response in the direction opposite to the stimulus. Prosaccades are triggered by the visual stimulus, but antisaccades require the selection of a motor programme (Reuter, Philipp, Koch, & Kathmann, 2006). Thus, in the antisaccade task two opposing saccade programmes need to be coordinated: the prepotent prosaccade towards the stimulus onset needs to be inhibited, and the less potent antisaccade away from the stimulus needs to be selected. Therefore, when participants fail to make a correct antisaccade response, the reason could either be a failure to inhibit the prosaccade response or a failure to select the antisaccade response. The relative contribution of each component has not been examined so far and it is unknown in how far a failure to select the correct antisaccade response contributes to higher error rates made by the elderly. The goal of the present experiment was to investigate these issues. Four possible outcomes can be envisioned. Poorer antisaccadic performance in the aged adult might occur because of (1) a failure to inhibit the prosaccade response, (2) a failure to select the antisaccade response, (3) both factors, which contribute independently to antisaccadic deficits, and (4) both factors, which combine in an interactive manner.

In order to estimate the contribution of saccade inhibition, we employed a go/no-go task that requires—like the antisaccade task—the inhibition of a prepotent prosaccade response to the visual onset stimulus, but it does not demand the selection of an opposing saccade response. Rather, in this task participants are instructed to either look at a peripheral stimulus (go-signal) or to maintain central fixation and not to look at a peripheral stimulus (no-go signal). Like in the antisaccade task participants are required on occasion to inhibit a prosaccade towards a peripheral visual signal, but unlike in the antisaccade task there is no competing saccadic response, i.e., the successful inhibition of a prosaccade response *is* the correct response on a no-go trial.

To test the potential role of a failure to select the correct response we ran conditions in which antisaccades were required instead of no-go responses. By replacing no-go trials with antisaccade trials we introduced the response selection component. On each antisaccade trial the competing antisaccade response had to be selected instead of the prepotent prosaccade. A comparison of the error rates between the conditions requiring no-go or antisaccade responses, informs us of the contribution of response selection. If error rates are the same, then there is no basis on which to argue that antisaccade response selection contributes significantly to antisaccade performance. But if the error rate is higher in the antisaccade task than in the no-go task, this would suggest that the selection of a saccadic response makes a meaningful contribution to antisaccade performance. Of course, inhibiting a prepotent prosaccade involves response selection as well, but this is shared in both the no-go and antisaccade trials. Only in the antisaccade task, however, is an additional stage involved, i.e., the selection of a saccadic movement response. This is what we mean by response selection, that is, response selection is defined as the selection of a *saccadic* response either towards or away from the stimulus.

Importantly though, the comparison of the error rates alone is not sufficient. An alternative explanation for a similarity or difference in error rates between tasks could be that inhibition is imposed differently in the two tasks. In order to assess inhibition, we measured the effect of inhibition on the prosaccadic go response in the go/no-go task by manipulating the proportion of no-go trials, i.e., when there were few no-go trials in an experimental block there should be little inhibition in place, and when there were many no-go trials inhibition should increase. In five blocks there were 0%, 10%, 30%, 50%, or 100% no-go trials. Thus, by systematically manipulating the proportion of no-go trials from 0% to 100%, we could titrate the effect of inhibition when a competing saccadic response did not have to be selected. Based on behavioural work showing that saccadic reaction time (saccadic RT) is significantly longer in a condition that requires the maintenance of fixation (no-go) on 80% of the trials compared to only 20% of the trials (Machado & Rafal, 2000), we expected that prosaccadic response time would increase as the percentage of no-go trials and thereby inhibition imposed by the participants were increased.

In the same way we manipulated the proportion of antisaccade trials from 0% (low inhibition) to 100% (high inhibition) in the pro/antisaccade conditions, expecting that the more trials require inhibition of a prosaccade, the slower prosaccade RT should become. This expectation dovetails with neurophysiological evidence that fixation cell activity is increased as prosaccade inhibition and response time increase (Everling, Dorris, Klein, & Munoz, 1999). In the study by Everling et al. (1999) the colour of the central fixation stimulus instructed a prosaccade or an antisaccade before the peripheral stimulus appeared. Activity of fixation cells was found to be higher and stimulus-related and saccade-related activity were reduced in antisaccade compared to prosaccade trials, a finding interpreted in terms of attenuation of preparatory activity in the superior colliculus to prevent erroneous prosaccades. In our task participants were informed of the percentage of trials that would require the inhibition of a prosaccade in the upcoming experimental block, thus we reason that the more trials require a no-go or an antisaccade response, the more inhibition should be placed on the oculomotor system, being reflected in higher activity of fixation cells and higher inhibition of saccade-related cells. Thus, in the condition consisting of 50% no-go or antisaccade trials and 50% prosaccades fixation cell activity should be higher than in a condition requiring only 30% or 10% no-go or antisaccade responses (and 70% or 90% prosaccades). This activation pattern should be mirrored in the prosaccade reaction time data. The comparison of the inhibition functions obtained from prosaccade RT in the no-go conditions with prosaccade RT in the pro/antisaccade conditions will enable us to determine whether inhibition is imposed similarly in both tasks.

In keeping with the literature, we expected that older participants would respond more slowly and commit more errors than younger participants in the antisaccade task. If their worse performance is best explained as an inhibition deficit, then error rates should not differ between the no-go and the antisaccade tasks or if they differ, an increase in the error rate in the antisaccade task should be reflected in a change in the inhibition placed on prosaccades compared between the no-go and the antisaccade tasks. If, however, more errors are made on antisaccade trials than on no-go trials but the inhibition functions measured by prosaccade reaction times in the no-go and the antisaccade tasks remain the same, this would indicate that deficiencies in the selection of the antisaccade response contribute to the higher error rates.

METHOD

Participants

Eleven young (mean age: 23 years, ranging from 18 to 36 years of age; five males, six females) and ten elderly participants (mean age: 65 years, ranging from 53 to 73 years of age; six males, four females) with normal or corrected vision gave informed consent and were paid for their participation.

Stimuli and procedure

Displays were generated and presented on a personal computer with a 17-inch VGA monitor. Example displays are shown in Figure 1. The display consisted of a fixation dot (diameter of 0.5°) surrounded by eight placeholder dots (diameter of 0.2°) (see Figure 1). The distance between fixation and the inner placeholder dots was 3° and between fixation and the outer placeholder dots was 6° of visual angle. Stimuli were black and presented on a white background.

Nine conditions, each run in a separate block, comprised the experiment. A target dot (diameter of 0.5°) appeared equally often at each of the eight possible placeholder locations. A green target dot always signalled for the execution of a prosaccade. Depending on the condition, a red target dot either instructed participants to maintain fixation (no-go task) or to execute an antisaccade (antisaccade task).

The percentage of trials requiring the inhibition of a prosaccade was manipulated between conditions by varying the ratio of green and red peripheral target stimuli within a block. The 100% prosaccades condition consisted of 64 trials, in which the target dot was always green and the task was to execute a prosaccade to the green dot on every trial. The 100% no-go

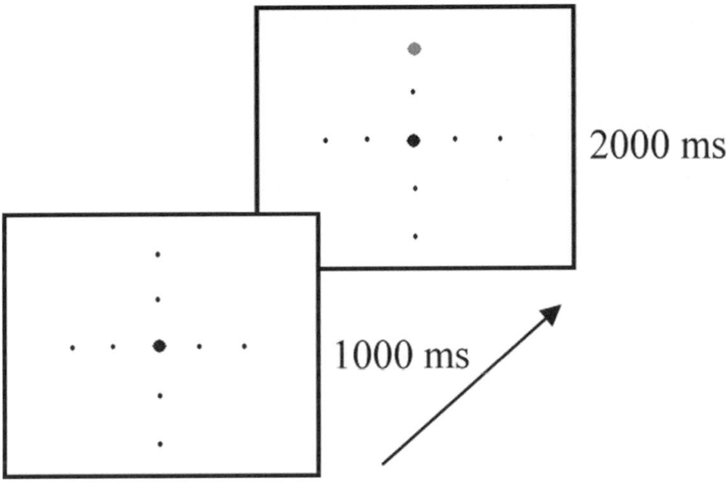

Figure 1. Example display. At the beginning of each trial a fixation display was shown. After 1000 ms a large peripheral dot (here shown in grey) instructed the type of response. If the large peripheral dot was green a prosaccade towards it was required. If the large peripheral dot was red it indicated either that central fixation had to be maintained (no-go) or an antisaccade response to the mirror-opposite location was required. The coloured stimuli appeared with the same probability at any of the eight locations that were marked with placeholder dots (small dots in the display). Displays were shown for 2000 ms. Note that displays are not drawn to scale.

condition and the 100% antisaccades condition consisted of 16 trials each in which the target dot was always red. In these conditions inhibition of a reflexive prosaccade was required on every trial. Three conditions consisted of 80 trials each with either 10% no-go/90% prosaccades, 30% no-go/70% prosaccades and 50% no-go/50% prosaccade trials. Three further conditions comprised 10% antisaccades/90% prosaccades, 30% antisaccades/70% prosaccades and 50% antisaccades/50% prosaccade trials. Note, that the displays of the no-go and antisaccade conditions were visually the same. The conditions merely differed in the task that had to be completed in response to the red dot.

Before each experimental block participants were informed about the ratio of green and red stimuli and whether a no-go or antisaccade response was required in response to the red dots. A fixation dot was presented at the beginning of each trial until fixation was stable and the trial began. The next frame showed the fixation dot together with the eight placeholder dots for 1000 ms after which the red or green target dot appeared for 2000 ms. The distance between the eyes and the screen was 57 cm. Participants' heads rested on a chinrest.

The design was a within-subjects design. Every participant completed each condition. Half of the participants began with the no-go conditions (in randomised order) and then completed the antisaccade conditions (in randomised order). The other half of participants first completed the antisaccade conditions followed by the no-go conditions.

Eye movement recording and analysis

Eye movements were recorded with the EyeLink I and II eyetrackers (SMI Germany, SR Research Canada) using the centre of the pupil as well as the corneal reflection technique to define pupil position. A testing session was preceded by a 9-point grid calibration and validation for which participants were instructed to saccade to a black circle (0.5°) on a white background, which appeared sequentially at nine points in a square array. Eye movements were recorded at 250 Hz sample rate at a spatial resolution, typically, of 0.3°. Saccade onset was defined as a change in eye position with a minimum velocity of 30°/s or a minimum acceleration of $8000°/s^2$. Participants viewed the displays with both eyes, but only data of the eye with the best spatial accuracy was analysed, as indicated by the calibration and validation results.

In the subsequent data analysis, trials were rejected if (1) a blink or recording error occurred, (2) the initial fixation location at the start of the trials was not within 1° around the centre of the fixation point, or (3) if saccadic reaction times (SRT) were shorter than 80 ms. These criteria led to an exclusion of 10.2% of trials. A trial was coded as a saccade trial if the saccade endpoint was at least 1° from central fixation.

RESULTS

Antisaccades

We first analysed antisaccade reaction times and saccade direction errors in order to establish whether the older participants responded more slowly and showed higher error rates than the younger participants, as would be expected based on the literature. The significance of main effects and interactions involving repeated measures were assessed using a Greenhouse-Geisser adjustment to the degrees of freedom where appropriate.

Antisaccade reaction times. Mean SRT of antisaccades that were executed correctly in the direction opposite to the target dot were subjected to an ANOVA with the factors age (young vs. elderly) and condition (90% pro/10% antisaccades, 70% pro/30% antisaccades, 50% pro/50% antisaccades, 100% antisaccades). For the older group, only the data from seven participants could be included in this analysis, as three participants did not

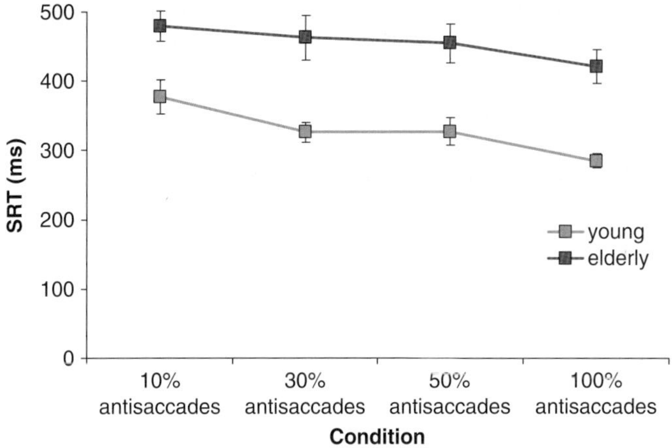

Figure 2. Saccadic reaction times (SRT) in ms of antisaccades for younger and older participants separately for each antisaccade condition. Error bars represent standard errors.

perform any correct antisaccades in the condition that contained only 10% antisaccade trials. This exclusion of participants points towards more difficulties of the older group with the execution of antisaccades in the correct direction, which will be analysed in more detail later. With respect to saccadic reaction times, as can be seen in Figure 2, SRT decreased with an increasing percentage of trials requiring the inhibition of a prosaccade and the execution of an antisaccade, $F(3,\ 48) = 9.37$, $MSE = 1744.34$, $p < .001$. All paired-comparisons (t-tests) between conditions were significant (all $ps < .014$) with the exception of the comparison of the 30% versus 50% antisaccades conditions. Young participants responded faster than elderly participants, $F(1,\ 16) = 23.30$, $MSE = 11587.96$, $p < .001$, but the condition × age interaction was not significant, $F(3,\ 48) = 0.65$, demonstrating that in both age groups SRT was affected similarly by the varying percentages of antisaccade trials. The older group benefited as much from an increase of antisaccade trials as the younger group.[1]

Accuracy on antisaccade trials. The ANOVA on the mean percentages of correctly directed antisaccades with the factors condition and age group indicates an increase of correct antisaccades with an increasing percentage of antisaccade trials, $F(3,\ 57) = 28.06$, $MSE = 175.62$, $p < .001$. When direction errors occurred, the majority (93.3%) of erroneous saccades were prosaccades made towards the stimulus. This was true for both groups

[1] An analysis considering the required amplitude of the antisaccade to be made (3° vs. 6°) showed no effect of amplitude on saccadic reaction times.

(93.3% for the younger and 93.29% for the older participants). As can be seen in Figure 3a, the younger participants committed less errors than the older participants, $F(1, 19) = 7.26$, $MSE = 1372.78$, $p < .02$. Importantly, the error pattern across conditions was modulated by age, as the age × condition interaction reached significance, $F(3, 57) = 3.74$, $p < .02$. For young participants paired comparisons confirmed significant differences between all conditions (all $ps < .009$; apart from 30% vs. 50% antisaccades: $p < .05$), showing that the more trials requested antisaccades the fewer errors occurred. In the condition with only 10% antisaccades performance of the younger participants was at its worst with correct responses occurring only about half the time. However, performance

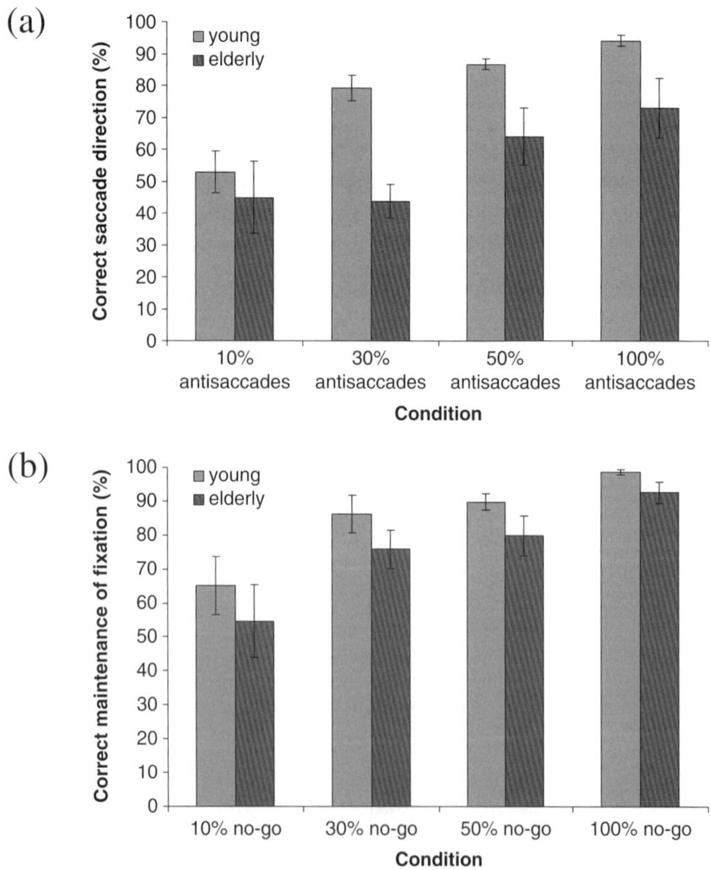

Figure 3. Percentage of trials with (a) correctly directed antisaccades and (b) correctly inhibited saccades (maintenance of fixation) on no-go trials. Error bars represent standard errors.

improved considerably when 30% of trials required an antisaccade with correct responses occurring now on 79% of the trials. This was not the case for the older participants though, that is, their high error rate remained unchanged as the percentage of antisaccade trials changed from 10% to 30% (44.9% and 43.7% correct responses, respectively). Older participants required at least 50% antisaccade trials in order to improve significantly. And importantly, even if 100% of the trials were antisaccade trials, older participants still only executed about 73% correct antisaccades. These observations were confirmed statistically: For older participants the comparisons between all conditions were significant (all $ps < .02$), apart from the comparisons between 10% versus 30% ($p > .85$) and 100% versus 50% antisaccade trials ($p > .15$).

Inhibition

The antisaccade data–slower SRT and higher error rates for older participants–replicate previous reports. Additionally, we found that varying the percentage of antisaccade trials affected the error rates of older participants differently than the error rates of younger participants. In order to explore whether a failure to inhibit underlies the low performance of older participants, we analysed the effect of inhibition on prosaccade reaction times. As outlined in the introduction, the more trials require a no-go or an antisaccade response, the more inhibition should be placed on the oculomotor system and the slower prosaccades should be executed. To assess the inhibition functions in the no-go and antisaccade conditions, and how they compare, we measured prosaccade reaction times in the prosaccade/no-go condition against those in the prosaccade/antisaccade condition. If inhibition is imposed differently in the two tasks then the inhibition functions should differ between tasks and if the older group differs in how well they impose inhibition in one or both of these tasks then the inhibition functions should differ between groups.

Prosaccade reaction times. Mean saccadic reaction times (SRT) for target-directed prosaccades in the "prosaccade/no-go conditions" were subjected to a repeated measures ANOVA with the factors condition (100% prosaccades, 90% pro/10% no-go, 70% pro/30% no-go, and 50% pro/50% no-go) and age group (young vs. elderly). As illustrated in Figure 4b, older participants responded more slowly overall than younger participants, $F(1, 19) = 7.70$, $MSE = 8525.21$, $p < .02$, and SRT increased gradually with an increase in the percentage of no-go trials (i.e., an increase in the percentage of trials requiring inhibition of prosaccades), $F(3, 57) =$

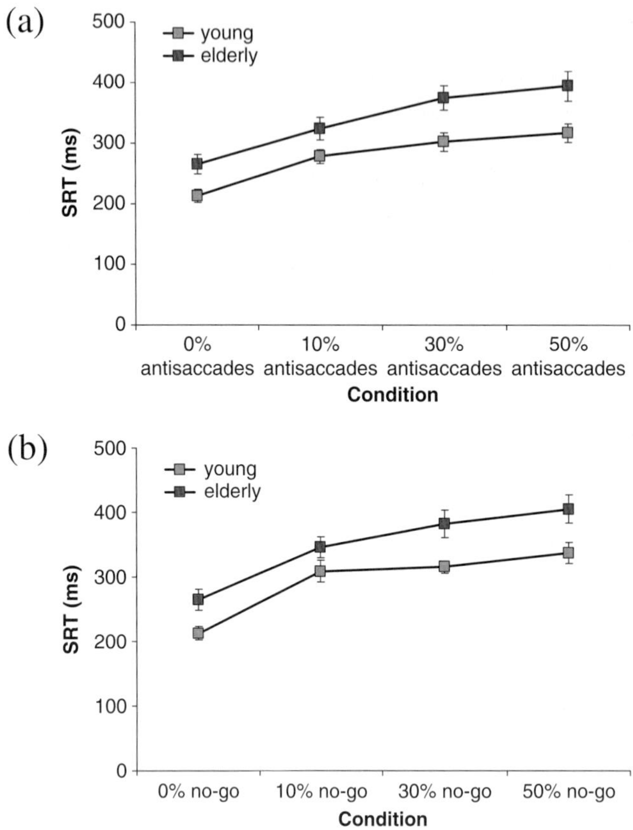

Figure 4. Saccadic reaction times (SRT) in ms of correct prosaccades for prosaccade trials from (a) prosaccade/antisaccade conditions and (b) prosaccade/no-go conditions. Error bars represent standard errors.

75.71, $MSE = 931.39$, $p < .001$.[2] Paired *t*-tests revealed a marginal difference between the 10% no-go and 30% no-go conditions ($p < .07$) but highly significant differences between all other conditions (all $p < .005$). Importantly, the

---

[2] By varying the percentage of no-go trials and antisaccade trials between conditions, the amount of trials on which participants have to switch between prosaccade and no-go (or antisaccade) trials may vary as well. Further ANOVAs were calculated on the SRT of prosaccades, errors on prosaccade trials, and errors on no-go trials, including nonswitch trials only, i.e., prosaccade trials preceded by a prosaccade trial. In each ANOVA the same effects were observed as in the ANOVAs described in the Results section, indicating that the SRT increase between conditions cannot be explained by task switching. For antisaccade trials an ANOVA including only nonswitch trials was not possibly to conduct, as splitting up the data resulted frequently in less than $N = 5$ nonswitch trials per participant.

two factors age and condition did not interact, $F(3, 57) = 1.14$, indicating that the older group increased inhibition across conditions in a manner that paralleled the younger group.

In a similar fashion mean SRT of target-directed prosaccades in the prosaccade/antisaccade conditions were subjected to a repeated measures ANOVA with the factors condition (100% prosaccades, 90% pro/10% antisaccades, 70% pro/30% antisaccades, and 50% pro/50% antisaccades) and age group (young vs. elderly). Older participants responded more slowly than younger participants, $F(1, 19) = 8.71$, $MSE = 9245.86$, $p < .009$, and SRT increased with an increase in the percentage of antisaccade trials (i.e., an increase in the percentage of trials requiring inhibition of prosaccades), $F(2.038, 38.720) = 66.83$, $MSE = 1225.47$, $p < .001$. Paired t-tests revealed significant differences between all conditions (all ps $< .02$). The age $\times$ condition interaction did not reach significance, $F(2.038, 38.720) = 1.45$, indicating that the older group increased the amount of inhibition gradually and as much as the younger participants. The results are illustrated in Figure 4a.

Both analyses of prosaccade reaction times show that the older group increased inhibition as much as the younger group. Figure 4 further suggests that the inhibition functions of both sets of prosaccades (from no-go and from antisaccade conditions) are parallel. In order to test this and to evaluate whether inhibition is imposed and increased between conditions in a similar or dissimilar manner in both tasks, we compared RTs of prosaccades from both tasks. If inhibition increased in a dissimilar way, then the condition $\times$ task interaction should reach significance. And if older participants increased inhibition differently than younger participants across conditions in the tasks, then there should be task $\times$ age, and condition $\times$ task $\times$ age interactions. The repeated measures ANOVA with the factors condition (10% prosaccades vs. 30% prosaccades vs. 50% prosaccades), task (no-go vs. antisaccades), and age (young, elderly) revealed that inhibition was in fact imposed and increased in a similar manner in both tasks, condition $\times$ task, $F(2, 38) = 0.88$, $MSE = 782.03$, and that this was not modulated by age, task $\times$ age, $F(1, 19) = 0.32$; condition $\times$ task $\times$ age, $F(2, 38) = 0.02$. Importantly, the lack of these interactions occurred despite of significant main effects of task, $F(1, 19) = 6.4$, $MSE = 1591.27$, $p < .03$, condition, $F(2, 38) = 44.99$, $MSE = 567.95$, $p < .001$, and age, $F(1, 19) = 7.87$, $MSE = 14945.12$, $p < .02$, with slower SRT for prosaccades from no-go conditions, with an increasing amount of trials requiring inhibition and for the older group. That the interactions were insignificant despite of these main effects highlights that the older group imposed inhibition in a similar manner to the younger group.

Selecting the saccadic response

Having found that the older group increases inhibition on the oculomotor system as much and in similar steps as the younger group, we now turned to estimate the potential contribution of a failure to select the correct saccadic response. To do so, we first calculated error rates on prosaccade trials, both from conditions in which prosaccades were randomised with no-go trials and randomised with antisaccade trials. The error rates indicate how well participants were able to select the response "prosaccade". We then calculated the error rates on no-go trials, indicating how often participants failed to inhibit the response and compared those to the antisaccade direction errors. The latter comparison indicates how well participants are able to select the response "antisaccade".

Error rates on prosaccade trials. We first analysed the error rates on prosaccade trials derived from the pro/no-go conditions. An ANOVA with the factors condition (100% prosaccades/0% no-go, 90% prosaccades/10% no-go, 70% prosaccades/30% no-go, and 50% prosaccades/50% no-go) and age (young, elderly) on the percentages of erroneously inhibited prosaccades showed an effect of condition, $F(1.937, 36.810) = 6.64$, $MSE = 28.04$, $p < .005$. *T*-tests clarified that significantly fewer errors were made in the condition requiring 100% prosaccades compared to conditions randomising prosaccade and no-go trials (all $ps < .004$). Moreover, fewer errors occurred in the condition with 90% prosaccade trials compared to 50% prosaccade trials ($p < .05$). These results suggest that the more trials require a prosaccade the easier it is to select a prosaccade as the correct response. Importantly, age did not modulate the results. No main effect of age, $F(1, 19) = 1.99$, $MSE = 66.21$, and no age × condition interaction, $F(1.937, 36.810) = 0.26$, were observed, showing that the elderly were as efficient at selecting correct prosaccades as the younger group. Error rates are given in Table 1. It is apparent that prosaccade reaction times and error rates increased together, ruling out a speed–accuracy tradeoff.

Second, an analysis of saccade direction errors on prosaccade trials from the prosaccade/antisaccade conditions was conducted. The ANOVA with the factors condition (100% prosaccades/0% antisaccades, 90% prosaccades/10% antisaccades, 70% prosaccades/30% antisaccades, and 50% prosaccades/50% antisaccades) and age (young, elderly) showed an increase of errors with an increase of antisaccade trials, $F(1.297, 24.641) = 23.39$, $MSE = 33.52$, $p < .001$. All conditions differed significantly from each other (all $ps < .002$). Although error rates for each location were too few to allow a detailed analysis, the vast majority (i.e., over 87%) of the incorrectly directed saccades were made in the opposite direction to the stimulus

TABLE 1
Mean error rates on prosaccade trials for no-go and antisaccade conditions (standard deviations in parentheses)

	Inhibition errors on prosaccade trials (pro/no-go conditions)		*Saccade direction errors on prosaccade trials (pro/antisaccade conditions)*	
	Young	*Elderly*	*Young*	*Elderly*
50% prosaccades	5.26 (8.81)	7.72 (6.95)	9.18 (9.51)	9.40 (5.13)
70% prosaccades	3.26 (3.89)	6.77 (8.06)	6.55 (5.89)	3.50 (2.76)
90% prosaccades	1.71 (2.33)	4.53 (5.12)	2.55 (1.86)	1.30 (1.42)
100% prosaccades	0.34 (0.75)	1.58 (2.29)	0.00 (0.00)	0.20 (0.63)

(i.e., erroneous antisaccades). The age groups did not differ from each other, $F(1, 19) = 0.48$, $MSE = 41.35$, and age did not interact with condition, $F(1.297, 24.641) = 0.86$, showing that the older group was as able as the younger group to select a prosaccade towards the visual stimulus. The error rates are given in Table 1.

Comparing error rates between tasks in an ANOVA with the factors condition (100% prosaccades, 10% prosaccades, 30% prosaccades and 50% prosaccades), type of error (inhibition error, saccade direction error), and age (young, elderly) showed that there were as many incorrect inhibition errors as saccade direction errors overall, $F(1, 19) = 0.04$, $MSE = 42.68$, but the error rates varied across conditions, $F(1.361, 25.854) = 19.50$, $MSE = 47.0$, $p < .001$, and there was a tendency for a type of error × condition interaction, $F(1.716, 32.613) = 3.19$, $MSE = 18.93$, $p = .07$. Importantly though, older participants did not show more errors than younger participants, $F(1, 19) = 0.38$, $MSE = 64.88$, indicating that selecting the correct response was not harder for the older group when the correct response was to make a saccade towards the visual stimulus, or in other words, to select a response that is supported by the visual environment.

Accuracy on no-go and antisaccade trials. Both no-go and antisaccade trials require the inhibition of a prosaccade. To estimate the contribution of the failure to select the antisaccadic response to antisaccade errors, we first assessed how well both groups of participants were able to inhibit a prosaccade towards a stimulus and then compared the results to the performance on antisaccade trials.

For the no-go trials the percentage of trials on which participants correctly refrained from executing a saccade was calculated and compared between conditions and age groups. As illustrated in Figure 3b, the ability to correctly inhibit a saccade increased with the percentage of trials requiring inhibition, $F(1.576, 29.951) = 20.52$, $MSE = 435.65$, $p < .001$.[3] All paired comparisons between conditions were significant as assessed with paired-sample t-tests (all $ps < .001$), with the exception of the comparison between 30% and 50% no-go trials. Although older participants failed numerically more frequently to suppress a saccade on a no-go trial, the factor age group did not reach significance, $F(1, 19) = 2.07$, $MSE = 859.4$, $p = .167$, and did not interact with condition, $F(1.576, 29.951) = 0.096$, $MSE = 435.65$, $p = .864$.

We then compared accuracy on no-go and antisaccade trials. In the ANOVA with the within-factors condition (100% inhibition [either 100% no-go or 100% antisaccades], 10%, 30%, and 50%) and task (no-go vs. antisaccades) and the between-factor age group (young, elderly), the main effects of condition, $F(1.784, 33.895) = 35.95$, $MSE = 440.137$, $p < .001$, and age group, $F(1, 19) = 5.19$, $MSE = 1941.55$, $p < .04$, reached significance, confirming our previous results. Further, the main effect of task was significant, $F(1, 19) = 24.44$, $MSE = 290.63$, $p < .001$, showing that more errors were committed in the antisaccade compared to the no-go task. This latter finding, coupled with our observation of equivalency in the ability to impose inhibition between age groups, supports the conclusion that antisaccade errors cannot be explained by inhibition failures but that antisaccade response selection is an important factor to consider when evaluating performance in the antisaccade task. Importantly, the task × age interaction reached significance, $F(1, 19) = 5.72$, $p < .03$, and the three-way condition × task × age interaction was marginally significant, $F(2.160, 41.044) = 2.38$, $p < .08$, suggesting that the difference between the age groups differs across the two tasks. In order to clarify this matter, two separate ANOVAs for each age group with the factors condition and task were conducted and confirmed for both groups significant main effects of condition, young: $F(1.6, 15.996) = 25.5$, $MSE = 418.88$, $p < .001$; elderly: $F(3, 27) = 13.6$, $MSE = 304.37$, $p < .001$, and task, young: $F(1, 10) = 6.54$, $MSE = 152.04$, $p < .03$; elderly: $F(1, 9) = 16.8$, $MSE = 444.62$, $p < .004$, but only for the group of older participants did the condition × task interaction show a significant effect, young: $F(1.466, 14.662) = 0.62$, MSE $= 292.79$; elderly: $F(3, 27) = 3.2$, $MSE = 142.49$, $p < .05$. This finding reveals that for the elderly group the change of performance across conditions did not follow

[3] In order to test whether the pattern of increasing prosaccade reaction times and decreasing error rates on no-go trials is indicative of a speed–accuracy tradeoff, we compared the reaction times of saccades made in prosaccade trials and saccades erroneously made on no-go trials. T-test comparisons showed that erroneously made saccades on no-go trials were not made significantly faster than saccades on prosaccade trials in any of the conditions, inconsistent with a speed–accuracy tradeoff. The comparison between the prosaccade only condition and no-go only condition even showed longer SRT for saccades made in the no-go condition, $t(7) = 2.5$, $p = .04$.

the same pattern in the no-go task as in the antisaccade task. The no-go task performance improved as the percentage of no-go trials increased from one condition to the next, but for antisaccades the improvement of performance began only when at least 50% of the trials required an antisaccade.

DISCUSSION

Our results are in line with previous research showing that older persons respond more slowly and make more erroneous prosaccades towards the stimulus in the antisaccade task. This decline in performance has been explained in terms of a decline in the ability to inhibit prepotent responses with age (e.g., Hasher & Zacks, 1988). But considering that in the antisaccade task two response options–a saccade towards the stimulus and a saccade away from the stimulus–are in competition and the less potent saccade away from the visual stimulus has to be selected, the present experiment sought to assess the contribution of inhibition failure and saccadic response selection failure to decreased performance in the antisaccade task in older persons.

We had envisioned four potential outcomes. Poorer performance could be explained by inhibition failure only, by response selection deficits only, by a separate contribution of both factors or by an interactive contribution of both factors.

Our data clearly revealed that poorer performance is not due to inhibition failure only. To estimate the contribution of inhibition we varied the proportion of no-go trials or antisaccade trials and measured the effect of inhibition on prosaccades and compared the inhibition functions between both tasks and age groups, allowing us to assess whether similar amounts of inhibition were imposed in both tasks and importantly, whether the inhibition functions differed between age groups. In our task inhibition had to be placed on the oculomotor system on every trial because the peripheral stimulus instructed which response was required. But as participants were informed about the percentage of no-go and antisaccade trials, they should be able to place more tonic inhibition on the oculomotor system in a condition in which such responses are frequent than in a condition in which such responses are infrequent. The data showed that the inhibition functions were the same between tasks and also between groups. Overall, elderly participants responded more slowly but they were able to titrate and to strategically place top-down inhibition in each block gradually and in similar steps as the younger participants. Prosaccade reaction times increased gradually and in an equivalent manner for both groups with an increasing percentage of trials requiring inhibition, irrespective of the kind of task (no-go or antisaccade). This finding suggests that the group of older participants imposed as much inhibition on the oculomotor system as the younger group. We also found that prosaccade reaction times were slower in the no-go task than in the antisaccade task. This effect is likely due to more inhibition being placed on the oculomotor system in the no-go task than the antisaccade task because in the no-go task participants have to refrain from making any saccadic eye movement.[4] But, importantly, the elderly participants were as good at imposing this inhibition as the younger participants because the inhibition functions are similar for both groups.

Second, we compared performance in the antisaccade task with performance in the no-go task. In both the inhibition of a prosaccade is required but in the latter, no saccade in the opposite direction has to be selected. Participants committed significantly more errors when an antisaccade had to be made than when fixation had to be maintained, hinting at the important contribution of the selection of the antisaccadic response to the error rates. The increase in error rates from no-go to antisaccade conditions occurred for both groups and also the error rates increased for no-go and antisaccade responses as the percentage of prosaccades increased for both groups. But importantly, whereas for the no-go trials the numeric difference between the groups remained the same across conditions, this was not the case for the antisaccade error rates as indicated by a significant Condition × Age group interaction. For both groups more antisaccade errors occurred when antisaccades were rare, but this was more pronounced for the older group. For young participants performance started to improve when 30% of the trials were antisaccade trials, whereas for elderly participants the error rates were still below chance in that condition. Their performance only started to improve when half of the trials were antisaccade trials. And notably, even if all trials were antisaccade trials, their performance was still quite poor with an error rate of 27%. Further, when performance between no-go and antisaccade conditions was compared, the condition × task interaction reached significance only for the elderly group, underlining that their error pattern differed between no-go and antisaccade conditions. This finding shows that a failure to select the correct saccadic response affected the performance of the older group more than the performance of the younger group, especially when antisaccade responses were rare. This in turn leads to the conclusion that a failure to select the

[4] We acknowledge that faster prosaccades in the prosaccade/antisaccade conditions than in the prosaccade/no-go conditions could also hint at more "oculomotor readiness" in the prosaccade/antisaccade conditions. However, we see "oculomotor readiness" as a complementary concept of "inhibition" because at the neural level, oculomotor readiness must also involve inhibition, i.e., high inhibition of fixation cells that occurs together with high activation of saccade-related cells and the mutual inhibition via inhibitory interneurons between fixation and saccade-related cells.

correct antisaccade response contributed significantly to the higher error rates for older persons.

The conclusion that a failure to select the correct antisaccade response contributed to the higher error rates for the older group leads to the question of whether this factor alone can possibly explain our results. In other words, if aged adults merely have a response selection deficit, then we should observe that the elderly are generally worse in selecting correct responses, also in prosaccade trials. To address this, we turned towards the error rate data of prosaccade trials. Those data highlight that the older group did not show more errors than the younger group on prosaccade trials, indicating that there are situations in which the elderly do not show difficulties in selecting the correct response, namely, when a prosaccadic response had to be selected, that is, a prepotent response supported by the visual environment. Thus a failure of response selection *in general* cannot explain the poorer performance on the antisaccade task by older adults.

The lack of significant deficits in inhibition and in response selection per se also renders the third possibility that we had envisioned unlikely–a separate contribution of both factors.

Our data suggest that error rates increase particularly for the elderly in specifically such situations in which two saccadic response alternatives compete and the less potent and rare response away from the stimulus has to be selected (the antisaccade) while the prepotent response (the prosaccade) has to be suppressed, supporting the fourth envisioned outcome: the interactive contribution of both factors. In other words, elderly participants may perform quite well when they are requested to only inhibit (e.g., no-go trials) or to only select a prepotent response (e.g., prosaccade), but when a situation requires inhibition of a prepotent response *and* the selection of a less potent response at the same time, their performance is impaired. And this impairment is especially evident when the less potent response is rare.

But what may be the reason as to why the elderly fail to select the less potent antisaccade response in a competition situation? Considering that antisaccades are volitional in nature, could a reduced ability of older persons to make volitional saccades be responsible, assuming that such a reduced ability may have the effect that they have to put more effort into making volitional saccades? This is unlikely for at least two reasons. First, Pratt, Dodd, and Welsh (2006) clearly demonstrated that aged adults are not impaired with respect to the execution of volitional saccades. Second, in our experiment we observed that as the percentage of trials demanding a volitional antisaccade increased, the faster these saccades were executed, and this benefit was demonstrated by both groups. Although the older group executed antisaccades more slowly in all conditions, SRT decreased in similar gradations for both groups, indicating that the older group was able to execute antisaccades efficiently once they had been selected.

A very different potential explanation is that older adults' decline in oculomotor performance in the antisaccade task reflects an increase in the demands placed on their working memory capacity which, in turn, decreases the efficiency of their inhibitory control (Eenshuistra et al., 2004; Roberts et al., 1994). Although working memory load may well have effects on antisaccade performance, the results of our experiment cannot be explained by this because there was neither an additional working memory task nor should demands on working memory with respect to saccade inhibition have been especially higher in the antisaccade conditions than in the no-go conditions. Further, we found that inhibition alone did not account for our results, so the idea that deficiencies in inhibitory control that are mediated by demands on working memory can be excluded as a viable explanation. For a similar reason the concept of "goal neglect" can also be ruled out. Goal neglect has been broadly defined as "the disregard of a task requirement even if it has been understood" (de Jong, 2001, p. 72) and it has been suggested that it may lead to worse performance because participants are not fully and consistently using their inhibitory capabilities (de Jong, 2001). Elderly persons may show more goal neglect or goal decay (Colcombe et al., 2003; Ryan et al., 2006) and this can result in a deficit in inhibitory control in the antisaccade task. Although a decrease in the activation of the goal to inhibit a response in the no-go and antisaccade conditions may in general contribute to increased error rates as the percentage of no-go and antisaccade trials decreased across conditions, inhibitory deficits due to goal neglect cannot account for our result of differences between the no-go and antisaccade error patterns for the elderly as the inhibitory functions were equivalent for both groups and in the two tasks. However, goal neglect could also refer to difficulties in *activating* a certain response. To the extent that goal neglect may vary between the no-go and the antisaccade task (e.g., the goal to activate an antisaccade response may be more effortful than the goal to activate a no-go response), goal neglect may be involved in poorer performance in the antisaccade task. Further, it is possible that the elderly may experience more difficulties in activating the goal to select the less potent antisaccadic response in a competition situation than the young participants.

In conclusion, our data indicate that elderly participants experience pronounced difficulties when a situation requires the selection of a rare, less potent saccadic response that competes with a prepotent saccadic response that has to be inhibited. Inhibition failure or response selection failure alone could not explain our results but it seems that the requirement of response selection in the context of inhibition leads to high error rates. Considering current models of saccade generation that state the parallel programming of saccades (Godijn & Theeuwes, 2002; Massen, 2004; Walker & McSorley,

2006) and the resolution of competition between these saccades, it may be the case that the older participants are less able to resolve the competition in favour of the antisaccade. Top-down signals reinforcing antisaccade generation and the activation of an antisaccade response may be weaker in the aged adult or these commands may be given too slowly to avoid the execution of the faster erroneous prosaccade (Hutton & Ettinger, 2006). A future avenue for research may thus be the investigation of differences in eye movement control in younger and older participants with a focus on the involvement of brain areas such as the frontal eye fields (FEF), supplementary eye fields (SEF), and dorsolateral prefrontal cortex (dlPFC) (Olk et al., 2006; Pierrot-Deseilligny, Milea, & Müri, 2004; Pierrot-Deseilligny et al., 1991; Ro, Henik, Machado, & Rafal, 1997; Schlag-Rey, Amador, Sanchez, & Schlag, 1997), in particular in tasks, such as those used here, that enable investigators to separate the contribution of saccade inhibition and response selection.

REFERENCES

Abel, L. A., & Douglas, J. (2007). Effects of age on latency and error generation in internally mediated saccades. *Neurobiology of Aging*, *28*, 627–637.

Bojko, A., Kramer, A. F., & Peterson, M. S. (2004). Age equivalence in switch costs for prosaccade and antisaccade tasks. *Psychology and Aging*, *19*, 226–234.

Butler, K. M., & Zacks, R. T. (2006). Age deficits in the control of prepotent responses: Evidence for an inhibitory decline. *Psychology and Aging*, *21*, 638–643.

Butler, K. M., Zacks, R. T., & Henderson, J.M. (1999). Suppression of reflexive saccades in younger and older adults: Age comparisons on an antisaccade task. *Memory and Cognition*, *27*, 584–591.

Colombe, A. M., Kramer, A. F., Irwin, D. E., Peterson, M. S., Colcombe, S., & Hahn, S. (2003). Age-related effects of attentional and oculomotor capture by onsets and color singletons as a function of experience. *Acta Psychologica*, *113*, 205–225.

De Jong, R. (2001). Adult age differences in goal activation and goal maintenance. *European Journal of Cognitive Psychology*, *13*, 71–89.

Eenshuistra, R. M., Ridderinkhof, K. R., & van der Molen, M. W. (2004). Age-related changes in antisaccade task performance: Inhibitory control or working-memory engagement? *Brain and Cognition*, *56*, 177–188.

Everling, S., Dorris, M. C., Klein, R. M., & Munoz, D.P (1999). Role of primate superior colliculus in preparation and execution of anti-saccades and pro-saccades. *Journal of Neuroscience*, *19*, 2740–2754.

Everling, S., & Fischer, B. (1998). The antisaccade: A review of basic research and clinical studies. *Neuropsychologia*, *36*, 885–899.

Faust, M. E., & Balota, D. A. (1997). Inhibition of return and visuospatial attention in healthy older adults and individuals with dementia of the Alzheimer type. *Neuropsychology*, *11*, 13–29.

Godijn, R., & Kramer, A. F. (2006). Prosaccades and antisaccades to onsets and color singletons: Evidence that erroneous prosaccades are not reflexive. *Experimental Brain Research, 172*, 439–448.

Godijn, R., & Theeuwes, J. (2002). Programming of endogenous and exogenous saccades: Evidence for a competitive integration model. *Journal of Experimental Psychology: Human Perception and Performance, 28*, 1039–1054.

Hasher, L., & Zacks, R. T. (1988). Working memory, comprehension, and aging: A review and a new view. In G. H. Bower (Ed.), *The psychology of learning and motivation* (Vol. 22 pp. 193–225). New York: Academic Press.

Hasher, L., Zacks, R. T., & May, C. P. (1999). Inhibitory control, circadian arousal, and age. In D. Gopher & A. Koriat (Eds.), *Attention and performance XVII: Control of cognitive performance* (pp. 653–675). Cambridge, MA: MIT Press.

Hutton, S. B., & Ettinger, U. (2006). The antisaccade task as a research tool in psychopathology: A critical review. *Psychophysiology, 43*, 302–313.

Klein, C., Fischer, B., Hartnegg, K., Heiss, W. H., & Roth, M. (2000). Optomotor and neuropsychological performance in old age. *Experimental Brain Research, 135*, 141–154.

Kramer, A. F., Hahn, S., Irwin, D. E., & Theeuwes, J. (2000). Age differences in the control of looking behavior: Do you know where your eyes have been? *Psychological Science, 11*, 210–217.

Machado, L., & Rafal, R. D. (2000). Strategic control over saccadic eye movements: Studies of the fixation offset effect. *Perception and Psychophysics, 62*, 1236–1242.

Massen, C. (2004). Parallel programming of exogenous and endogenous components in the antisaccade task. *Quarterly Journal of Experimental Psychology: Human Experimental Psychology, 57A*, 475–498.

Nieuwenhuis, S., Ridderinkhof, K. R., de Jong, R., Kok, A., & van der Molen, M. W. (2000). Inhibitory inefficiency and failures of intention activation: Age-related decline in the control of saccadic eye movements. *Psychology and Aging, 15*, 635–647.

Olincy, A., Ross, R. G., Young, D. A., & Freedman, R. (1997). Age diminishes performance on an antisaccade eye movement task. *Neurobiology of Aging, 18*, 483–489.

Olk, B., Chang, E., Kingstone, A., & Ro, T. (2006). Modulation of antisaccades by transcranial magnetic stimulation over the human frontal eye field. *Cerebral Cortex, 16*, 76–82.

Olk, B., & Kingstone, A. (2003). Why are antisaccades slower than prosaccades? A novel finding using a new paradigm. *NeuroReport, 14*, 151–155.

Pierrot-Deseilligny, C., Milea, D., & Müri, R. M. (2004). Eye movement control by the cerebral cortex. *Current Opinion in Neurology, 17*, 17–25.

Pierrot-Deseilligny, C., Rivaud, S., Gaymard, B., & Agid, Y. (1991). Cortical control of reflexive visually-guided saccades. *Brain, 114*, 1473–1485.

Pratt, J., Dodd, M., & Welsh, T. (2006). Growing older does not always mean moving slower: Examining aging and the saccadic motor system. *Journal of Motor Behavior, 38*, 373–382.

Reuter, B., Philipp, A. M., Koch, I., & Kathmann, N. (2006). Effects of switching between leftward and rightward pro- and antisaccades. *Biological Psychology, 72*, 88–95.

Ro, T., Henik, A., Machado, L., & Rafal, R. (1997). Transcranial magnetic stimulation of the prefrontal cortex delays contralateral endogenous saccades. *Journal of Cognitive Neuroscience, 9*, 433–440.

Roberts, R. J., Hager, L. D., & Heron, C. (1994). Prefrontal cognitive processes—working memory and inhibition in the antisaccade task. *Journal of Experimental Psychology: General, 123*, 374–393.

Ryan, J. D., Shen, J., & Reingold, E. M. (2006). Modulation of distraction in ageing. *British Journal of Psychology, 97*, 339–351.

Schlag-Rey, M., Amador, N., Sanchez, H., & Schlag, J. (1997). Antisaccade performance predicted by neuronal activity in the supplementary eye field. *Nature, 390*, 398–401.

Sweeney, J. A., Rosano, C., Berman, R. A., & Luna, B. (2001). Inhibitory control of attention declines more than working memory during normal aging. *Neurobiology of Aging*, *22*, 39–47.

Walker, R., & McSorley, E. (2006). The parallel programming of voluntary and reflexive saccades. *Vision Research*, *46*, 2082–2093.

EUROPEAN JOURNAL OF COGNITIVE PSYCHOLOGY
2009, 21 (2/3), 428–444

Psychology Press
Taylor & Francis Group

The role of interference in identification of emotional facial expressions in normal ageing and dementia

Beatriz García-Rodríguez

Universidad Nacional de Educación a Distancia, Department of Basic Psychology II, Madrid, Spain

Heiner Ellgring

Julius Maximilian Universität, Würzburg, Germany

Anna Fusari

Universidad Nacional de Educación a Distancia, Department of Basic Psychology II, Madrid, Spain

Ana Frank

Hospital Universitario La Paz, Department of Neurology, Madrid, Spain

In normal daily life, the identification of emotional facial expressions (EFEs) usually takes place simultaneously with other demands, requiring working memory resources. In the current study, the authors investigate the role of the interference caused by a secondary task in emotional facial identification. The decline in performance in a given task when adding a secondary task may be one of the strongest variables differentiating between normal and pathological ageing. The goal of the current study was to assess to what extent processing of EFEs is affected when cognitive resources are experimentally (over)loaded. Three groups of participants (Alzheimer's patients, healthy older adults, and healthy young adults) had to identify six basic emotions under two conditions: identification-only and identification with a visual secondary task. The results showed a decrease in performance of EFEs identification when the processing of this mental image was interfered by another visual stimulus, for all groups. When computing the dual-task costs, AD patients showed higher costs than older and young adults, revealing that dementia but not ageing itself, is more vulnerable to interference effects. This study reveals further data supporting the hypothesis of a top-down control in emotional processing and offers a new approach to understand EFEs identification in analogous real-life conditions and reveals how this processing is differentially affected by ageing and dementias.

Correspondence should be addressed to Beatriz García Rodríguez, Facultad de Psicología, UNED, Juan del Rosal, 10, 28040 Madrid, Spain. E-mail: bgarcia@psi.uned.es

http://www.psypress.com/ecp DOI: 10.1080/09541440802475793

Keywords: Facial expression identification; Dual-task; Working memory; Ageing; Alzheimer's disease.

Within the area of cognitive functions, processing speed, episodic memory, and working memory (WM) undergo the largest age-related declines, being especially impaired in early Alzheimer's disease (AD). Emotional processing is another domain where impairments with age are a common result. Several studies have shown a decline in the identification of emotions in normal ageing (for a review, see Sullivan & Ruffman, 2004) as well as in AD (Cadieux & Greve, 1997; Hargrave, Maddock, & Stone, 2002; Koff, Zaitchik, Montepare, & Albert, 1999).

A theoretical approach of emotional processing has proposed that emotional stimuli are automatically processed, and that discrete emotions are supported by distinct brain areas, offering evidence that in ageing and in AD patients, impairments in the identification of fear and other negative emotions are caused by atrophy and neuropathological changes in the amygdala (Adolphs & Tranel, 2004; Adolphs et al., 1999; LeDoux, 1996), a part of the basal ganglia critically involved in computing the emotional significance to events or stimuli. LeDoux (1996) points to a "low route" as a pathway that allows emotional stimulus processing without cortical influence. The issue that the amygdala responds very rapidly to emotional stimuli has suggested that emotional processing could be automatic or requiring scarce attentional resources (Globisch, Hamm, Esteves, & Öhman, 1999; Öhman, Esteves, & Soares, 1995; Vuilleumier, Armony, Driver, & Dolan, 2001), even in absence of conscious awareness. However, there is further evidence showing that the "low route" cannot discriminate emotional versus nonemotional stimuli without cortical involvement (Duvel, Smith, Talk, & Gabriel, 2001; Komura et al., 2001). Another area involved in emotional processing and particularly sensitive to the effects of ageing is the prefrontal cortex (Bechara, Damasio, & Damasio, 2000; Phillips, Drevets, Rauch, & Lane, 2003), revealing its crucial role in the processing of emotions in complex social situations (Damasio, 1997). In this sense, Adolphs (2002) suggested that the identification of a fearful expression requires a processing network of various brain structures, the visual cortex, amongst other areas. However, although age-related neuropathological alterations underlying emotional behaviour have been described in discrete brain regions, the functional consequences of such changes are less clear.

Behavioural studies propose that visual processing of emotional facial expressions (EFEs) does not occur automatically, and that age-related impairments partially depend on the type of task (identification, categorisation, or matching). In a recognition task, Bucks and Radford (2004) showed that AD patients correctly recognised most of EFEs, although their performance on cognitive tasks was impaired when compared with that of healthy older adults. Similarly, in Burnham and Hogervorst's (2004) study, AD patients showed difficulties to match EFEs, whereas their performance on recognition and classification tasks did not differ from that of controls. The authors suggested that a visuospatial dysfunction was more likely than an impaired emotional processing the cause of deficits in patients' performance. It has been suggested (Suzuki, Hoshino, Shigemasu, & Kawamura, 2007) that all different types of face recognition, including facial expressions identification, first require visuospatial processing. Adolphs (2002) remarks that processing and recognising EFEs require first the visual cortex to grossly identify the face, then to determine whether the face contains an expression or not. Others studies (for a review, Grady, McIntosh, Horwitz, & Rapoport, 2000) have shown that ageing affects both visuospatial processing of faces and neural responses to faces. Pessoa, McKenna, Gutiérrez, and Ungerleider (2002), reported that healthy adults have difficulties identifying EFEs when their resources are engaged in a selective attention task and showed that all brain regions involved, including the amygdala, responded to emotional faces only when disposing of sufficient attentional resources for the visual processing of stimuli. Their conclusion was that this kind of processing is not automatic, but top-down directed. Taken together, these data suggest that a correct identification of EFEs necessarily requires the involvement of cognitive resources. We (García-Rodríguez, Ballesteros, Rodríguez, Reales, & Fusari, 2006; García-Rodríguez, Fusari, & Ellgring, 2008), as well as others (Gazzaley & D'Esposito, 2007; Pessoa et al., 2002; Storbeck & Clore, 2007) suggest that EFEs should be studied using cognitive paradigms to understand the mental processes underlying emotional identification. Traditional behaviour studies did not regard emotion as a cognitive process. However, current empirical researches are being undertaken to examine the role of cognition in emotional identification, integrating cognitive science and neuropsychology to understand how the brain implements emotional-processing functions and how these can be altered when the functional systems involved are damaged. It is not conceivable to identify a structure or brain region involved exclusively in cognition or emotion with no interactions with other processes.

Identification of EFEs is a fundamental part of normal daily life and social interaction. Ekman (2003) regards emotional facial identification as a key signal system always on and ready to process. One of the functions of this system is to bear additional information to help the interpretation of other people's words and actions. Furthermore, interpersonal communication takes place simultaneously with other activities, having to process various sources of information at the same time (i.e., decoding the emotional facial expression, connecting it to verbal information, etc.). This continuous flow of information requires a network of processes in order to manipulate, evaluate, and select alternatives, currently defined as WM. Of all WM components, the visuospatial sketchpad is most directly concerned with face processing. Visuospatial ability has been consistently related to facial expression recognition, as this task is considered visuospatial in nature (Buitelaar, van der Wees, Swaab-Barneveld, & van der Gaag, 1999; Haxby, Hoffman, & Gobbini, 2000). Moreover, several studies have shown the special role of visual components of WM in face perception. Maurer, Le Grand, and Mondloch (2002) suggested that WM is highly specialised in face processing. More concretely, these authors found that upright faces are processed more configurally (holistic) than inverted faces or other objects. Curby and Gauthier (2007) proposed that this configural processing allows more faces to be stored in WM than other objects of similar visual complexity. Moreover, a recent study (Morgan, Klein, Boehm, Shapiro, & Linden, 2008) has provided evidence of neural mechanisms of WM for faces, suggesting that higher order visual areas play an important role in WM for faces. All these findings show that visual WM is closely linked to perceptual processes engaged when seeing faces.

Working memory is typically tested by concurrent performance of two simultaneous tasks or by the inclusion of a secondary task introduced in the processing time of the primary task. The decline in performance in a given task when adding a secondary task may be one of the strongest variables differentiating between normal and pathological ageing (Baddeley, 1986). From lesion studies, it is accepted that the simultaneous performance of two tasks partially depends on the integrity of the dorsolateral prefrontal cortex. Regions of the prefrontal cortex appear to be particularly sensitive not only to ageing effects (Hedden & Gabrieli, 2004), but to degeneration in early and preclinical stages of AD, where neurons containing intracellular neurofibrillary tangles have been localised in areas of the neocortex (Bussire et al., 2003). Therefore, processing tasks that require the involvement of this region are very sensitive to detect subtle impairments related to disease (Hedden & Gabrieli, 2004). It can be expected that AD patients will have more difficulties than healthy older adults when decoding and identifying EFEs when simultaneously attending to other sources of information.

Experimentally, the dual-task paradigm has been used to study the interference of one task over another (Baddeley, Della Sala, Papagno, & Spinnler, 1997; MacPherson, Della Sala, Logie, & Wilcock, 2007). The attentional demands of the secondary task decrease performance in the primary task, causing interference in its processing. This effect is also evident when the secondary task is inserted during the processing time of the primary task (Murdock, 1982). The amount of interference depends mainly on whether the two tasks are of similar or different nature, producing a major impairment in the first case (Salway & Logie, 1995). Another factor that affects performance is the level of difficulty of the two tasks. Several studies (Allport, Antonis, & Reynolds, 1972; Park & Mason, 1982) have measured performance of a primary task with different levels of difficulty, using a secondary task of standard difficulty level. In all cases, the primary task was clearly interfered by the presence of the secondary task. The dual-task paradigm has been frequently used in studies on automaticity, revealing that an automatic process does not affect processing capacity (Naveh-Benjamin, 1987; Schneider, Dumais, & Shiffrin, 1984; Schneider & Shiffrin, 1987). Whether a process is automatic or controlled will be determined by the absence/presence of interference caused by one task over another (Fisk & Schneider, 1983; Naveh-Benjamin & Jonides, 1986; Schneider & Shiffrin, 1977). In the study of emotional processing, a double-task paradigm can help to understand to what extent EFEs identification is an automatic process or whether is mediated by cognitive resources.

In line with these findings, the main objective of the current study has been to investigate whether EFEs identification in AD patients is more impaired than that of healthy older and young adults when adding a secondary task. More precisely, we sought to investigate the effects of (1) dementia versus health, and (2) ageing, in facial emotional identification under a dual-task paradigm. The ability to identify EFEs was assessed under two conditions: identification-only and identification with a secondary task. In contrast to a rich literature on emotional processing, no studies have examined, so far, the involvement of WM on EFEs identification. To this purpose, we have used the six basic emotions (Ekman & Friesen, 1978) in order to get some generality of the emotion variable, with no ambition to dwell on differences between discrete emotions. The results obtained by this study may help to understand how EFEs are decoded, specifically whether a bottom-up (data-driven) or a top-down (schema-driven) approach is more appropriate to explain decoding of emotions from facial expression and its implications on ageing and dementias. This question was based on previous studies of double processing (Baddeley, Baddeley, Bucks, & Wilcock, 2001; Baddeley, Bressi, Della Sala, Logie, & Spinnler, 1991; MacPherson et al., 2007) that showed an impaired performance of AD patients in a dual-task with respect to healthy older adults. These studies reveal that a decreased functioning of the WM system is attributed to pathological conditions and not to ageing effects. Moreover, there is no evidence that performance on dual tasks is affected by ageing when different cognitive resources are involved, and when their levels of difficulty are being adjusted to compare performance of groups. Similarly, our predictions in the current study are that differences in dual-task performance of the current study will be related to dementia and not to ageing effects.

METHODS

Participants

A total of 48 adults volunteered to participate in this study. We tested 12 probable AD patients (six males, mean age 77.14 years, $SD = 5.20$; six females, mean age 79.52, $SD = 4.98$), 18 healthy older adults (nine males, mean age 72.56 years, $SD = 7.02$; nine females, mean age 76.76, $SD = 5.45$) and 18 young adults (nine males, mean age 30.78, $SD = 4.70$; nine females, mean age 32.88 years, $SD = 5.20$). Participants in the AD group were diagnosed with probable mild AD by a neurologist of the University Hospital La Paz of Madrid, attending NINCDS-ADRDA criteria and screened by a test of global function (Mini Mental State Examination–MMSE; Folstein, Folstein, & McHughs, 1975; 35 item version). The mean MMSE score in this test was of 20.6 for AD patients. Older participants were recruited from a public Centre for the Elderly of Madrid. Their mean MMSE score was of 31.8. Young participants were graduate students and clerical workers of the University. No cognitive screening was done with this group. All participants had normal or corrected-to-normal vision by self-report.

Experimental design

The experimental design for the analysis of dementia versus health consisted of a mixed factorial design with 2 (group: AD patients, healthy older adults) × 2 (condition: identification-only, identification with secondary task) factors. Condition was the within-subjects variable, and group was the between-subjects variable. The same design was used to assess the ageing effect with 2 (older and young adults) × 2 (condition) factors. In both cases, the dependent variable was the number of correct responses given to all emotional faces.

Experimental tasks

Primary task: Emotional identification. As a test of facial expression identification, a forced-choice recognition task was used. Participants were presented with the facial expressions of virtual actors enacting the six basic emotions, one at a time. In each trial they were asked to identify, from a set of six response alternatives, the emotion that best described the target stimulus.

Each trial started with a 1500 ms fixation cross with an acoustic signal. The acoustic signal was the tone "F" with a frequency of 500 Hz and duration of 150 ms. The visual signal was a grey coloured cross (the sign +) presented simultaneously with the acoustic signal. A 600 ms black screen followed. After that, the emotional stimulus was displayed within a square of

16 × 16 cm for 1500 ms, followed by another 600 ms black screen. Next, participants had to identify the emotional expression from the set of six emotion words as response alternatives. The number of correct identifications was the dependent variable. This score could vary between 0 and 12 within each emotion. The maximum number of correct answers was 72. "Correctness" was defined by an answer corresponding to the label given according to the Facial Action Units. Chance level would be two correct answers for a single emotion and 12 for the whole set of 72 items. The duration of the whole task was of approximately 20–30 min.

The facial stimuli used in this task were full colour emotional faces expressing the six basic emotions (happiness, sadness, anger, fear, surprise, disgust) with facial surface changes as described in the handbook of the Facial Action Coding System (FACS; Ekman & Friesen, 1978; Ekman, Friesen, & Hager, 2002, p. 174). These emotions were enacted by six virtual actors (three male and three female avatars), created by a 3-D image technique (POSER 6 program; Curious Labs, Santa Cruz, CA). The enactment of the expressions was done by an experienced FACS coder (JHE) by activating virtual muscles with respect to single Action Units (AUs) with the programme (Table 1). Male and female versions were created by using the standard deformers in Poser 6.

Using avatar faces of emotional expressions has been shown to elicit facial electromyographical reactions (Weyers, Mühlberger, Hefele, & Pauli, 2006) as well as amygdala activation (Moser et al., 2007) comparable to pictures of real faces and can thus be regarded as a valid method for producing standardised expressions of emotions for the assessment of emotion recognition.

Identification rates of the target emotions by young adults were 71.0%, far above the 16.6% to be expected by chance (see also Figure 3). Facial

TABLE 1
Number of single Action Units (AUs) from Facial Action Coding System for the six basic emotions

Emotion	*Facial Action Units*
Happiness	6+12+26
Sadness	1+4+15
Surprise	1+2+5+26
Disgust	4+9+10+15
Anger	4+5+24
Fear	1+4+5+20+26

Description of the Facial Action Units (FACS) corresponding to the emotions used in this study: 1 = inner brow raiser, 2 = outer brow raiser, 4 = brow lowerer, 5 = upper lid raiser, 6 = cheek raiser, 9 = nose wrinkler, 10 = upper lip raiser, 12 = lip corner puller, 15 = lip corner depressor, 20 = lip stretcher, 24 = lip pressor, 26 = jaw drop.

expressions were presented on a 17-inch computer screen. The total number of stimuli was 72, such that each emotional face was presented twice during the task. Images were presented in random order to each participant. Examples of the stimuli are shown in Figure 1, and Table 1 includes a description of each emotion on terms of facial Action Units according to FACS. Action Units represent the muscular activity that produces changes in facial expressions.

Secondary task: Corsi block. As secondary task, a variant of the Corsi blocks was used, composed of nine circles (eight white, one red) displayed in horizontal and vertical position (Figure 2) within a square of 16 × 16 cm on a 17-inch LCD computer monitor. In each trial, the static image of the nine circles was displayed for 600 ms. Next, participants had to report the location of the target (one red circle). The one-circle variant (Figure 2) is considered a control condition, as it contains only a sensorimotor element, not involving WM resources.

A key prerequisite of this study was to assure a standard difficulty level of the Corsi block task to equate performance of young, healthy older adults, and AD patients, as disproportional dual-task effects can be expected when a secondary task requires cognitive processes to a high degree. This issue can be controlled using simple tasks in order to equate performance (Baddeley, 1986). To assess an equal performance in the Corsi block task, we previously tested a small sample of young adults, older adults and AD patients. We decided to use the one-circle condition on the basis of two criteria: (1) to assure a standard difficulty level of the Corsi block task, by equating performance of the three groups, and (2) to assure that all participants could solve the secondary task during the 600 ms time interval.

Emotional stimuli examples

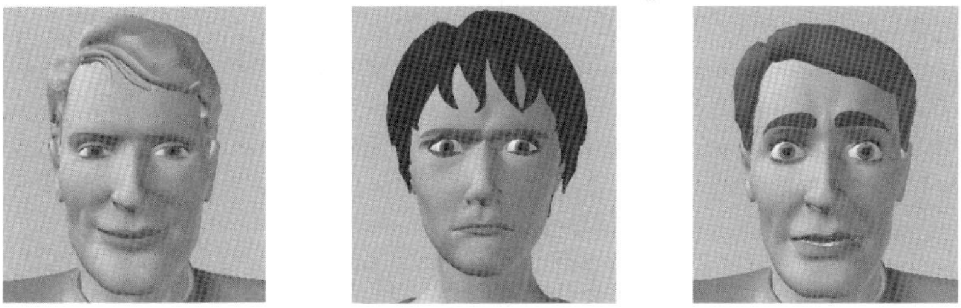

Happiness **Anger** **Fear**

Figure 1. Some stimuli examples. From left to right, happiness, anger, and fear portrayed by three virtual actors. The emotional expressions were based on the facial surface changes of the Facial Action Coding System (FACS; Ekman & Friesen, 1978). The virtual actors were created by a 3-D image technique (POSER 6 program, Curious Labs, Santa Cruz, CA) by using the standard deformers in Poser 6.

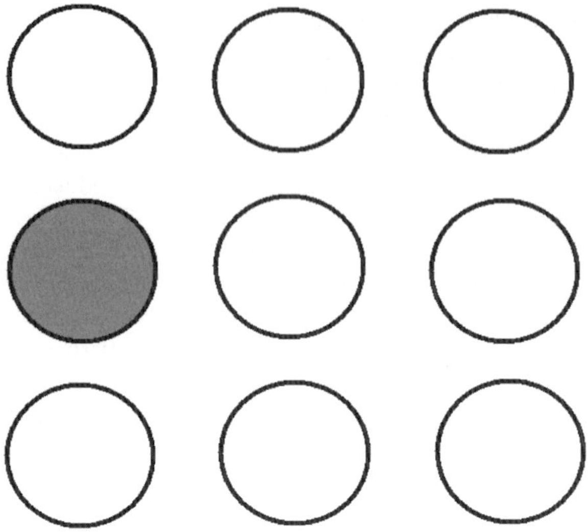

Figure 2. A Corsi block trial used in the identification with secondary task.

Procedure

All participants were tested individually in a quiet room. At the beginning of the experiment, the nature of the study was explained to each participant and written informed consent was obtained. The order of the two tasks was counterbalanced and, in order to avoid learning effects, performance was assessed in two separate sessions. In one session, the identification-only task was completed as referenced earlier. In a different session, participants were presented with the identification with secondary task. In this task, each trial started with a 1500 ms fixation cross and an acoustic signal, such as in the identification-only task. After a 600 ms black screen, an emotional face was displayed for 1500 ms. Next, the Corsi block trial was displayed for 600 ms (the time interval of the second black screen of the identification-only task). Then, participants had to mark the location of the target circle and name the emotional expression, in this order. Responses from facial expressions were recorded by the experimenter.

RESULTS

First, to examine to what extent the level of difficulty of the Corsi blocks affected performance on EFEs facial identification, we analysed the number of correct responses obtained from Corsi block task by the three groups. The univariate ANOVA did not show significant differences in the Corsi block scores between AD patients, healthy older, and young adults, $F(2, 47) = 2.52$,

$MSE = 0.09$, $p > .05$. Although AD patients' performance was below that of older and young adults, the effect was not statistically significant. These data reveal that the secondary task assured an equivalent performance of the three groups ($M = 71.75$, 71.89, and 72.00 for AD, healthy older, and younger adults, respectively).

Second, the results of the emotional identification tasks were analysed on the basis of the two main independent variables studied: dementia/health and ageing. Analysis on dementia/health was computed with results from AD patients and healthy older adults, whereas analysis on ageing was carried out with results from older and younger adults.

Data analysis as a function of dementia/health: Identification rates by AD patients and healthy older adults

The total number of correct identifications of EFEs in the two identification tasks showed that, overall, AD patients performed below the level of healthy older adults in the identification-only task ($M = 23.92$ and 32.39, respectively) as well as in the identification with secondary task ($M = 19.50$ and 31.33, respectively) (Figure 3).

In order to assess differences in EFEs identification, between task conditions, a 2 (group: AD patients vs. healthy older adults) × 2 (condition: identification-only and identification with secondary task) ANOVA was carried out, revealing a lower number of responses with dementia, $F(1, 28) = 13.27$, $MSE = 111.79$, $p < .005$. AD patients, on average, identified less emotional stimuli than healthy older adults (ms = 3.61 and 5.31 over 12, respectively). Condition was also significant, $F(1, 28) = 21.57$, $MSE = 4.99$, $p < .001$, showing that all participants identified more emotional stimuli in the identification-only task ($M = 4.69$) than when they had to additionally perform a secondary task ($M = 4.23$), revealing a decreased performance in emotional identification when a secondary task was included. A significant

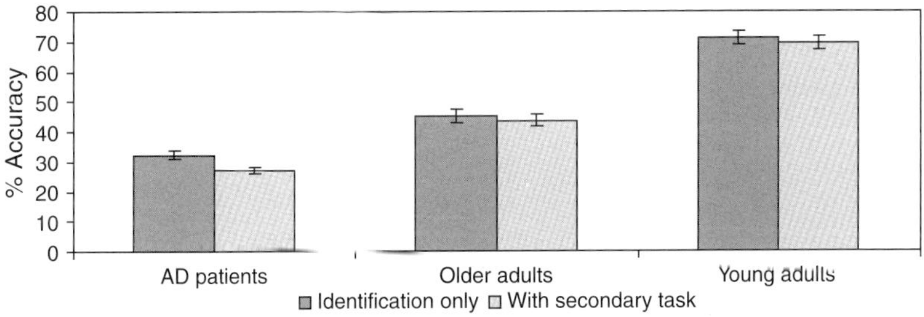

Figure 3. Accuracy rates for EFEs identification obtained in the identification-only and in the identification with secondary task, as a function of dementia status and ageing.

interaction was revealed between condition and group, $F(1, 28) = 8.13$, $MSE = 40.66$, $p < .01$. To consider if differences in dual-task performance could be attributed to effects already present at baseline or to tasks interaction, proportional dual-task costs (DTC) were computed for accuracy data, DTC = [(ACC single – ACC dual)/ACC single] * 100 (Salthouse, Fristoe, Lineweaver, & Coon, 1995). This dual-task approach is focused on assessing cognitive resources shared by tasks from different domains, calculating proportional age or dementia differences, as it has been shown by studies with older adults and dementia patients (Baddeley, 1986; Baddeley et al., 1991, 2001). In WM conditions, when tasks share stimulus modality or cognitive control, disproportional dual-task effects are revealed more precisely with this approach, showing differences in age or dementia. The dementia/health effects were analysed by a one-way ANOVA. The results showed a main effect of group, $F(1, 28) = 12.43$, $MSE = 1984.17$, $p < .005$, revealing that in the condition that included WM elements, DTC were significantly larger in AD patients than in healthy older (Figure 4). Specifically, AD patients, on average, incremented about 18.97% DTC, whereas older adults, on average, incremented about 2.37% DTC when facial emotional identification required WM resources. In conclusion, results of AD patients and healthy older show that, overall, patients identified less emotional expressions than healthy older and their performance was especially impaired when they had to identify EFEs in a WM condition.

Data analysis as a function of ageing: Identification rates by younger and older adults

The analysis of the correct identification rates of EFEs showed that younger identified more emotional expressions than older in the identification-only

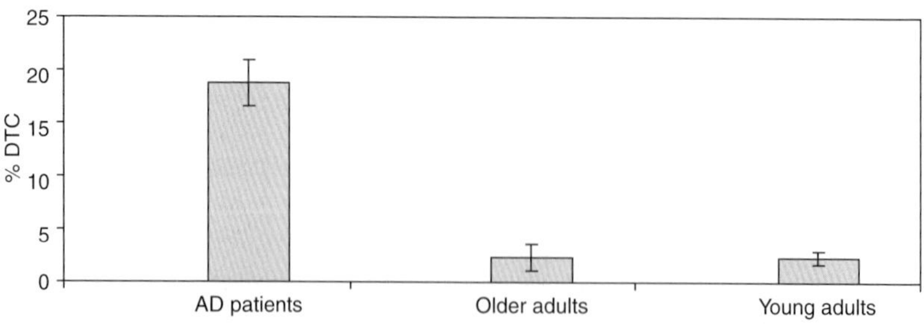

Figure 4. Differences in proportional dual-task costs as a function of dementia status and ageing, computed on rates of EFEs identification between task conditions in which a working memory load was included or not.

task ($M = 51.11$ and 32.39, respectively) as well as in the identification with secondary task ($M = 49.94$ and 31.33, respectively) (Figure 3).

A two-factor mixed ANOVA conducted on correct identifications with condition (identification-only and identification with secondary task) as the within-subject variable, and group (younger vs. older) as between-subjects variable was computed. The main effect of group, $F(1, 34) = 48.88$, $MSE =$ 128.30, $p < .001$, revealed a better performance of younger with respect to older adults. The mean identification rate of older was of 5.31 versus 8.42 of younger adults (over 12). Condition was statistically significant, $F(1, 34) =$ 5.36, $MSE = 4.13$, $p < .05$, showing that the introduction of a secondary task negatively affected EFEs identification ($M = 6.95$ and 6.77 for identification-only and identification with secondary task, respectively). The condition by group interaction was not significant, $F(1, 34) = 0.013$, $MSE = 0.05$, $p <$ .001. Finally, in order to compute differences in proportional DTC as a function of ageing, a one-way ANOVA was carried out, revealing similar DTC in younger and older adults, $F(1, 34) = 0.00$, $MSE = 0.03$, $p > .05$. This last data shows that ageing is not particularly affected by DTC in emotional identification tasks (Figure 4). Younger and older adults incremented similarly DTC when emotional identification was processed in a higher demanding condition (2.31% and 2.37% for younger and older, respectively). In sum, these results reveal that older identify less emotional expressions than younger adults, and their performance is not more affected than that of younger participants by the inclusion of the secondary task.

DISCUSSION

The current study had a main objective, to investigate whether EFEs identification in AD patients is more negatively affected than in healthy older and young adults when requiring visual WM resources and to assess specific dual-task deficits associated to dementia/health and ageing. With regard to this question, whether AD patients identify less emotional expressions than healthy older and young adults in a dual-task condition, the results obtained confirmed our hypothesis. As predicted, performance was negatively affected by dementia/health but not by ageing. In line with our hypothesis, dual-task decrements in EFEs identification when adding a secondary task were higher in AD patients than in healthy older and young adults. These results show that AD patients have more difficulties to identify emotional expressions than older and young adults, and that DTC are exacerbated when patients have to identify with an increased working memory load. These data reveal that in Alzheimer's disease, emotional identification is negatively affected by an increase of memory load, as confirmed by results on dual-task performance and are in line with other studies of dual-tasks showing that disproportional performance decrements are more evident in AD patients than in older adults (Hedden & Gabrieli, 2004; Petrides, 1995). With regard to the other studied variable, ageing, similar performance of younger and older adults revealed that both groups of participants did not accrue larger DTC in the emotional identification task when a secondary task was added. Several studies have also reported an absence of dual-task costs in performance of older adults (for a review, see Logie & Della Sala, 2001), and others (e.g., Nyberg, Nilsson, Olofsson, & Bäckman, 1995) have shown that, after correcting scores under dual-task conditions for differences in single task performance, age did not predict performance.

With respect to whether emotional identification is an automatic or controlled process, our data provide further evidence that identification of emotional stimuli is not independent from cognitive processing, revealing the role of cognition in emotional processing (Adolphs & Damasio, 2001; Barnard, Duke, Byrne, & Davidson, 2007; Storbeck & Clore, 2007). Although a great corpus of empirical studies have used the double-task paradigm to assess age-related differences in several cognitive processes, no studies have attempted, as far as we know, to investigate age- or health-related differences in EFEs identification. The current work offers a broader understanding of emotional processing for two reasons. First, nonverbal communication of emotions can be expressed in different ways (facial expressions, body contact, looks, body gestures, etc.) and they all are useful and helpful to repeat, contradict, substitute, complete, increase or regulate other's people behaviour, and this implies a double processing of information. The study of EFEs identification by a double processing paradigm adds new and remarkable knowledge to the current understanding of emotional processing. Second, the analysis of the ability to identify emotions by a WM task offers a theoretical explanation on the type of processing involved in the behaviour of emotional facial identification. A highly debated question has been if EFEs identification does not require attentional resources, thus implying an automatic process. The double-task paradigm is frequently used in most of the studies on automaticity. The basic assumptions that support theories on automaticity are that an automatic process not only does not decrease the processing capacity, but also it does not require processing resources, in contrast to a controlled processing that decreases the processing capacity, demanding and consuming processing resources (LaBerge, 1981; Naveh-Benjamin, 1987; Naveh-Benjamin & Jonides, 1986; Schneider & Shiffrin, 1987; Shiffrin, Dumais, & Schneider, 1981; Zacks, Hasher, Alba, Sanft, & Rose, 1984). Therefore, the automatic or controlled characteristic of a given task will be determined by the possible interference that will cause the processing of one task over the other: Whereas a task of controlled characteristic always causes interference, an automatic task does not, although it affects, to some extent, the processing of a concurrent task (Logan, 1979; Naveh-Benjamin & Jonides, 1986; Schneider & Shiffrin, 1977). The results obtained in our experiment allow us to conclude that the processing of emotional facial expressions is not as automatic as previous studies have proposed (Globisch et al., 1999; Öhman et al., 1995; Vuilleumier et al., 2001; Wells & Matthews, 1994). A major goal in the field of affective neuroscience is to describe the elementary mental operations of emotion and to relate them to the corresponding brain regions, as cognitive neuroscience has achieved in recent years within cognitive processes.

Another contribution of this study has been the development of a new approach to study the complexity of EFEs identification in analogous real-life conditions. An important suggestion offered by Adolphs (2002) is the need to develop stimuli and tasks of more ecological validity. In this pursuit, we suggest that new methodological approaches should be implemented to be able to generalise from observed behaviour in the laboratory to natural behaviour, in order to enrich our understanding of emotional processing. In daily life, when we identify emotions, we do not express judgements about basic emotions shown in pictures of single faces. Instead, both facial expression and other signals encounter together in a social background supported by the individual's cognitive resources. This issue is extremely important for clinical diagnosis and rehabilitation training. Some neuro-degenerative disorders, such as AD, involve alterations in the ability to perceive, recognise, express, or experience emotions, which explain the difficulties patients experience in performing basic daily life activities, such as identifying other people's facial expressions. This study offers a broader understanding of emotional processing in Alzheimer's disease, revealing the difficulties patients experience when they attempt to identify emotions from other people's faces. The functional consequences of such impairments have scarcely been studied, although the social life of AD patients is heavily affected by pathology.

REFERENCES

Adolphs, R. (2002). Recognizing emotion from facial expressions: Psychological and neurological mechanism. *Behavioral and Cognitive Neuroscience Reviews*, *1*, 21–62.

Adolphs, R., & Damasio, A. (2001). The interaction of affect and cognition: A neurobiological perspective. In J. P. Forgas (Ed.), *Handbook of affect and social cognition* (pp. 27–49). Mahwah, NJ: Lawrence Erlbaum Associates, Inc.

Adolphs, R., & Tranel, D. (2004). Impaired judgments of sadness but not happiness following bilateral amygdala damage. *Journal of Cognitive Neuroscience*, *16*, 453–462.

Adolphs, R., Tranel, D., Hamann, S., Young, A. W., Calder, A. J., Phelps, E., et al. (1999). Recognition of facial emotion in nine individuals with bilateral amygdala damage. *Neuropsychologia, 37*, 1111–1117.

Allport, D. A., Antonis, B., & Reynolds, P. (1972). On the division of attention: A disproof of the single channel hypothesis. *Quarterly Journal of Experimental Psychology, 24*, 225–235.

Baddeley, A. D. (1986). *Working memory*. Oxford, UK: Clarendon Press.

Baddeley, A. D., Baddeley, H. A., Bucks, R. S., & Wilcock, G. K. (2001). Attentional control in Alzheimer's disease. *Brain, 124*(8), 1492–1508.

Baddeley, A. D., Bressi, S., Della Sala, S., Logie, R., & Spinnler, H. (1991). The decline of working memory in Alzheimer's disease: A longitudinal study. *Brain, 114*, 2521–2542.

Baddeley, A. D., Della Sala, S., Papagno, C., & Spinnler, H. (1997). Dual-task performance in dysexecutive and nondysexecutive patients with a frontal lesion. *Neuropsychology, 11*, 187–194.

Barnard, P. J., Duke, D. J., Byrne, R. W., & Davidson, I. (2007). Differentiation in cognitive and emotional meanings: An evolutionary analysis. *Cognition and Emotion, 21*, 1155–1183.

Bechara, A., Damasio, H., & Damasio, A. (2000). Emotion, decision making and the orbitofrontal cortex. *Cerebral Cortex, 10*(3), 295–307.

Bucks, R. S., & Radford, S. A. (2004). Emotion processing in Alzheimer's disease. *Aging and Mental Health, 8*(3), 22–232.

Buitelaar, J. K., van der Wees, M., Swaab-Barneveld, H., & van der Gaag, R. J. (1999). Verbal memory and performance IQ predict theory of mind and emotion recognition ability in children with autistic spectrum disorders and in psychiatric control children. *Journal of Child Psychology and Psychiatry and Allied Disciplines, 20*, 869–881.

Burnham, H., & Hogervorst, E. (2004). Recognition of facial expressions of emotion by patients with dementia of the Alzheimer type. *Dementia and Geriatric Cognitive Disorders, 18*, 75–79.

Bussire, T., Gold, G., Kvari, E., Giannakopoulos, P., Bouras, C., Perl, D. P., et al. (2003). Stereologic analysis of neurofibrillary tangle formation in prefrontal cortex area 9 in aging and Alzheimer's disease. *Neuroscience, 117*(3), 577–592.

Cadieux, N. L., & Greve, K. W. (1997). Emotion processing in Alzheimer's disease. *Journal of the International Neurological Society, 3*, 411–419.

Curby, K. M., & Gauthier, I. (2007). A visual short-term memory advantage for faces. *Psychonomic Bulletin and Review, 14*, 620–628.

Damasio, A. R. (1997). Towards a neuropathology of emotion and mood. *Nature, 386*, 769–770.

Duvel, A., Smith, D., Talk, A., & Gabriel, M. (2001). Medial geniculate, amygdalar and cingulated cortical training-induced neuronal activity during discriminative avoidance learning in rabbits with auditory cortical lesions. *Journal of Neuroscience, 21*, 3271–3281.

Ekman, P. (2003). *Emotions revealed*. London: Weidenfeld & Nicolson.

Ekman, P., & Friesen, W. V. (1978). *The Facial Action Coding System*. Palo Alto, CA: Consulting Psychologists Press.

Ekman, P., Friesen, W. V., & Hager, J. C. (2002). *Facial Action Coding System: Investigator's guide*. Salt Lake City, UT: Research Nexus.

Fisk, A. D., & Schneider, W. (1983). Category and word search: Generalising search principles to complex processing. *Journal of Experimental Psychology: Learning, Memory, and Cognition, 10*(2), 181–197.

Folstein, M., Folstein, S., & McHughs, P. (1975). The "Mini Mental State": A practical method for grading the cognitive state of patients for the clinician. *Journal of Psychiatric Research, 12*, 189–198.

García-Rodríguez, B., Ballesteros, S., Rodríguez, B., Reales, J. M., & Fusari, A. (2006). Implicit memory of emotional facial expressions in AD patients and healthy older adults. In S. Ballesteros (Ed.), *Ageing, cognition, and neuroscience* (pp. 293–305). Madrid, Spain: UNED.

García-Rodríguez, B., Fusari, A., & Ellgring, H. (2008). Procesamiento emocional de las expresiones faciales en el envejecimiento normal y patológico. *Revista de Neurología, 46*, 609–617.

Gazzaley, A., & D'Esposito, M. (2007). Top-down modulation and normal aging. *Nature Neuroscience, 8*(10), 1928–1300.

Globisch, J., Hamm, A. O., Esteves, F., & Öhman, A. (1999). Fear appears fast: Temporal course of startle reflex potentiation in animal fearful subjects. *Psychophysiology, 36*, 66–75.

Grady, C. L., McIntosh, A. R., Horwitz, B., & Rapoport, S. I. (2000). Age-related changes in the neural correlates of degraded and nondegraded face processing. *Cognitive Neuropsychology, 17*, 165–186.

Hargrave, R., Maddock, R. J., & Stone, V. (2002). Impaired recognition of facial expressions of emotion in Alzheimer's disease. *Journal of Neuropsychiatry and Clinical Neurosciences, 14*, 64–71.

Haxby, J. V., Hoffman, E. A., & Gobbini, M. I. (2000). The distributed human neural system for face perception. *Trends in Cognitive Sciences, 4*, 223–233.

Hedden, T., & Gabrieli, J. D. E. (2004). Insights into the ageing mind: A view from cognitive neuroscience. *Nature Reviews Neuroscience, 5*, 87–96.

Koff, E., Zaitchik, D., Montepare, J., & Albert, M. S. (1999). Emotion processing in the visual and auditory domains by patients with Alzheimer's disease. *Journal of the International Neuropsychological Society, 5*, 32–40.

Komura, Y., Tamura, R., Uwano, T., Nishijo, H., Kaga, K., & Ono, T. (2001). Retrospective and prospective coding for predicted reward in the sensory thalamus. *Nature, 412*, 546–549.

LaBerge, D. (1981). Automatic information processing: A review. In J. Long & A. Baddeley (Eds.), *Attention and performance IX* (pp. 173–186). Hillsdale, NJ: Lawrence Erlbaum Associates, Inc.

LeDoux, J. (1996). *The emotional brain: The mysterious underpinnings of emotional life.* New York: Simon & Schuster.

Logan, G. D. (1979). On the use of a concurrent memory load to measure attention and automaticity. *Journal of Experimental Psychology: Perception and Performance, 5*(2), 189–207.

Logie, R. H., & Della Sala, S. (2001). Theoretical and practical implications of dual-task performance in Alzheimer's disease. *Brain, 124*, 1479–1481.

MacPherson, S. E., Della Sala, S., Logie, R. H., & Wilcock, G. K. (2007). Specific AD impairment in concurrent performance of two memory tasks. *Cortex, 43*, 858–865.

Maurer, D., Le Grand, R., & Mondloch, C. J. (2002). The many faces of configural processing. *Trends in Cognitive Sciences, 6*, 255–260.

Morgan, H. M., Klein, C., Boehm, S. G., Shapiro, L., & Linden, D. E. J. (2008). Working memory load for faces modulates P300, N170, and N250r. *Journal of Cognitive Neuroscience, 20*(6), 989–1002.

Moser, E., Demtl, E., Robinson, S., Fink, B., Gur, R. C., & Grammer, K. (2007). Amygdala activation at 3T in response to human and avatar facial expressions of emotions. *Journal of Neuroscience Methods, 161*, 126–133.

Murdock, B. B. (1982). A theory for the storage and retrieval of item and associative information. *Psychological Review, 89*, 609–626.

Naveh-Benjamin, M. (1987). Coding of spatial location information: An automatic process? *Journal of Experimental Psychology: Learning, Memory, and Cognition, 12*, 378–386.

Naveh-Benjamin, M., & Jonides, J. (1986). On the automaticity of frequency coding: Effects of competing task load, encoding strategy and intention. *Journal of Experimental Psychology: Learning, Memory, and Cognition, 12*, 378–386.

Nyberg, L., Nilsson, L.-G., Olofsson, U., & Bäckman, L. (1997). Effects of division of attention during encoding and retrieval on age differences in episodic memory. *Experimental Aging Research, 23*, 137–143.

Öhman, A., Esteves, F., & Soares, J. J. F. (1995). Preparedness and preattentive associative learning: Electrodermal conditioning to masked stimuli. *Psychophysiology, 9*(2), 99–108.

Park, D. C., & Mason, D. A. (1982). Is there evidence for automatic processing of spatial and colour attributes present in pictures and words? *Memory and Cognition, 10*, 76–81.

Pessoa, L., McKenna, M., Gutiérrez, E., & Ungerleider, L. G. (2002). Neural processing of emotional faces requires attention. Proceedings of the National Academy of Sciences. *USA, 99*, 11458–11463.

Petrides, M. (1995). Functional organization of the human frontal cortex for mnemonic processing: Evidence from neuroimaging studies. *Annals of the New York Academy of Science, 769*, 85–96.

Phillips, M. L., Drevets, W. C., Rauch, S. L., & Lane, R. (2003). Neurobiology of emotion perception I: The neural basis of normal emotion perception. *Biological Psychiatry, 54*, 504–514.

Salthouse, T. A., Fristoe, N. M., Lineweaver, T. T., & Coon, V. E. (1995). Aging of attention: Does the ability to divide decline? *Memory and Cognition, 23*(1), 59–71.

Salway, A. F. S., & Logie, R. H. (1995). Visuospatial working memory, movement control and executive demands. *British Journal of Psychology, 86*, 253–269.

Schneider, W., Dumais, S. T., & Shiffrin, R. M. (1984). Automatic and control processing and attention. In R. Parasunaman (Ed.), *Varieties of attention* (pp. 1–27). New York: Academic Press.

Schneider, W., & Shiffrin, R. M. (1977). Automatic and controlled information processing in vision. In D. LaBerge & J. Jonides (Eds.), *Basic processes in reading: Perception and comprehension* (pp. 127–154). Hillsdale, NJ: Lawrence Erlbaum Associates, Inc.

Schneider, W., & Shiffrin, R. M. (1987). Controlled and automatic human information processing: I. Detection, search and attention. *Psychological Review, 84*(1), 1–66.

Shiffrin, R. M., Dumais, S. T., & Schneider, W. (1981). Characteristics of automatism. In J. Long & A. Baddeley (Eds.), *Attention and performance IX* (pp. 223–238). Hillsdale, NJ: Lawrence Erlbaum Associates, Inc.

Storbeck, J., & Clore, G. L. (2007). On the interdependence of cognition and emotion. *Cognition and Emotion, 21*(6), 1212–1237.

Sullivan, S., & Ruffman, T. (2004). Emotion recognition deficits in the elderly. *International Journal of Neuroscience, 114*, 403–432.

Suzuki, A., Hoshino, T., Shigemasu, K., & Kawamura, M. (2007). Decline or improvement? Age-related differences in facial expression recognition. *Biological Psychology, 74*, 75–84.

Vuilleumier, P., Armony, J., Driver, J., & Dolan, R. (2001). Effects of attention and emotion on face processing in the human brain: An event-related fMRI study. *Neuron, 30*(3), 829–841.

Wells, A., & Matthews, G. (1994). *Attention and emotion: A clinical perspective*. Hove, UK: Lawrence Erlbaum Associates Ltd.

Weyers, P., Mühlberger, A., Hefele, C., & Pauli, P. (2006). Electromyographic responses to static and dynamic avatar emotional facial expressions. *Psychophysiology, 43*, 450–453.

Zacks, R. T., Hasher, L., Alba, J. W., Sanft, H., & Rose, K. C. (1984). Is temporal order encoded automatically? *Memory and Cognition, 12*, 387–394.

EUROPEAN JOURNAL OF COGNITIVE PSYCHOLOGY
2009, 21 (2/3), 445–472

Psychology Press
Taylor & Francis Group

Do age differences between young and older adults in inhibitory tasks depend on the degree of activation of information?

Erika Borella

Faculty of Psychology and Educational Sciences, University of Geneva, Geneva, Switzerland, and Faculty of Psychology, University of Padova, Padova, Italy

Christophe Delaloye

Faculty of Psychology and Educational Sciences, University of Geneva, and Department of Psychiatry, University Hospitals of Geneva, Geneva, Switzerland

Thierry Lecerf and Olivier Renaud

Faculty of Psychology and Educational Sciences, University of Geneva, Geneva, Switzerland

Anik de Ribaupierre

Faculty of Psychology and Educational Sciences, and Center for Interdisciplinary Gerontology, University of Geneva, Geneva, Switzerland

Three inhibition/interference tasks (Stroop colour, Negative priming embedded within the Stroop colour, and Hayling) were administered to young and older adults, with two main objectives, each of which embedded within a developmental perspective: First manipulate the level of activation of the irrelevant information, and second, assess the number of individuals presenting a reliable effect rather than analyse the results only at the group level. For each task, two versions were used, corresponding to two levels at which the irrelevant information was likely to be

Correspondence should be addressed to Erika Borella, Department of General Psychology, Via Venezia, 8, 35131 Padova, Italy. E-mail: erika.borella@unipd.it

The present study was supported by the Swiss National Research Fund (grants numbers 1114052565.97 and 1213065020.01). Partial results were presented at the 2002 Cognitive Ageing Conference, Atlanta, 18–21 April. We thank Nathalie Aguilar-Louche, Frédérique Bozon, Christian Chicherio, and Céline Jouffray for their help in running the experiments and scoring data. Our thanks go particularly to all persons who agreed to participate in this very long experiment.

http://www.psypress.com/ecp DOI: 10.1080/09541440802613997

activated. Analyses were conducted on relative difference scores rather than on raw response times. Results indicated that age differences in the magnitude of an interference effect were small and even null in the Negative priming task, independently of the salience of the irrelevant information. A bootstrap procedure showed that whereas the majority of both young and older adults presented a reliable interference effect in the Stroop colour and in the Hayling tasks, it was not the case in the Negative priming task. Moreover, correlations between the indices of interference/inhibition were very weak questioning the dimensionality of inhibition. Altogether these findings suggest that highly activated versions of the inhibitory tasks used do not really influence age-related differences in inhibitory control. It is also recommended to use bootstrap procedures more frequently instead of restricting analyses at a group level.

Keywords: Ageing; Bootstrap; Inhibition.

Within the past 20 years, interest in the concepts of inhibition and interference control has dramatically increased, and these concepts have become central in psychology, explaining several cognitive activities and behaviours as well as development and ageing. The objective of the present paper is to contribute to better understand these constructs and their possible change with age by adding two important methodological issues, namely to control that the irrelevant information, which is supposed to require inhibition, is really processed, and an analysis of the effects at the level of individuals rather than, as is most usually done in the field, at the group level. We will also question, like a number of other studies, the generality of these constructs by analysing whether different tasks supposed to measure inhibitory efficacy do indeed correlate.

Inhibition is generally defined as an attentional processes that acts in actively suppressing irrelevant information, clearing irrelevant action or thoughts, reducing interference from competing distractors in order to maintain the task goals or to ensure a coherent and organised behaviour (Friedman & Miyake, 2004). Despite this general view of inhibition, it is worth mentioning that the meaning of the term inhibition is broad and inconsistent across authors, and that several definitions have been proposed particularly because cognitive inhibition is less clearly observable in experimental psychology than it is in neuroscience, for instance within the brain, or at a cellular level (see for a review Aron, 2007). At an empirical level, the question of the nature of inhibition has also been raised by the recurrent observation of low or nonsignificant correlations between widely used inhibition tasks (e.g., Borella, Carretti, & de Beni, 2008; Delaloye et al., in press; Rabbitt, Lowe, & Shilling, 2001; Salthouse & Meinz, 1995; Shilling, Chetwynd, & Rabbitt, 2002). Therefore, several authors (e.g., Bjork, 1989; Harnishfeger, 1995; Nigg, 2000) proposed to distinguish different types of inhibition. For instance, Hasher and Zacks (1988) suggested three inhibitory functions to explain age-related decline in working memory content that are aimed at: determining which activated representations gain entrance into working memory (access function), suppressing representations that are irrelevant or no longer relevant to the current goal (deletion function), and preventing predominant but inappropriate responses (restraint function). Presently, inhibition is largely viewed as a family of functions rather than as a single unitary construct (Bjork, 1989; Harnishfeger, 1995; Nigg, 2000; Lustig, Hasher, & Tonev, 2001).

Despite these theoretical efforts to precise the nature of inhibition, correlations among tasks supposed to measure a same type of inhibition remain relatively weak. For instance, de Ribaupierre (2001), using structural equation modelling on a sample of younger and older adults, observed that the latent variable labelled inhibition accounted for almost no variance in the observed inhibitory variables.

Even if inhibition is still not clearly defined, it should be distinguished from interference. These two terms are often used interchangeably in the literature; although they can not be considered as synonymous. Interference refers to the susceptibility to distracting stimuli, leading to a decrement in performance; it does not necessarily involve an active suppression of processes or contents. Inhibition, in contrast, is a suppression process that keeps irrelevant information from entering and cluttering working memory. The distinction between interference and inhibition is difficult to operationalise, as one usually relies on the amount of interference to draw conclusions about the efficacy of inhibition; interference is less marked when irrelevant information can be efficiently suppressed. Thus, a relatively high level of interference might reflect not only a particular sensitivity to distraction, but also less than optimal inhibitory processes. Reciprocally, a relatively small effect of interference may be due either to efficient inhibition or simply to a lesser sensitivity to distractors, whether because these are not very salient or because of individual differences. Furthermore, interference and inhibition probably take place at different moments of processing information; but this is still more difficult to demonstrate.

In the field of selective attention, classical inhibitory measures that require a controlled inhibition are the following: the Stroop colour test, inhibition of overlearned processes of reading names of colours, the Hayling task, inhibition of the most obvious and familiar word that comes to mind, and the Negative priming task, inhibition of distracting information selectively to respond to a target stimulus.

The interference effect in the Stroop colour test (Stroop, 1935) refers to an increase in response latency to name the colour of a word, when the word and the colour in which it is written are incongruent (e.g., "red" written in blue) relative to a congruent or a control condition (e.g., "red" written in red or "strong" written in yellow). This increase in response times has been interpreted as the time needed to suppress actively the irrelevant information (i.e., the name of the word), that is automatically activated (highly prepotent). The amount of interference in this task is considered an index of the efficiency of inhibition; a larger interference effect reflects a decreased efficiency of inhibition.

The interference effect in the Hayling task refers to an increase in the time needed to complete high-cloze sentences (e.g., The captain wanted to stay with the sinking…) when an unexpected ending has to be provided; for instance in a condition that requires to complete them with words that make the sentences meaningless (e.g., peanut) compared to a condition that requires to complete them with words that make the sentences meaningful (e.g., ship). This response latency increase has been postulated to represent the time necessary to inhibit the prepotent and automatic response (ship). Thus, the Hayling task is very similar to the Stroop colour test because both require inhibition of highly prepotent responses (restrain function) in order to respect the instructions.

In the Negative priming task, information presented as distracting at encoding on the prime trial (n) becomes the target information to which participants have to respond on the probe trial ($n+1$) (e.g., Tipper, 1985). The selection of the relevant stimulus during the prime trial can be accomplished only if this relevant stimulus is activated and if at the same time the distractor (irrelevant stimulus) is efficiently inhibited. It is hypothesised that an attentional mechanism blocks (inhibits) the representation of the distractor stimulus on the prime trial from access to the response system (Hasher & Zacks, 1988); consequently, when the distractor becomes a target on the subsequent trial (probe trial), one has to suppress previous inhibition, which requires some additional time. Thus, an explanation of the negative priming effect is that the internal representation of the distractor should be inhibited during the prime trial. However, when the next trial is processed (i.e., the probe trial), the irrelevant stimulus becomes relevant. The internal representation of this stimulus should be "reactivated", and one has to "suppress" inhibition; this results in longer response times (May, Kane, & Hasher, 1995; Tipper, 2001). In contrast with the two previously mentioned tasks, longer latencies (negative priming effect) reflect a more efficient inhibition of the distractor (e.g., Lavie & Fox, 2000).

Whereas the Stroop colour and the Hayling tasks are, in the proper sense, two paradigms for investigating susceptibility to interference, the Negative priming paradigm is supposed to assess more directly inhibition (or more precisely disinhibition).

With ageing, performance in a large number of cognitive domain declines (e.g., Park & Schwarz, 2000). Because some of these performance decrements are intercorrelated (Verhaeghen & Salthouse, 1997), it has been suggested that a limited number of mechanisms (cognitive primitives) are involved. Inhibitory processes have been suggested to be such a cognitive primitive (Hasher, Lustig, & Zacks, 2007; Hasher & Zacks, 1988; Lustig, Hasher, & Zacks, 2007), as they are known to influence performance in various cognitive domains (Amieva, Philipps, Della Salla, & Henry, 2004), and to change with age (Persad, Abeles, Zacks, & Denburg, 2002). Data on cognitive ageing on the efficiency of inhibition suggest a specific deficit in inhibitory processes in older adults (Rowe, Valderrama, Hasher, & Lenartowicz, 2006). Some authors have observed an impairment of inhibitory functioning with ageing in some classical inhibitory tasks such as the Stroop colour test (Schelstraete & Hupet, 2002; Spieler, Balota, & Faust, 1996; West & Alain, 2000), the Hayling test (e.g., Burgess & Shallice, 1996), and the Negative priming task (e.g., Hasher, Stoltzfus, Zacks, & Rypma, 1991; May et al., 1995; Neill, Valdes, & Terry, 1995). Indeed, longer response times in the incongruent condition compared to the neutral one in the Stroop colour test (Davidson, Zacks, & Williams, 2003; Hartley, 1993; Salthouse & Meinz, 1995), longer completion times in the inhibition condition of the Hayling task (Andrés & van der Linden, 2000), and failure to produce negative priming effects (Kane, Hasher, Stoltzfus, Zacks, & Connelly, 1994) have been interpreted as a reduction of the efficiency of inhibitory processing during ageing. Other studies also found a steep decline of inhibition in later adulthood (quadratic effect of age; Borella et al., 2008; Persad et al., 2002). However, some experiments have also reported that age differences were minimal, if not nonexistent, once other variables were controlled for. Indeed the poor performance of older adults on those tasks may also reflect other types of cognitive deficit such as age-related decline in speed of processing. With respect to the Stroop colour test, for instance, Verhaeghen and de Meersman (1998a), in their meta-analysis, reported that age effects were related to developmental changes in processing speed rather than to changes in inhibitory mechanisms. The same conclusion was suggested by Uttl and Graff (1997), who used structural equations modelling. Thus, longer response times for older adults could be expected primarily because of reduction in processing speed, which has been shown to be a strong mediator of age differences in cognition (see Salthouse, 1996, for a review; Bugg, DeLosh, Davalos, & Davis, 2007). As regards the Hayling test, no age difference was observed when processing speed or baseline condition were controlled for (Andrés & van der Linden, 2000). Finally, as concerns Negative priming measures, Verhaeghen and de Meersman (1998b) also conducted a meta-analysis, and showed that older adults have more difficulty inhibiting irrelevant aspects of a stimulus than younger adults, but again less than it was initially suggested. Gamboz, Russo, and Fox (2002) in a meta-analysis on age differences in the identity Negative priming, concluded that the effect was not different between young and old adults (see also Sullivan & Faust, 1993). One possible explanation for this discrepancy in results is that, rather than presenting less efficient inhibitory processes, older adults are more susceptible to irrelevant information. That is, prepotent, irrelevant information might be more highly activated in older than in young adults.

It is interesting to note that few studies have ensured that irrelevant information is indeed processed before concluding that inhibition is at work or is deficient. Yet, one can wonder what need there would be for inhibition in any of the tasks mentioned so far (e.g., the Stroop colour or the Hayling tasks) if irrelevant information is not activated (e.g., Neill et al., 1995). It is therefore crucial, when evaluating susceptibility to interference with ageing, to make sure that the irrelevant information has been previously activated (Hedden & Park, 2001). In some tasks, such as in the classical Stroop colour test, the activation of the irrelevant information is almost obligatory (at least for good readers); such irrelevant information is also probably more highly activated and/or faster to activate than relevant information, because of the over learned response that is required (automatic reading process), whereas the relevant information (colour to name) is itself activated only by the instruction. This asymmetry in activation is why the highly activated, erroneous response is referred to as prepotent, or misleading (e.g., Pascual-Leone, 1969). This asymmetry in the level of activation of the relevant and irrelevant information, respectively, is probably not identical in all inhibitory tasks. Some of the controversial results might, thereby, be due to the fact that, in some tasks, the level of activation of the distractors is too low for inhibition to be necessary. Young adults, for example, might process only the relevant information, resulting in no interference; they would therefore not need to inhibit irrelevant information. In contrast, older adults might process both types of information, relevant and irrelevant. Consequently, they may have to inhibit irrelevant information, which implies more processing than young adults; this would, in turn, generate longer response times.

It is of course not possible to measure the level of activation of information, or to equate it across tasks and across ages. This is one of the reasons why the level of activation at the level of the task was manipulated in the present study, by using two versions of a same task. Therefore, two versions of the Stroop colour test (see also Hartley, 1993), which embedded two Negative priming tasks, and two versions (i.e., phases) of the Hayling task (Burgess & Shallice, 1996) were created. The two versions of each task differ in the salience or degree of activation of the irrelevant information: Observing a difference in the effect of interference between the two versions, which are identical in all other respects (e.g., instructions, type of stimuli, etc.) makes it possible to insure that irrelevant information has been attended to.

In the integrated version of the Stroop colour, called the "highly activated" version (the colour-word task in Hartley's experiment, i.e., the most frequently task used within the Stroop family of tasks), the relevant and the irrelevant information is embedded in the same stimulus (e.g., "red" written in blue); thus irrelevant information should be highly activated because it cannot remain unattended. In the spatially dissociated Stroop colour ("less activated" version), the task consists in naming the colour of a colour patch with the colour word being placed above or below the patch (the colour-block task in Hartley's experiment; for instance a blue patch with the word "red" written above). The relevant and the irrelevant stimuli are spatially and temporally dissociated; although it cannot be totally ignored, the irrelevant stimulus should be less salient (Hartley, 1993; Schooler, Neumann, Caplan, & Roberts, 1997). A Negative priming condition was also embedded in each version of the Stroop colour test (Negative priming tasks). As concerns the Hayling task, participants first had to complete a series of sentences with their very probable ending (which insured that the highly probable word was activated at some point), before producing an ending that made no sense. Participants had also to complete another series of sentences, presented only once, with an improbable ending. The difference, if observed, between the two versions of the Hayling task would indicate that irrelevant information was activated and that some inhibition would be required. Thus, we hypothesised that larger interference effects would be observed in the highly activated versions compared to the less ones, and that this could be particularly true for older adults, leading to an Age × Version (highly vs. less activated version) interaction (e.g., Hartley, 1993).

As already mentioned, the question of the generality of inhibition remains an unresolved issue particularly in the ageing field. By this term, we refer both to across-task generality (i.e., do the tasks correlate?) and to individual differences (i.e., independently of the group effects, do all the individuals show inhibition or interference effects?). One way to operationalise this question is to study correlations between tasks supposed to measure inhibition. High correlations would attest to some stability across the tasks in terms of interindividual differences, on the basis of which a certain amount of generality across tasks can be inferred. Supposing that both the Stroop colour and the Hayling tasks are misleading tasks, and if there is some generality to the construct, moderate to high correlations should be observed, at least between the highly activated versions (Pascual-Leone, 1969; see also Johnson, Im-Bolter, & Pascual-Leone, 2003). As stated previously, correlations between different inhibitory measures have generally been found to be quite low (Kramer, Humphreys, Larish, Logan, & Strayer, 1994; Rabbitt et al., 2001; Salthouse & Meinz, 1995). In particular, it was observed for the Stroop colour tasks, that correlations computed between differences scores instead of raw scores were also low (Salthouse & Meinz,

1995). It has been advanced sometimes that the lack of correlation could be due to a lack of reliability, particularly when difference scores are used. In the cognitive literature, it is often assumed, albeit implicitly and based on group effects, that all or almost all individuals show the expected effect, as soon as there is a significant effect; this is, however, not always the case, even within non pathological populations (Amieva et al., 2004; Della Sala, Logie, Marchetti, & Wynn, 1991). Testing the generality of the effect at the level of individuals was therefore an additional objective of the present study. It is not straightforward to assess whether a given individual presents a reliable effect. Indeed, due to measurement errors, it is certainly not sufficient to compute a difference in response time or a ratio and to decide that a difference of a few milliseconds reflects an effect. Thus, in order to assess both intra-individual stability and the reliability of the effects in each task, we used a formal test procedure for each individual. Because of the interference score calculated (relative difference), a bootstrap procedure was used, which allows for nonstandard distribution.

To summarise, the present study pursued several objectives. First, it was intended to further examine whether young and older adults differ in their inhibitory efficiency, using three classical tasks: the Stroop colour test, the Hayling task, and the Negative priming task (the Negative priming was embedded within the Stroop colour task). Second, by using two versions for each task, differing from one another in the salience of irrelevant information (more highly activated vs. less highly activated), it was aimed at studying whether age differences vary with the level of activation of the irrelevant information. Third, the stability and reliability of intra-individual performance was estimated by a bootstrap procedure. This procedure allowed also to assess whether effects were observed in all individuals and similarly so for young or older adults. This issue is of particular interest as older adults are a more heterogeneous group than young adults (Nelson & Dannefer, 1992). Fourth, it was meant to address the question of the dimensionality of inhibitory processes, by studying the correlations across the tasks; we hypothesised that correlations would be higher for the more highly activated than for the less highly activated versions.

METHOD

Participants

A total of 150 young adults (79% of women), ranging from 19 to 35 years of age, and of 130 older adults (71% of women), ranging from 60 to 88 years of age, participated in the study. The mean age was 22.28 ($SD = 3.05$) for the young adults and 71 ($SD = 6.16$) for the older adults. Younger adults were University students, who participated to the experiment as part of course credit. Older adults were community dwelling and mainly recruited from the University for the Third Age of the University of Geneva; they were paid back for their travelling costs to the laboratory. None of the older adults, as shown by a large battery of tasks administered (de Ribaupierre et al., 2004), presented an incipient dementia. All participants were French native speakers or very fluent in French. From Table 1, it can be seen that the average level of education was quite high for both groups (more than 13 years). Moreover, performance on the Mill Hill task was higher for the older adults, than for the young adults, $F(1, 278) = 36.18$, $MSE = 10.61$, $p < .001$, $\eta^2 = .12$. Older adults had also a significantly poorer performance than younger ones on tasks assessing fluid intelligence, the Raven test (PM38; Raven, 1988), $F(1, 278) = 213.44$, $MSE = 49.65$, $p < .001$, $\eta^2 = .43$, and speed of processing, the Letter Comparison test (e.g., de Ribaupierre et al., 2004, adapted from Salthouse & Babcock, 1991), $F(1, 278) = 266.41$, $MSE = 834.84$, $p < .001$, $\eta^2 = .49$. Finally, as concerns health level, measured with a subjective Health questionnaire, there was no significant difference between young and older adults. These findings are in line with the literature that shows an age-related increase in vocabulary skills, or at least maintenance, and a decline in fluid intelligence measures, in processing speed (e.g., Park et al., 2002).

Materials

As part of a large battery of cognitive tasks, participants completed two versions of three computerised tasks: Stroop colour, Negative priming, and Hayling task. All tasks were run on an I-Mac with a voice key, linked to a button box, and the applications were created using PsyScope. The voice key was used to record reaction times (RTs). Response accuracy was manually recorded by the experimenter.

TABLE 1
Sample description and demographics variables (standard deviations)

	Young	*Elderly*
N	150	130
Mill Hill	36.71 (2.71)	39.06 (3.79)
Fluid intelligence	53.12 (4.29)	40.78 (9.26)
Raven Test (PM38)		
Processing speed		
Letter comparison (s)	104.87 (23.67)	161.38 (33.94)
Health	1.82 (0.55)	1.87 (0.63)
Years of education	>13 years	13.36 (3.12)

Stroop colour test. Two versions of the task were used. The highly activated (integrated) Stroop colour task consisted of the classical version of the task, in which the relevant and the irrelevant information are embedded in the same stimulus. That is, participants had to name the colour in which words or word-like stimuli (row of four or five typographical signs) were presented. All stimuli appeared in the centre of the screen.

In the less activated (dissociated) version, a colour patch was presented, together with a word (or a row of typographical signs) written in a neutral colour. Participants had to report the colour of the patch and thus had to ignore the word (or sign). The word was presented above or below the patch, with a distance of 2 cm between the centre of the word and the centre of the patch, both stimuli being equidistant from the centre of the screen. Following the procedure used by Schooler et al. (1997), a fixed stimulus–onset asynchrony (SOA) of 100 ms—the time at which the maximal interference was observed in Schooler's and colleagues experiment—was used. The colour patch was presented first, followed by a colour word written in white. In both versions, the stimulus remained on the screen until the response was emitted. Because the irrelevant information is embedded with the relevant one in the integrated version, it should be more difficult to disregard. Therefore, this version was considered as a "highly activated" condition, whereas the dissociated one was considered a "less activated" condition.

Five conditions were used in the two tasks: two neutral conditions, one congruent, one incongruent, and one Negative priming (prime and probe). Four colours were used: "rouge" ["red"], "bleu" ["blue"], "jaune" ["yellow"], and "vert" ["green"]. In the "signs" neutral condition, the task was to name the colour of rows of signs (four signs were used: + + + +, ****, ““““““, ^^^^). In the "words" neutral condition, the task was to name the colour of noncolour words. The four words were "grave" ["serious"], "neuf" [new"], "plein" ["full"], "fort" ["strong"], presented in the four colours mentioned earlier, i.e., all adjectives, with the same number of letters as the colour words with a surface frequency of at least 5000 (according to the Brulex database). In the congruent condition, the task was to name the colour of a word written in the same colour (e.g., the word red written in red). In the incongruent condition, the meaning of the colour words and the colour in which they were written was incongruent (e.g., the word "red" shown in blue). In the Negative priming condition, the colour word to be inhibited in the prime display was of the same colour as the target in the subsequent probe display (e.g., the word "red" written in blue followed by the word "yellow" written in red). In other words, the colour to be named on item "*n*" was the same as the name of the colour word on item "$n-1$". In the present study, only the results for the incongruent, "signs" neutral, and the Negative priming conditions will be reported.

In both versions of the Stroop colour task, that contain Negative priming conditions, the stimulus list consisted of 144 trials. Twenty-four trials were administered in each condition (12 pairs in the Negative priming condition), and the different conditions were randomly distributed throughout the task, but the order was identical for all participants; colours appeared an equal number of times across trials. Half of the trials (72) were incongruent, including the negative priming pairs. Positive priming and consecutive presentation of more than two trials belonging to the same condition were avoided.

For both versions of the Stroop colour task, and thus for the Negative priming condition, each trial began with a fixation point at the centre of the screen, presented for 1000 ms, followed by the target word (signs), for the highly activated version, or colour patch, for the less activated version, to be named, which remained on the screen until response. After the response was given, there was an 800 ms delay until the next ready signal appeared. In the less activated version of Stroop colour, the colour patch was presented first, followed 100 ms later by a colour word written in white. Timing of response latency and accuracy were recorded. Latencies reflected time from stimulus onset to response onset. The experimenter recorded accuracy manually.

The Hayling task. This task was adapted from Burgess and Shallice (1996). It consisted of 30 high-cloze sentences in which the final word was omitted; a pilot study was first conducted, on a larger number of sentences to assess whether they were high cloze, and 30 sentences with a probability of completion of at least .98 were retained. Sentences were also selected on the basis of: the number of syllables, the starting phonemes and length of the target word. These 30 sentences were assigned to one of two groups of 15 sentences to be used in the first and the third phase (A and AP) or in the second phase (B) of the task. The two sets of sentences were counterbalanced across participants.

In the first phase (A), participants had to find as quickly as possible the word that best completed the sentence (e.g., We sleep in a . . . [bed]). In the second phase (B), which was conducted immediately after Phase A, the basic task was to provide an ending which made no sense at all in the context of the sentence, while still grammatically correct (e.g., Most cats see well at . . . [conversation]). In the third phase (AP), the 15 sentences of Phase A were presented again, but, like in Phase B, the task was to provide an ending which made no sense at all (e.g., We sleep in a . . . [fish]). For this phase (highly activated version), it was assumed that the expected ending (i.e., an ending providing sense) would be more highly activated than in Phase B (less activated version), because it had been generated in Phase A. Therefore, Phase B will be considered as a "less activated" condition, whereas Phase AP will be considered as a "highly activated" condition. A practice phase (five sentences) was presented before each test condition. Each sentence remained on the screen until response. The experimenter manually recorded accuracy, and the computer recorded the response time latencies.

Procedure

Participants were tested individually. The Stroop colour, the Negative priming, and the Hayling tasks were administered on different sessions; the interval between each session was at least 2 days. One of the Stroop colour tasks, and therefore one of the Negative priming tasks, as it is part of the Stroop colour test, was administered during the first session, the Hayling task during the second session, and the other Stroop colour test with the Negative priming during the third session. The order of presentation of the highly and less activated version of the Stroop colour task (including Negative priming) was counterbalanced across participants. A brief control of vision was also administered, which enabled the experimenter to insure that all stimuli could be identified and the colours discriminated. Each task started with some practice trials.

RESULTS

Design of the analyses

Results will be reported as follows: first, reliability of the measures at the group level, then analyses on the effect of age and version (highly vs. less activated), and their possible interaction; second, in order to take into account intra-individual variability, a confidence interval for each subject was computed on the relative indices of interference for the Stroop colour, Hayling, and Negative priming, to determine the presence or not of an effect, based on a bootstrapping procedure; and third, correlations across the tasks, whether on the whole sample, or only on those participants presenting a reliable effect.

For each of the three tasks a similar design was adopted for the analyses. With respect to latencies, all RTs associated with errors (voice key and other errors) were eliminated. RTs less than 200 ms for the Stroop colour test, with the Negative priming, and 400 ms for the Hayling task were also eliminated. As concerns the Hayling task, a superior threshold was also fixed after a visual inspection of RTs distributions: RTs greater than 7000 ms were excluded (in order to be sure of measuring inhibition and not lapses of attention). The different thresholds used for the two tasks were due to the different nature of the stimuli: for the Stroop colour test and the Negative priming, words or signs had to be named, while sentences were completed in the Hayling task. Moreover, following Friedman and Miyake's (2004) suggestions on data cleaning, RTs for trials immediately following errors were also excluded. The percentage of trials eliminated because of various errors or because they followed an error was less than 11% in the two Stroop tasks. Interference indices in the Stroop colour test were based on the relative difference between RTs in the incongruent and RTs in the "signs" neutral condition (that is: [RT incongruent − RT signs]/RT signs). The relative difference is often used in the literature to control for individual differences in baseline performance (e.g., de Frias, Dixon, & Struss, 2006). We used the "signs" neutral condition as control, because we considered that the interference effect reflects the efficiency of suppressing a prepotent word-reading response (Davidson et al., 2003; see Salthouse, Atkinson, & Berisch, 2003). The Negative priming indices were based on the relative difference in RTs between the probe and the prime conditions. Finally, indices in the Hayling task were based on the relative difference in RTs between Phase AP and Phase A (highly activated), or between Phase B (less activated) and Phase A.

Task reliability

Reliability estimates were computed for the RTs by condition, using Cronbach's alpha for each task version (highly and less activated). Both versions of the Stroop colour task showed a very good reliability (signs, $\alpha =$ .94; incongruent, $\alpha = .94$; and for the Negative priming, prime, $\alpha = .95$; probe, $\alpha = .95$). With respect to the two versions of the Hayling tasks, reliability estimates were reasonable (Phase A, $\alpha = .78$, Phase B, $\alpha = .76$, Phase AP, $\alpha = .80$). Reliability coefficients were also computed for the indices (relative differences), using split half (odd-even) correlations with the Spearman-Brown correction. Reliability was acceptable for the Stroop colour and Hayling test in both versions (highly activated version: $r = .71$, and $r = .54$; less activated: $r = .51$, and $r = .58$, respectively). In contrast, for the Negative priming indices reliability was quite poor (highly version: $r = .12$, less activated version: $r = .33$).

The effects of age and version

Interference and Negative priming indices (relative differences) were submitted to a two-way, mixed analysis of variance with age (young vs. older adults) as a between-subject factor and version (highly vs. less activated) as a within-subject factor.[1] In order to allow for comparisons across tasks, effect sizes were computed and based on η^2, relating the variance due to age to the total between-subject variance. Analyses were first run on the RTs, using three-way Age × Version × Condition designs. They will not be reported here, for sake of space; however, it should be noted that results were congruent with many other studies in the field, showing an effect of age, and an interaction of age with the condition, pointing to a larger increase of RTs in the experimental (incongruent) condition in older adults.

Stroop colour tasks[2]

A two-way Age (2) × Version (2) mixed ANOVA was performed on interference indices. Results showed both a main effect of age, $F(1, 278) = 7.75$, $MSE = 0.02$, $p < .01$, $\eta^2 = .03$, and of version, $F(1, 278) = 57.23$, $MSE = 0.01$, $p < .001$, $\eta^2 = .17$. The Age × Version interaction was also significant, $F(1, 278) = 9.58$, $p < .01$, $\eta^2 = .04$ (Figure 1). Comparisons indicated a significant age difference in the less activated version, with older adults showing a larger interference effect compared to younger ones, $F(1, 278) = 22.07$, $p < .01$. However, in the highly activated version, the difference between both groups was not significant, $F(1, 278) < 1$. The effect size of age was almost null for the highly activated version, and equal to .07 in the less activated one. Finally, for both age groups, interference indices were higher in the highly activated version than in the less activated one.

[1] Because the distributions were significantly different from a normal one, we first computed median RTs for the correct trials. This technique is, indeed, more appropriate, as compared to other data transformations, because it is relatively uninfluenced by spuriously fast or slow RTs (Ulrich & Miller, 1994), and it is less sensitive to the number of extreme observations that is postulated to increase with age (Bunce, Warr, & Cochrane, 1993). We also calculated nonparametric Mann-Whiney statistics to assess the presence of age-related differences on the measures of interest. As results were comparable to those obtained with inferential parametric analyses, we reported only the latter ones, which made it easier to analyse the potential Age × Version interactions.

[2] Three-way Age (young vs. older adults) × Experimental conditions (signs vs. incongruent for the Stroop colour; prime vs. probe for the Negative priming; A vs. B and A vs. AP for the Hayling) × Version (highly vs. less activated) mixed analyses of variance (ANOVA) were performed on the median response times for the Stroop colour, Negative priming, and Hayling tasks. Age effects were found in all tasks, as long as the raw data were analysed. The size of the age effect was larger in the Stroop colour task ($\eta^2 = .35$), including the Negative priming condition ($\eta^2 = .32$), than in the Hayling task ($\eta^2 = .02$). An Age × Condition was found for the Stroop colour task only ($\eta^2 = .09$, greater interference effect for older adults than for young). In accordance with a number of studies, this pattern of results shows that older adults had more difficulty resisting interference and/or inhibiting efficiently the irrelevant information.

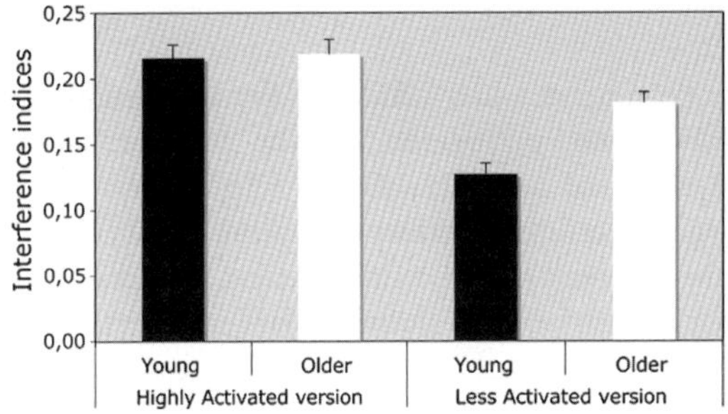

Figure 1. Stroop colour task. Interference indices by age and version (highly activated vs. less activated version). Bars represent one standard error.

Negative priming

An Age (2) × Version (2) mixed ANOVA was performed on the Negative priming indices (Figure 2). Results showed that the main effect of age was not significant, $F(1, 278) = 1.17$, $p = 28$. In contrast, the main effect of version was significant, $F(1, 278) = 6.78$, $MSE = 0.01$, $p < .01$, $\eta^2 = .03$. The Age × Version interaction was marginally significant, $F(1, 278) = 3.64$, $p = .06$, $\eta^2 = .01$. The effect size of age was null for the highly activated version, and equal to .02 in the less activated version.

The decomposition of the Age × Version interaction indicated that for young adults the Negative priming score was higher in the highly activated version than in the less activated version, $F(1, 278) = 10.95$, $p < .01$. For older adults, there was no difference between the highly activated and the less activated version. As concerns the comparison between young and older adults, results showed that Negative priming score was higher for older than for young adults in the less activated version, $F(1, 278) = 4.57$, $p < .05$; the difference was not significant in the highly activated version.

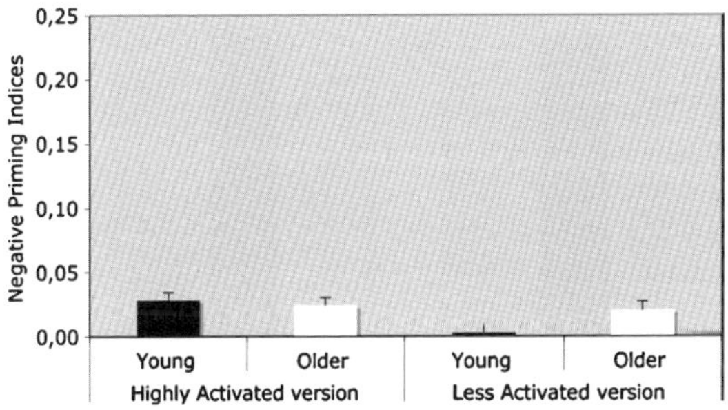

Figure 2. Negative priming task. Inhibitory/interference indices by age and version (highly activated vs. less activated version). Bars represent one standard error.

Hayling task

A two-way Age (young vs. older adults) × Version (highly activated vs. less activated) ANOVA was performed on the interference indices. Results showed a main effect of age, $F(1, 278) = 3.86$, $MSE = 0.35$, $p < .05$, $\eta^2 = .02$, due to a larger interference effect for young adults than for older adults (1.04 vs. 0.94, respectively), and a main effect of version, $F(1, 278) = 5.2$, $MSE = 0.11$, $p < .05$, $\eta^2 = .02$, showing larger interference effect in the highly activated version (A vs. AP) than in the less activated one (1.02 vs. 0.96, respectively). The Age × Version interaction was not significant, $F(1, 278) = 1.28$, $p = .26$.

Individual stability and reliability: Bootstrap procedure

A second main objective of the present study was to assess the stability and the reliability of the effects (interference effect and Negative priming effect) at the level of the individuals and for the two different versions of the tasks. A nonparametric procedure, the bootstrap, allowed us to estimate a confidence interval for the different effects for each participant in each task (and in each version). The bootstrap procedure is, indeed, probably the best known resampling method for assessing the stability and the replicability of a given sample, as it estimates the distribution of the statistic of interest empirically, using information drawn from the sample of observations, and simulating new samples. This technique is meaningful for understanding how stable the results may be across related sample results. The nonparametric ABC bootstrap confidence interval was, thus, used (Davison & Hinkley, 1997) to estimate to what extent the experimental effect, reported at the level of the groups, was observed in each individual. The requirement for this method is that the specified statistic is a smooth

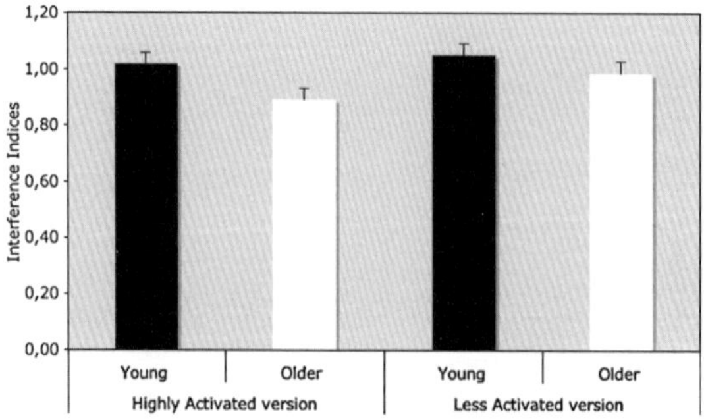

Figure 3. Hayling task. Interference indices by age and version (highly activated vs. less activated version). Bars represent one standard error.

function of the sample moments, which is the case here. Because it was not implemented in our statistical software packages, the program was created by one of us, and was then run on the statistical package S-Plus (2002). It is worth noticing that this procedure was conducted on RTs indices (and not on the raw RTs); because it concerns only individuals, a 68% confidence interval was used, as discussed previously.

It was therefore possible: to assess whether an effect is observed for each individual; to examine whether young and older adults differ in this respect; and, finally to determine whether those individuals presenting a reliable effect in one task also presented a reliable effect in another one. Table 2 reports the percentage of individuals showing a reliable effect in the expected direction, as well as those presenting an effect in the opposite direction or those for whom the effect was not reliable. As concerns the interference indices in the Stroop colour tasks, almost all participants showed a reliable effect of interference, for both versions. For the young adults, the number of individuals presenting a reliable effect was higher in the highly activated version than in the less activated one (93% vs. 79%, respectively), whereas

TABLE 2
Percentage of participants presenting reliable interference/inhibition indices (bootstrap procedure) by task

	Expected effect	*Inverse effect*	*No reliable effect*	*Expected effect*	*Inverse effect*	*No reliable effect*
	Stroop colour test					
	Highly activated version			*Less activated version*		
Young	0.93	<1%	0.07	0.79	0.00	0.21
Older	0.96	0.00	0.04	0.91	0.00	0.09
	Negative priming					
	Highly activated version			*Less activated version*		
Young	0.29	0.11	0.61	0.17	0.16	0.67
Older	0.29	0.12	0.58	0.21	0.09	0.70
	Hayling task					
	Highly activated version (Phase AP vs. A)			*Less activated version (Phase B vs. A)*		
Young	0.97	0.01	0.03	0.99	0.00	0.01
Older	0.94	0.00	0.07	0.98	0.00	0.01

An expected effect corresponds to a reliable effect in the expected direction, that is, to a measure of interference larger than zero (response time longer in the incongruent condition). An inverse effect was also considered reliable but with an unexpected direction, when the corresponding 68% bootstrap confidence interval was entirely below the value 0. If the interval contained the value 0, the effect was considered not reliable.

the difference between the two versions was lower for older adults (96% vs. 91%, respectively). Except for one young adult, no participant presented an inverse effect.

Results were strikingly different for the Negative priming indices. In the highly activated Stroop colour version, only 29% of participants, in both age groups, showed a reliable Negative priming effect; more than half of the individuals did not show any reliable effect, and about 11–12% showed even a reliable positive priming effect. In the less activated Stroop colour version, only 17% of young adults and 21% of older adults showed a reliable negative priming effect in the expected direction, whereas 67% of young and 70% of older adults did not show a reliable effect. It should be noted that, in the analyses run on RTs, the effect of condition was significant for both versions, pointing to a reliable negative priming effect at the group level. Moreover, as analysed previously, the effect of version was significant. Finally, the Hayling task behaved very similarly to the Stroop colour test. That is, almost all individuals presented a reliable effect, whether in the highly activated version (when comparing Phase A and AP; 97% and 94% for the young and the older adults, respectively), or in the less activated one (when comparing Phase B and A; 99% and 98%, respectively).

Table 3 reports the individuals who showed a same effect (or lack of effect) in both versions of the task. Not surprisingly, the percentage of individuals showing a reliable expected effect in both versions of the Stroop colour task or in both phases of the Hayling task was quite high. Thus, 77% of young and 84% of older adults showed a reliable effect in both versions of the Stroop colour test, that is in the highly and the less activated version. The proportion was even somewhat higher in the Hayling task, in which 97% of young and 93% of older adults showed an effect in both versions of the task. In the Negative priming task, in contrast, not only the percentage of participants showing an effect in either version was low, but few participants

TABLE 3

Bootstrap procedure and level of activation: across tasks percentage of participants presenting a reliable expected effect by version and age

	Less activated version					
	Stroop colour		*Hayling*		*Negative priming*	
Highly activated version	*Young*	*Older*	*Young*	*Older*	*Young*	*Older*
Stroop	**77**	**84**	*81*	*86*	*22*	*29*
Hayling	91	89	**97**	**93**	*31*	*32*
Negative priming	37	38	39	39	**13**	**14**

Below diagonal = highly activated versions; above diagonal = less activated version (in italics); diagonal = highly vs. less activated version of the same task (in bold).

showed the same effect for the two versions; thus, only 13% of young and 14% of older adults presented a reliable effect in both versions.

Between-task relationships

This study was also aimed at assessing the interindividual stability across tasks, which is one of the means to address the question of the generality of the processes. Directly following from the preceding section, the question was whether individuals presenting a reliable effect in one of the tasks also presented an effect in another task. Correlations were thus computed both for the total sample and for those individuals presenting a reliable effect.

Table 3 also reports the percentage of participants who showed a reliable effect in pairs of tasks, rather than within tasks. For the highly activated versions of the tasks, 91% of young adults and 89% of older adults showed a reliable effect in both the Hayling and the Stroop colour tasks. This is of course rather trivial, given the very high percentage of participants who showed an effect in either task; it would have been difficult not to observe an effect in both tasks. Similarly, some participants presenting an effect in the Negative priming task also showed an effect in the Stroop colour test (37% for young and 38% for older adults) and in the Hayling task (39% and 39%, respectively). With respect to the less activated version of the tasks, more than 80% of participants showed a reliable effect in both the Stroop colour and the Hayling tasks (81% of young and 86% of older adults); only 22% of young and 29% of older adults presented a reliable effect in both the Negative priming and the Stroop colour tasks, and 31% and 32% of young and older adults showed an effect for both the Negative priming and the Hayling tasks. This latter result could be due to the very low proportion of participants who showed an effect in the Negative priming task.

To circumvent this problem of low or high proportion of participants who showed an effect, another interesting statistic that binds the effects on two tasks (or two versions) is the phi coefficient (e.g., Howell, 1998) that can be viewed as a correlation coefficient between two dichotomous variables. This coefficient lies between -1 and 1, and values distant from 0 are evidence of (positive or negative) correlation/association. Assessing the interindividual stability across two tasks may be operationalised as assessing whether participants who present a reliable effect on one task have more chance of presenting a reliable effect on the other than participants who do not show a reliable effect. The test that corresponds to this hypothesis is the independence chi-square statistic based on the two-way contingency table (reliable effect or not on first task vs. reliable effect or not on second task). The phi coefficient is a direct function of this chi-square statistic and can be interpreted as a correlation coefficient. The phi coefficient computed between the two versions of the Hayling task was significant for both age groups (phi = .44, $p < .001$, and phi = .23, $p < .05$, for young and older adults, respectively). For these correlations, the null hypothesis can be rejected; the effect in one task was related to the effect in the other task. All other pairs of tasks (or versions) did not show evidence of stability (independence chi-square nonsignificant and associated phi below 0.1).

Table 4 presents the correlations across tasks for the total sample, and Table 5 only for the participants who showed reliable expected effects; in the latter case, obviously, the number of participants varied across pairs of tasks. In both sets of correlations, significant correlations were obtained between the two versions of the Stroop colour test ($r = .22$, $p < .001$), and between the two versions of the Hayling task ($r = .54$, $p < .001$). The pattern of these correlations partialled for age did not change (Stroop colour test: $r = .22$, $p < .001$; Hayling task: $r = .53$, $p < .001$).

These results were also found when analysing each age group separately (Stroop colour: young, $r = .61$, $p < .001$; older adults, $r = .37$, $p < .001$; Hayling: young, $r = .23$, $p < .01$; older adults, $r = .40$, $p < .001$). Moreover, the less activated version of the Stroop test and the Hayling task correlated significantly but weakly and negatively ($r = -.13$, $p < .05$); once controlled for age this pattern correlation did not change ($r = -.10$, $p < .05$). It is worth noticing that the Negative priming task did not correlate significantly with any other measures.

When analyses were run for participants with reliable effects only, results were similar; correlations were significant between the two versions of the Hayling task, between the versions of the Stroop colour test, and finally between the less activated version of the Stroop colour and the Hayling tasks (see Table 5). Moreover, a small significant correlation was obtained between the Stroop colour and the Negative priming in the highly activated version. It is noteworthy that we also ran partial correlation analyses controlling for

TABLE 4
Between-task correlations for the total sample

	Total sample		
	Less activated version		
Highly activated version	*Stroop*	*Hayling*	*Negative priming*
Stroop Colour	.22***	*−.13**	*−.01*
Hayling	−.02	.54***	*−.02*
Negative priming	.06	−.02	.06

Below diagonal = highly activated versions; above diagonal = less activated version (in italics); diagonal = highly vs. less activated version of the same task. $N = 280$. ***$p < .001$, *$p < .05$.

TABLE 5
Between-task correlations for participants with a reliable effect

	Reliable effect		
	Stroop	*Hayling*	*Negative priming*
Stroop	.31*** (.31***) (N = 223)	*−.18** (−.17**) (N = 232)*	*.02 (.02) (N = 70)*
Hayling	−.04 (N = 252)	.52*** (.51***) (N = 265)	*−.00 (.03) (N = 87)*
Negative priming	.18* (.17) (N = 105)	−.00 (.00) (N = 109)	.08 (.08) (N = 37)

Below diagonal = highly activated versions; above diagonal = less activated version (in italics); diagonal = highly vs. less activated version of the same task. (Correlation partialled out for age in parentheses). ***$p < .001$, **$p < .01$, *$p < .05$.

age. None of the significant correlations previously mentioned changed except for the one between the Stroop colour and the Negative priming that became nonsignificant ($r = .17$, $p = .08$).

GENERAL DISCUSSION

In summary, this study pursued the following objectives: examine age differences across three inhibitory tasks (Stroop colour, Negative priming, and Hayling tasks); study whether varying the level of activation of irrelevant information had an effect on age differences, and investigate the generality of interference effects both by means of across-task correlations and by assessing whether reliable effects could be observed at an intra-individual level, in a majority of individuals, in both age groups. This latter analysis was particularly novel; we do not know of any other study that has pursued the same objective in the field of inhibition and ageing. All analyses were performed on relative differences ([experimental condition − control condition]/control condition) (see de Frias et al., 2006) following the literature recommendation concerning the necessity to control for baseline because of the age-related decline in the speed of processing.

First, with respect to age differences, we found negligible effects. It is worth noticing that the pattern of results found with RTs (see Footnote 2) suggested an age-related difference in inhibitory efficacy, as in many other studies. Once performance in the control condition was controlled for (by means of the relative difference, used throughout the present paper), a significant age effect was observed only for the less activated version of the Stroop colour test, and for both versions of the Hayling test. These results are consistent with Verhaeghen and de Meersman's meta-analyses (1998a, 1998b), or with other studies (e.g., Kieley & Hartley, 1997; Salthouse & Meinz, 1995). It is therefore difficult to consider that there is a specific age deficit in susceptibility to interference or inhibition beyond a general slowing (controlled for in the interference indices used). It is intriguing that the interference effect in the Hayling task was larger for young than for older adults, again with processing speed controlled for. It could be that the larger size and accessibility of the knowledge base for older adults would represent an advantage for them. According to various findings (e.g., Baltes, 1987), knowledge is indeed well preserved in ageing. Thus, older adults may rely on preserved verbal abilities and/or larger background knowledge to compensate for a possible decline in processing speed. Delaloye (2004), for example, found a significant negative correlation between a verbal fluency score and response times in the Hayling test; this suggests that knowledge accessibility may play a role in this task. It is to note that most of the studies using the Hayling task considered the type of errors committed, which were not taken into consideration in the present study, and not response times. The present results would, in any case, suggest that other aspects than inhibition take place in this task (selection strategies, etc.).

Second, the manipulation of the level of activation of irrelevant information displayed the expected effect, because a main effect of version was observed in all tasks. However, the expected Age × Version interaction was only marginally significant in the Negative priming and not significant in the Hayling test, showing that in these two tasks, older adults were overall not more sensitive to increased interference. Curiously, also, older adults tended to show a somewhat higher negative priming effect than young adults in the less activated version, but no difference between the highly and the less activated version. Likewise, in the Stroop colour tasks, older adults showed a larger interference effect than young adults in the less activated version but not in the highly activated one. This result led us to speculate that older adults might present a lower threshold to interference than young adults. Note that it is not in agreement with Hartley's study (1993), in which a larger age effect was observed in the colour-word than in the colour-block condition, nor with West and Bell's study (1997) that replicated Hartley's results in the colour-block version. There are, however, a number of methodological differences. In particular, Hartley used different SOA; scores were also computed differently, as Hartley used a proportional score computed between the two versions. Perhaps, the SOA adopted in the present study, chosen on the basis of Schooler et al.'s study (1997) with young adults, made it particularly difficult for the older adults to avoid reading the word. In any case, it would be worth studying further this issue, and comparing young and older adults at various SOA.

Third, a bootstrap procedure was used to assess the reliability of the effects at the level of individuals taking into account intra-individual variability. Altogether, we would argue that this type of analysis is not used enough in cognitive psychology, with the result that many researchers consider, at least implicitly, that an effect reliable at the group level should be observed in all individuals. Della Sala et al. (1991), for instance, discovered with a certain surprise that a well known effect in the field of working memory, namely the word length effect, was not observed in a sizeable part of their sample, despite a clearly very significant effect at the level of the group. In the present study, as could be expected but rarely empirically demonstrated, almost all participants were subject to interference in the Stroop colour and in the Hayling tasks, for both versions, at least as long as the criterion for the confidence intervals is adapted to the intra-individual situation (i.e., 68%). No individual showed an inverse effect, except one young adult, and there were no significant age differences. It is nevertheless worth stressing that 21% of the young adults did not show a reliable effect in the dissociated version of the Stroop task. Results were very different for the Negative priming paradigm: Not even one-third of the participants showed a reliable effect in the highly activated version and about 20% in the less activated one. Moreover, more than 10% showed an inverse effect, that is, a reliable positive priming effect; as the different conditions were randomly distributed across the Stroop colour task (except for the two trials composing the pair of a negative priming trial), there was no advantage for the participants in consciously attending the distractor, a strategy observed sometimes when conditions are blocked. Once again, no age differences were observed with respect to the number of individuals presenting a reliable effect. According to the literature on Negative priming, we could have expected that older adults would be less numerous to present a reliable effect. Recall that a significant effect was observed at the group level (on response times, analyses not reported here); moreover, the sample was quite large. It is therefore difficult to consider that the results are simply due to an unreliability of the task.

We also asked whether younger and older adults presenting a reliable effect in one task also presented a reliable effect in another task. This was the case as concerns the Hayling and the Stroop colour tasks, both within each task (between the versions) and across the two tasks. Given the high percentage of individuals presenting a reliable effect, a different result would hardly have been possible. There were, however, few individuals not showing both effects. Once again, the picture was different as concerns the Negative priming task. That is, among those showing a reliable effect in the less activated version, only a modest percentage of both young and older adults also showed an effect in the highly activated version.

Thus, the present data highlight the importance of testing whether a group effect is observed in all or at least in most individuals; as already mentioned with respect to Della Sala et al.'s (1991) study, such analyses might reserve some surprise, even with respect to well established effects. The bootstrap procedure can also be a very useful method in clinical neuropsychological context to assess precisely the presence of an inhibitory impairment for one individual.

Across-task generality was also assessed by means of correlations. Correlations were very low for the interference/inhibition indices within each version (except for the Hayling task), as well as between tasks. Our initial hypothesis was that correlations would be stronger between highly activated versions of the tasks. This hypothesis was not supported, as the only significant correlation was between the two versions of the Hayling task; the phi coefficient also showed a significant, but modest, correlation between both versions of the Hayling task. Significant but small correlations were found between the less activated version of the Hayling task and of the Stroop colour test. With respect to highly activated task versions, weak or nonexistent correlations were found using both the phi correlations and the Pearson ones.

This pattern of results demonstrates, once more, after a number of other studies, that inhibition cannot be considered as a general mechanism. Referring to Hasher and Zacks' inhibitory processes, one could have expected that the Hayling and the Stroop colour tasks correlate more strongly because they both represent the ability to prevent predominant but inappropriate responses (restraint function) (Hasher & Zacks, 1988; Hasher et al., 2007), whereas the Negative priming task corresponds to the access function. Nonetheless, the pattern of correlations did not support this distinction, as correlations were significant for two tasks only, in their less activated versions. Results thus speak for multiple inhibitory processes (Nigg, 2000). Recent neuroimaging studies have also shown that different neural regions are responsible for the resolution of interference at different stages of processing and depending on the type of task administered (Nee, Wagner, & Jonides, 2007). Results obtained can be considered consistent with the view that inhibitory processes are not so strongly impaired in older adults. Nevertheless, the data showed some evidence that older adults as supposed were more sensitive to interference: Age differences were larger in the less activated version than in the highly activated version of the Stroop colour task; there was a slightly larger effect in the less activated Negative priming task, as if older adults had processed the distracting information when it was less salient, and could inhibit it more easily in this version than in the highly activated one, relative to young adults. Further studies are needed, however, before confirming our hypothesis that older adults have a general lower threshold to interference. The present study also suggested, in line with other studies, that Negative priming is not reliable at the level of both groups and participants, and does not provide a good index of inhibition (e.g., Kramer et al., 1994; Little & Hartley, 2000).

CONCLUSION

In the present study, experimental and correlational approaches in a large sample of young and older adults were combined and the salience of irrelevant information was manipulated. Overall, the data did not support either the hypothesis according to which the salience of irrelevant information determines age-related differences in inhibitory efficacy—although an interesting result was that older adults might be more sensitive to tasks presenting a lesser degree of interference—nor the postulate that inhibition is a general mechanism. Distinct and specific inhibitory processes seem to be involved in each task; inhibition cannot be considered a unitary process. In itself, this is not a novel result (e.g., Kramer et al., 1994). Friedman and Miyake (2004) also questioned this issue and suggested a fractionation of inhibitory processes. Their sample included only young adults, and those studies that have administered several inhibitory tasks to young and older adults are still rare. Our recommendation would be that, when investigators study age differences in inhibition, they analyse more in depth the task used and the type of inhibition it calls for. Further research is required to explore the different types of inhibition, and the corresponding age effects. We also recommend that inhibition mechanisms be analysed at the level of the individuals, and not only at a group level. It was the case, in the present study, that well known interference effects were not only replicated for the group but also observed at the level of individuals. But this could well not be observed in other tasks. Recall that a sizeable proportion of young adults did not show a reliable effect in the dissociated Stroop colour task. Such results point not to a lack of reliability, but to the possibility that different individuals use different strategies. It is now time to take such individual differences seriously.

REFERENCES

Amieva, H., Phillips, L. H., Della Sala, S., & Henry, J. D. (2004). Inhibitory functioning in Alzheimer's disease. *Brain*, *127*, 949–964.

Andrés, P., & van der Linden, M. (2000). Age related differences in supervisory attentional system functions. *Journal of Gerontology: Psychological Sciences*, *35*, 373–380.

Aron, A. R. (2007). The neural basis of inhibition in cognitive control. *The Neuroscientist*, *13*, 214–228.

Baltes, P. B. (1987). Theoretical propositions of lifespan developmental psychology: On the dynamics between growth and decline. *Developmental Psychology*, *23*, 611–626.

Bjork, R. A. (1989). Retrieval inhibition as an adaptive mechanism in human memory. In F. I. M. Craik & H. L. Roediger III (Eds.), *Varieties of memory and consciousness: Essays in honor of Endel Tulving* (pp. 309–330). Hillsdale, NJ: Lawrence Erlbaum Associates, Inc.

Borella, E., Carretti, B., & de Beni, R. (2008). Working memory and inhibition across the adult life-span. *Acta Psychologica, 128*, 33–44.

Bugg, J. M., DeLosh, E. L., Davalos, D. B., & Davis, H. P. (2007). Age differences in Stroop interference: Contributions of general slowing and task-specific deficits. *Aging, Neuropsychology, and Cognition, 14*, 155–167.

Bunce, D. J., Warr, P. B., & Cochrane, T. (1993). Blocks in choice responding as a function of age and physical fitness. *Psychology and Aging, 8*, 26–33.

Burgess, P. W., & Shallice, T. (1996). Response suppression, initiation and strategy use following frontal lobe lesions. *Neuropsychologia, 34*, 263–273.

Davidson, D. J., Zacks, R. T., & Williams, C. C. (2003). Stroop interference, practice and aging. *Aging, Neuropsychology, and Cognition, 10*, 85–98.

Davison, A. C., & Hinkley, D. V. (1997). *Bootstrap methods and their application*. Cambridge, UK: Cambridge University Press.

De Frias, C. M., Dixon, R. A., & Strauss, E. (2006). Structure of four executive functioning tests in healthy older adults. *Neuropsychology, 20*, 206–214.

Delaloye, C. (2004). *Mémoire de travail, inhibition et processus automatiques et contrôlés: Une analyse de leurs relations lors du vieillissement normal*. Thèse de Doctorat, FPSE, Université de Genève.

Delaloye, C., Moy, G., Baudois, S., de Bilbao, F., Dubois Remund, C., Hofer, C., et al. (in press). The contribution of aging to the understanding of the dimensionality of executive functions. *Archives of Gerontology and Geriatrics*.

Della Sala, S., Logie, R. H., Marchetti, C., & Wynn, V. (1991). Case studies in working memory: A case for single cases? *Cortex, 27*, 169–191.

De Ribaupierre, A. (2001). Working memory and attentional processes across the lifespan. In P. Graf & N. Otha (Eds.), *Lifespan development of human memory* (pp. 59–80). Cambridge, MA: MIT Press.

De Ribaupierre, A., Atzeni, T., Fagot, D., Jouffray, C., Lecerf, T., & Ludwig, C. (2004). *Dimensionalité de l'inhibition cognitive au travers du lifespan (final report)*. Geneva: University of Geneva.

Friedman, N. P., & Miyake, A. (2004). The relations among inhibition and interference control functions: A latent-variable analysis. *Journal of Experimental Psychology: General, 133*, 101–135.

Gamboz, N., Russo, R., & Fox, E. (2002). Age differences and the identity negative priming effect: An updated meta-analysis. *Psychology and Aging, 17*, 525–531.

Harnishfeger, K. K. (1995). The development of cognitive inhibition: Theories, definitions, and research evidence. In F. N. Dempster & C. J. Brainerd (Eds.), *Interference and inhibition in cognition*. San Diego, CA: Academic Press.

Hartley, A. A. (1993). Evidence for the selective preservation of spatial selective attention in old age. *Psychology and Aging, 8*, 371–379.

Hasher, L., Lustig, C., & Zacks, R. T. (2007). Inhibitory mechanisms and the control of attention. In A. A. Conway, C. Jarrold, M. J. Kane, A. Miyake, & J. N. Towse (Eds.), *Variation in working memory* (pp. 227–249). Oxford, UK: Oxford University Press.

Hasher, L., Stoltzfus, E. R., Zacks, R. T., & Rypma, B. (1991). Age and inhibition. *Journal of Experimental Psychology: Learning, Memory, and Cognition, 17*, 113–139.

Hasher, L., & Zacks, R. T. (1988). Working memory, comprehension, and aging: A review and a new view. In G. H. Bower (Ed.), *The psychology of learning and motivation: Advances in research and theory* (Vol. 22, pp. 193–225). San Diego, CA: Academic Press.

Hedden, T., & Park, D. C. (2001). Aging and interference in verbal working memory. *Psychology and Aging, 16*, 666–681.

Howell, D. C. (1998). *Méthodes statistiques en sciences humaines*. Brussels: De Boeck Université.

Johnson, J., Im-Bolter, N., & Pascual-Leone, J. (2003). Development of mental attention in gifted and mainstream children: The role of mental capacity, inhibition, and speed of processing. *Child Development*, *74*, 1594–1614.

Kane, M. J., Hasher, L., Stoltzfus, E. R., Zacks, R. T., & Connelly, S. L. (1994). Inhibitory attentional mechanisms and aging. *Psychology and Aging*, *9*, 103–112.

Kieley, J. M., & Hartley, A. A. (1997). Age-related equivalence of identity suppression in the Stroop color-word task. *Psychology and Aging*, *12*, 22–29.

Kramer, A. F., Humphreys, G. W., Larish, J. F., Logan, G. D., & Strayer, D. L. (1994). Aging and inhibition: Beyond a unitary view of inhibitory processing in attention. *Psychology and Aging*, *9*, 491–512.

Lavie, N., & Fox, E. (2000). The role of perceptual load in negative priming. *Journal of Experimental Psychology: Human Perception and Performance*, *26*, 1038–1052.

Little, D. M., & Hartley, A. A. (2000). Further evidence that negative priming in the Stroop color-word task is equivalent in older and younger adults. *Psychology and Aging*, *15*, 9–17.

Lustig, C., Hasher, L., & Tonev, S.T. (2001). Inhibitory control over the present and the past. *European Journal of Cognitive Psychology*, *13*, 107–122.

Lustig, C., Hasher, L., & Zacks, R. T. (2007). Inhibitory deficit theory: Recent developments in a "new view". In D. S. Gorfein & C. M. MacLeod (Eds.), *The place of inhibition in cognition* (pp. 145–162). Washington, DC: American Psychological Association.

May, C. P., Kane, M. J., & Hasher, L. (1995). Determinants of negative priming. *Psychological Bulletin*, *118*, 35–54.

Nee, D., Wagner, T. D., & Jonides, J. (2007). Interference resolution: Insight from a meta-analysis of neuroimaging tasks. *Cognitive, Affective, and Behavioral Neuroscience*, *7*, 1–17.

Neill, W. T., Valdes, L. A., & Terry, K. M. (1995). Selective attention and the inhibitory control of cognition. In F. N. Dempster & C. J. Brainerd (Eds.), *Interference and inhibition in cognition* (pp. 207–261). San Diego, CA: Academic Press.

Nelson, A. E., & Dannefer, D. (1992). Aged heterogeneity: Fact or fiction? The fate of diversity in gerontological research. *The Gerontologist*, *32*, 17–23.

Nigg, J. T. (2000). On inhibition/disinhibition in developmental psychopathology: Views from cognitive and personality psychology and a working inhibition taxonomy. *Psychological Bulletin*, *126*, 220–246.

Park, D. C., Lautenschlager, G., Hedden, T., Davidson, N. S., Smith, A. D., & Smith, P. K. (2002). Models of visuospatial and verbal memory across the adult life span. *Psychology and Aging*, *17*, 299–320.

Park, D. C., & Schwarz, N. (Eds.).(2000). *Cognitive aging: A primer*. New York: Psychology Press.

Pascual-Leone, J. (1969). *Cognitive development and cognitive style: A general psychological integration*. Unpublished doctoral dissertation, University of Geneva, Switzerland.

Persad, C. C., Abeles, N., Zacks, R. T., & Denburg, N. L. (2002). Inhibitory changes after age 60 and their relationship to measures of attention and memory. *Journals of Gerontology: Psychological Sciences and Social Sciences*, *57B*, 223–232.

Rabbitt, P., Lowe, C., & Shilling, V. (2001). Frontal tests and models for cognitive ageing. *European Journal of Cognitive Psychology*, *13*, 5–28.

Raven, J. C. (1998). *Raven's Progressive Matrices and Vocabulary Scales*. San Antonio, TX: Psychological Corporation.

Rowe, G., Valderrama, S., Hasher, L., & Lenartowicz, A. (2006). Attention disregulation: A long-term memory benefit. *Psychology and Aging*, *21*, 826–830.

Salthouse, T. A. (1996). The processing-speed theory of adult age differences in cognition. *Psychological Review*, *103*, 403–428.

Salthouse, T. A., Atkinson, T. M., & Berish, D. E. (2003). Executive functioning as a potential mediator of age-related cognitive decline in normal adults. *Journal of Experimental Psychology: General*, *132*, 566–594.

Salthouse, T. A., & Babcock, R. L. (1991). Decomposing adult age differences in working memory. *Developmental Psychology, 27*, 763–776.

Salthouse, T. A., & Meinz, E. J. (1995). Aging, inhibition, working memory, and speed. *Journals of Gerontology: Psychological Sciences and Social Sciences, 50b*, 297–306.

Schelstraete, M.-A., & Hupet, M. (2002). Cognitive aging and inhibitory efficiency in the Daneman and Carpenter's working memory task. *Experimental Aging Research, 28*, 269–279.

Schooler, C., Neumann, E., Caplan, L. J., & Roberts, B. R. (1997). A time course analysis of Stroop interference and facilitation: Comparing normal individuals and individuals with schizophrenia. *Journal of Experimental Psychology: General, 126*, 19–36.

Shilling, V. M., Chetwynd, A., & Rabbitt, P. M. A. (2002). Individual inconsistency across measures of inhibition: An investigation of the construct validity of inhibition in older adults. *Neuropsychologia, 40*, 605–619.

Spieler, D. H., Balota, D. A., & Faust, M. E. (1996). Stroop performance in healthy younger and older adults and in individuals with dementia of the Alzheimer's type. *Journal of Experimental Psychology: Human Perception and Performance, 22*, 461–479.

S-Plus 6.1 [Computer software]. (2002). Seattle, WA: Insightful Corporation.

Stroop, J. R. (1935). Studies of interference in serial verbal reactions. *Journal of Experimental Psychology, 18*, 643–662.

Sullivan, M. P., & Faust, M. E. (1993). Evidence for identity inhibition during selective attention in old adults. *Psychology and Aging, 8*, 589–598.

Tipper, S. P. (1985). The negative priming effect: Inhibitory priming by ignored objects. *Quarterly Journal of Experimental Psychology, 37A*, 571–590.

Tipper, S. P. (2001). Does negative priming reflect inhibitory mechanisms? A review and integration of conflicting views? *Quarterly Journal of Experimental Psychology, 54A*, 321–343.

Ulrich, R., & Miller, J. (1994). Effects of truncation on reaction time analysis. *Journal of Experimental Psychology: General, 123*, 34–80.

Uttl, B., & Graf, P. (1997). Color-word Stroop performance across the adult life span. *Journal of Clinical and Experimental Neuropsychology, 1*, 405–420.

Verhaeghen, P., & de Meersman, L. (1998a). Aging and the Stroop effect: A meta-analysis. *Psychology and Aging, 13*, 120–126.

Verhaeghen, P., & de Meersman, L. (1998b). Aging and the negative priming effect: A meta-analysis. *Psychology and Aging, 13*, 435–444.

Verhaeghen, P., & Salthouse, T. (1997). Meta-analyses of age-cognition relations in adulthood: Estimates of linear and nonlinear age effects and structural models. *Psychological Bulletin, 122*, 231–249.

West, R., & Bell, M. A. (1997). Stroop color-word interference and electroencephalogram activation: Evidence for age-related decline in the anterior attention system. *Neuropsychology, 11*, 421–427.

West, R. L., & Alain, C. (2000). Age-related decline in inhibitory control contributes to the increased Stroop effect observed in older adults. *Psychophysiology, 37*, 179–189.

Subject index